QUICK LOOK
DRUG BOOK

WILLIAMS & WILKINS

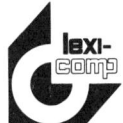

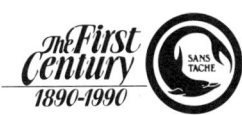

QUICK LOOK DRUG BOOK

WILLIAMS & WILKINS

Leonard L. Lance, R.Ph., B.S.
Senior Editor
Pharmacist
Lexi-Comp Inc
Hudson, Ohio

Charles Lacy, R.Ph., Pharm.D.
Editor
Drug Information Pharmacist
Cedars-Sinai Medical Center
Los Angeles, California

Flynn Warren, R.Ph., M.S.
Editor
Clinical Pharmacy Associate
College of Pharmacy
University of Georgia
Athens, Georgia

1991

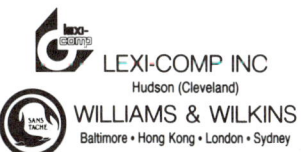

LEXI-COMP INC
Hudson (Cleveland)

WILLIAMS & WILKINS
Baltimore • Hong Kong • London • Sydney

Notice

This handbook is intended to serve the user as a handy quick reference and not as a complete drug information resource. It does not include information on every therapeutic agent available. The publication covers 1232 commonly used drugs and is specifically designed to present certain important aspects of drug data in a more concise format than is typically found in medical literature or product material supplied by manufacturers.

Although great care was taken to ensure the accuracy of the handbook's content when it went to press, the editors, contributors and publisher cannot be responsible for the continued accuracy of the supplied information due to ongoing research and new developments in the field. The manufacturer's most current product information or other standard recognized references should always be consulted for more detailed information.

The editors and contributors have written this book in their private capacities. No official support or endorsement by any federal agency or pharmaceutical company is intended or inferred.

This manual was produced using the FormuLex™ Program —
A complete publishing service of Lexi-Comp Inc.

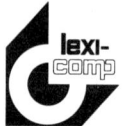

Lexi-Comp Inc.
P.O. Box 1633
Stow, Ohio 44224
(216) 650-6506

ISBN 0-683-07052-5

TABLE OF CONTENTS

PREFACE

Working with clinical pharmacists, hospital pharmacy and therapeutics committees, and hospital drug information centers, our panel of editors have assisted in developing hospital-specific formulary manuals for major medical institutions in the United States and Canada. These manuals provide pertinent details on medications used within the hospital, office and other clinical settings. The most current information on drugs and medications has been reviewed, coalesced, and cross-referenced to form the *Quick Look Drug Book*.

The Indications Index is an expedient mechanism for locating the medication of choice. This index helps the user to, with knowledge of the disease state, identify medications which are most commonly used in treatment. All disease states are cross-referenced to a varying number of medications with the most likely or best medications noted.

All generic and brand names or synonyms appear as individual entries in the alphabetical listing of drugs. Thus, there is no alphabetical index of drugs.

This handbook gives the user quick access to data on 1232 medications. A standard, concise format was developed to ensure consistent presentation of information. Selection of medications included in this handbook was based on an analysis of medications offered in a wide range of hospital formularies.

— L. L. Lance

ACKNOWLEDGMENTS

The *Quick Look Drug Book with Indications Index* exists in its present form as the result of the concerted efforts of many individuals. The publisher and president of Lexi-Comp Inc, Robert D. Kerscher, deserves much credit for bringing the concept of such a book to fruition. His dedication to the project, and his support and development of the many unique and innovative features included in the book, eg, format, internal cross-references and Indications Index, contribute substantially to the content and usefulness of the book.

Other members of the Lexi-Comp staff whose contributions were invaluable and whose patience with the editors' enumerable drafts, revisions, deletions, additions, and enhancements was inexhaustible include: Lynn Coppinger and Barbara F. Kerscher, production managers, Alexandra Hart, Jil Neuman, Jeanne Eads, and Deborah Burns, production assistants, Jeff J. Zaccagnini and Brian B. Vossler, sales managers, Edmund A. Harbart, vice-president, custom publishing division, and Jack L. Stones, vice-president, reference publishing division. The complex computer programming required for the typesetting of the book was provided by Dennis P. Smithers and Jay I. Katzen, system analysts, under the direction of Thury L. O'Connor, vice-president, and David K. Ream, vice-president, development.

In addition, sincere appreciation to Vaughn W. Floutz, PhD and Priscilla Jane Frank, MT(ASCP) who served as editorial consultants.

FDA PREGNANCY CATEGORIES

Throughout this book there is a field labeled Pregnancy Risk Factor (PRF) and the letter A, B, C, D or X immediately following which signifies a category. The FDA has established these five categories to indicate the potential of a systemically absorbed drug for causing birth defects. The key differentiation among the categories rests upon the reliability of documentation and the risk:benefit ratio. Pregnancy Category X is particularly notable in that if any data exists that may implicate a drug as a teratogen and the risk:benefit ratio is clearly negative, the drug is contraindicated during pregnancy.

These categories are summarized as follows:

A   Controlled studies in pregnant women fail to demonstrate a risk to the fetus in the first trimester with no evidence of risk in later trimesters. The possibility of fetal harm appears remote.

B   Either animal-reproduction studies have not demonstrated a fetal risk but there are no controlled studies in pregnant women, or animal-reproduction studies have shown an adverse effect (other than a decrease in fertility) that was not confirmed in controlled studies in women in the first trimester and there is no evidence of a risk in later trimesters.

C   Either studies in animals have revealed adverse effects on the fetus (teratogenic or embryocidal effects or other) and there are no controlled studies in women, or studies in women and animals are not available. Drugs should be given only if the potential benefits justify the potential risk to the fetus.

D   There is positive evidence of human fetal risk, but the benefits from use in pregnant women may be acceptable despite the risk (eg, if the drug is needed in a life-threatening situation or for a serious disease for which safer drugs cannot be used or are ineffective).

X   Studies in animals or human beings have demonstrated fetal abnormalities or there is evidence of fetal risk based on human experience, or both, and the risk of the use of the drug in pregnant women clearly outweighs any possible benefit. The drug is contraindicated in women who are or may become pregnant.

USE OF THE QUICK LOOK DRUG BOOK WITH INDICATIONS INDEX

The *Quick Look Drug Book* is organized into a drug information section, an appendix and several very useful indices.

The drug information section of the handbook, wherein all drugs are listed alphabetically, details information pertinent to each drug. Extensive cross referencing is provided by brand name and synonyms.

Drug information is presented in a consistent format and for quick reference will provide the following:

Generic Name	U.S. Adopted Name
Pronunciation Guide	
Brand Names	Common trade names
Synonyms	
Use	Information pertaining to appropriate use of the drug
Restrictions	According to DEA classification (see descriptions in appendix)
Pregnancy Risk Factor	Five categories established by the FDA to indicate the potential of a systemically absorbed drug for causing birth defects (See detailed explanation on page iv.)
Usual Dosage	The amount of the drug to be typically given or taken during therapy

Appendix

The appendix offers a compilation of tables, guidelines and conversion information which can often be helpful when considering patient care.

Indications Index

This index provides a listing of accepted drugs for various disease states thus focusing attention on selection of medications most frequently prescribed in relation to a clinical diagnosis. Diseases may have other nonofficial drugs for their treatment and this indications index should not be used by itself to determine the appropriateness of a particular therapy. The listed indications may encompass varying degrees of severity and, since certain medications may not be appropriate for a given degree of severity, it should not be assumed that the agents listed for specific indications are interchangeable.

ALPHABETICAL LISTING OF DRUGS

A-200™ Pyrinate [OTC] *see* Pyrethrins *on page 309*

A and D™ Ointment [OTC] *see* Vitamin A and Vitamin D
on page 377

Aarane® *see* Cromolyn Sodium *on page 91*

A-ase *see* Asparaginase *on page 30*

Abbokinase® *see* Urokinase *on page 370*

Abbott HTLV III EIA *see* Diagnostic Test for Virus
on page 108

Absorbable Cotton *see* Cellulose, Oxidized *on page 65*

Absorbable gelatin sponge *see* Gelatin, Absorbable
on page 156

Accurbron® *see* Theophylline *on page 348*

Accusens T® *see* Diagnostic Test for Taste Function
on page 108

Accutane® *see* Isotretinoin *on page 194*

Acebutolol Hydrochloride (a se byoo' toe lole)
Brand Names Sectral®
Use Treatment of hypertension; ventricular arrhythmias
Pregnancy Risk Factor B
Usual Dosage 400-800 mg/day in two divided doses

Acetaminophen (a set a mee' noe fen)
Brand Names Anacin-3® [OTC]; Dorcol® [OTC]; Fevernol™ [OTC]; Pana-
dol® [OTC]; Tylenol® [OTC]
Synonyms APAP; N-Acetyl-P-Aminophenol; Paracetamol
Use Treatment of mild to moderate pain and fever, does not have antirheu-
matic effects
Pregnancy Risk Factor B
Usual Dosage

Adult: 325-650 mg every 4-6 hours or 1000 mg 3-4 times daily

Children: May repeat doses 4-5 times daily; do not exceed five doses in
24 hours. See table.

Acetaminophen

Age	Dosage (mg)	Age	Dosage (mg)
0–3 mo	40	4–5	240
4–11 mo	80	6–8	320
1–2 y	120	9–10	400
2–3 y	160	11	480

Acetaminophen and Codeine
Brand Names Phenaphen® #3; Tylenol® With Codeine
Synonyms Codeine and Acetaminophen
Use Relief of mild to moderate pain
Restrictions C-III
Pregnancy Risk Factor B
Usual Dosage Should be adjusted according to severity of pain and response of the patient. Adult doses of 60 mg and higher fail to give commensurate relief of pain but merely prolong analgesia and are associated with an appreciably increased incidence of side effects.

Adult: Oral:
Antitussive: (15-30 mg/dose) every 4-6 hours
Analgesic: Based on codeine (30-60 mg/dose) every 4-6 hours
One or two tablets every four hours with a maximum of 12 tablets per 24 hours

Children:
3-6 years of age: 5 mL 3-4 times daily
7-12 years: 10 mL 3-4 times daily
< 3 years: Safe dosage has not been established

Acetaminophen and Hydrocodone see Hydrocodoné and
Acetaminophen *on page 173*

Acetaminophen and Isometheptene Mucate
Brand Names Midrin®
Use Relief of migraine and tension headache
Pregnancy Risk Factor B
Usual Dosage Adult: Oral: Take 2 capsules at first sign of headache, followed by one capsule every 60 minutes until relieved, up to 5 capsules in a 12 hour period

Acetaminophen and Oxycodone see Oxycodone and
Acetaminophen *on page 264*

Acetaminophen and Phenyltoloxamine
Brand Names Percogesic® [OTC]
Use Relief of mild to moderate pain
Pregnancy Risk Factor B
Usual Dosage Adult: Oral: Take one or two tablets every 4 hours

Acetaminophen, Chlorpheniramine and Pseudoephedrine
Brand Names Sinutab® [OTC]
Use Temporary relief of sinus symptoms
Pregnancy Risk Factor B
Usual Dosage Adult: Oral: Take two tablets every six hours

Acetazolamide (a set a zole' a mide)
Brand Names Diamox®
Use Lower intraocular pressure to treat glaucoma, also as a diuretic, adjunct treatment of refractory seizure and acute altitude sickness
(Continued)

Acetazolamide *(Continued)*

Pregnancy Risk Factor C
Usual Dosage

Adult:

Glaucoma: Oral: 250-1000 mg in 1-4 divided doses, or 500 mg sustained release capsule twice daily; I.M.: 250-500 mg; may repeat in 2-4 hours

Edema: Oral, I.M., I.V.: 250-375 mg once daily

Epilepsy: Oral: 8-30 mg/kg in 1-4 divided doses

Altitude sickness: Oral: 250 mg every 8-12 hours

Children:

Glaucoma: Oral: 8-30 mg/kg/24 hours in divided doses every 6-8 hours; I.M., I.V.: 20-40 mg/kg/24 hours in divided doses

Edema: Oral, I.M., I.V.: 5 mg/kg/24 hours or 150 mg/m^2/24 hours once daily

Epilepsy: Oral: 8-30 mg/kg/24 hours in 2-4 divided doses; maximum: 1 gram per day

Acetest® [OTC] *see* Diagnostic Test for Acetone in Urine
on page 106

Acetic Acid (a see' tik)

Brand Names VōSol®; Vōsol-HC®
Synonyms Ethanoic Acid
Use For continuous or intermittent irrigation of the bladder; treatment of superficial bacterial infections of the external auditory canal and vagina
Pregnancy Risk Factor C
Usual Dosage

Irrigation: For continuous irrigation of the urinary bladder with 0.25% acetic acid irrigation, the rate of administration will approximate the rate of urine flow; usually 500-1500 mL per 24 hours. For periodic irrigation of an indwelling urinary catheter to maintain patency, about 50 mL of 0.25% acetic acid irrigation is required. (Note dosage of an irrigating solution depends on the capacity or surface area of the structure being irrigated.)

Otic: Insert saturated wick; keep moist 24 hours; remove wick and instill five drops 3-4 times daily

Acetohexamide (a set oh hex' a mide)

Brand Names Dymelor®
Use As an adjunct to diet for the management of mild to moderately severe, stable, noninsulin-dependent (type II) diabetes mellitus
Pregnancy Risk Factor C
Usual Dosage 250 mg-1.5 g daily

Acetophenazine Maleate (a set oh fen' a zeen)

Brand Names Tindal®
Use Management of manifestations of psychotic disorders
Pregnancy Risk Factor C
Usual Dosage 20 mg three times a day up to 40-80 mg/day

Acetoxymethylprogesterone *see* Medroxyprogesterone Acetate
on page 216

Acetylcholine Chloride (a se teel koe' leen)

Brand Names Miochol®

Use To produce complete miosis in cataract surgery, hematoplasty, iridectomy and other anterior segment surgery where rapid miosis is required

Pregnancy Risk Factor C

Usual Dosage 0.5-2 mL of 1% injection (5-20 mg) instilled into anterior chamber before or after securing one or more sutures

Acetylcysteine (a se teel sis' tay een)

Brand Names Mucomyst®

Synonyms *N*-Acetylcysteine; *N*-Acetyl-L-cysteine

Use Adjunctive therapy in patients with abnormal or viscid mucous secretions in acute and chronic bronchopulmonary diseases; pulmonary complications of surgery and cystic fibrosis; diagnostic bronchial studies; antidote for acute acetaminophen toxicity

Pregnancy Risk Factor B

Usual Dosage

Acetaminophen poisoning: Children and Adult: Oral: 140 mg/kg; followed by 17 doses of 70 mg/kg every four hours or until acetaminophen assay reveals nontoxic levels; repeat dose if emesis occurs within 1 hour of administration

Inhalation: *N*-Acetylcysteine 10% and 20% solution (Mucomyst®) (Dilute with water):
Infants: 2 mL of 5% solution until nebulized 3-4 times/day
Children: 3-5 mL of 5-10% solution until nebulized 3-4 times/day
Adolescents: 5-10 mL of 5-10% solution until nebulized 3-4 times/day
Note: Patients should receive an aerosolized bronchodilator 10-15 minutes prior to acetylcysteine

Meconium Ileus equivalent: Children and Adult: 100-200 mL of 5-10% solution by irrigation or orally

Acetylsalicylic Acid *see* Aspirin *on page 30*

Achromycin® *see* Tetracycline *on page 346*

Achromycin® V *see* Tetracycline *on page 346*

Aciclovir *see* Acyclovir *on next page*

Acid Mantle® *see* Aluminum Acetate *on page 14*

Acidulin® [OTC] *see* Glutamic Acid Hydrochloride
on page 159

A-Cillin® *see* Amoxicillin *on page 21*

Aclovate® *see* Alclometasone Dipropionate *on page 11*

ACTH *see* Corticotropin *on page 89*

Acthar® *see* Corticotropin *on page 89*

Actidose-Aqua® [OTC] *see* Charcoal *on page 68*

Actidose® With Sorbitol [OTC] *see* Charcoal *on page 68*

Actifed® *see* Triprolidine and Pseudoephedrine *on page 365*

Actifed® With Codeine *see* Triprolidine, Pseudoephedrine and Codeine *on page 365*

Actigall™ *see* Ursodiol *on page 370*

Actinomycin D *see* Dactinomycin *on page 96*

Activase® *see* Alteplase *on page 14*

Activated Carbon *see* Charcoal *on page 68*

Activated Dimethicone *see* Simethicone *on page 324*

Activated Ergosterol *see* Ergocalciferol *on page 132*

Acutrim® Precision Release® [OTC] *see* Phenylpropanolamine Hydrochloride *on page 283*

ACV *see* Acyclovir *on this page*

Acycloguanosine *see* Acyclovir *on this page*

Acyclovir (ay sye' kloe ver)
Brand Names Zovirax®
Synonyms Aciclovir; ACV; Acycloguanosine
Use Treatment of initial and prophylaxis of recurrent mucosal and cutaneous herpes simplex (HSV-1 and HSV-2) infections
Pregnancy Risk Factor C
Usual Dosage

Adult:

Oral: Initially 200 mg every four hours while awake (five times daily) for prophylaxis, 200 mg three times daily

Topical: 1/2 inch ribbon of ointment every three hours (six times daily)

Mucocutaneous HSV infection: 750 mg/m^2/day every 8 hours in 3 divided doses or 15 mg/kg/day every 8 hours in 3 divided doses for 5-10 days

HSV encephalitis: 1500 mg/m^2/day every 8 hours in 3 divided doses or 30 mg/kg/day every 8 hours in 3 divided doses for 10 days

Neonatal HSV infection: 1500 mg/m^2/day every 8 hours in 3 divided doses or 30 mg/kg/day every 8 hours in 3 divided doses for 10-14 days

Varicella-zoster virus infection: 1500 mg/m^2/day every 8 hours in 3 divided doses or 30 mg/kg/day every 8 hours in 3 divided doses for 5-10 days

Adalat® *see* Nifedipine *on page 252*

Adapin® *see* Doxepin Hydrochloride *on page 122*

Adenine Arabinoside *see* Vidarabine *on page 375*

Adenocard® *see* Adenosine *on this page*

Adenosine (a den' oh seen)
Brand Names Adenocard®
Use Treatment of paroxysmal supraventricular tachycardia (PSUT)
Usual Dosage Adult: I.V.: 6 mg, if the dose is not effective within one to two minutes, a rapid I.V. dose of 12 mg may be given

ADH *see* Vasopressin *on page 373*

Adipex-P® *see* Phentermine Hydrochloride *on page 280*

ADR *see* Doxorubicin Hydrochloride *on page 123*

Adrenalin® *see* Epinephrine *on page 131*

Adrenaline *see* Epinephrine *on page 131*

Adriamycin PFS™ *see* Doxorubicin Hydrochloride *on page 123*

Adriamycin RDF™ *see* Doxorubicin Hydrochloride *on page 123*

Adrucil® *see* Fluorouracil *on page 151*

Adsorba® 300 C [OTC] *see* Charcoal *on page 68*

Adsorbent Charcoal, Activated Charcoal *see* Charcoal *on page 68*

Adsorbocarpine® *see* Pilocarpine Hydrochloride *on page 285*

Adsorbonac® [OTC] Ophthalmic *see* Sodium Chloride *on page 327*

Advance® [OTC] *see* Diagnostic Test for Pregnancy *on page 108*

Advil® [OTC] *see* Ibuprofen *on page 181*

AeroBid® *see* Flunisolide *on page 149*

Aerolate® *see* Theophylline *on page 348*

Aerolate III® *see* Theophylline *on page 348*

Aerolate JR® *see* Theophylline *on page 348*

Aerolate SR® S *see* Theophylline *on page 348*

Aerolone® *see* Isoproterenol *on page 193*

Aerosporin® *see* Polymyxin B Sulfate *on page 290*

Afrin® Nasal Solution [OTC] *see* Oxymetazoline Hydrochloride *on page 265*

Afrinol® [OTC] *see* Pseudoephedrine *on page 307*

Aftate® [OTC] *see* Tolnaftate *on page 357*

Agar, Mineral Oil (a' gar)
  Brand Names Agoral® Plain
  Use Temporary relief of hyperacidity
  Usual Dosage Adult: Oral: 7.5 mL-30 mL at bedtime with a full glass of water

Agoral® Plain *see* Agar, Mineral Oil *on this page*

AHF *see* Antihemophilic Factor, Human *on page 26*

A-hydroCort® *see* Hydrocortisone *on page 174*

Akarpine® *see* Pilocarpine Hydrochloride *on page 285*

AK-Chlor® *see* Chloramphenicol *on page 69*

AK-Con® *see* Naphazoline Hydrochloride *on page 246*

AK-Dilate® Ophthalmic Solution *see* Phenylephrine Hydrochloride *on page 282*

Akineton® *see* Biperiden Hydrochloride *on page 45*

AK-Nefrin® Ophthalmic Solution *see* Phenylephrine Hydrochloride *on page 282*

Akne-Mycin® *see* Erythromycin, Topical *on page 135*

AK-Pred® *see* Prednisolone *on page 294*

AK-Tate® *see* Prednisolone *on page 294*

AK-Tracin® *see* Bacitracin *on page 35*

Albalon® Liquifilm® *see* Naphazoline Hydrochloride *on page 246*

Albuminar®-25 *see* Albumin Human *on this page*

Albumin Human (al byoo' min)
Brand Names Albuminar®-25; Albumisol®
Synonyms Normal Human Serum Albumin; Normal Serum Albumin (Human)
Use Plasma volume expansion and maintenance of cardiac output in the treatment of certain types of shock or impending shock
Pregnancy Risk Factor C
Usual Dosage

Adult: Depends on condition of patient, usual adult dose is 25 g; no more than 250 g should be administered within 48 hours

Children: Emergency initial dose 25 g, nonemergencies 25-50% of the adult dose
Hypoproteinemia: I.V.: 0.5-1 g/kg/dose; repeat every 1-2 days as calculated to replace ongoing losses
Hypovolemia: I.V.: 0.5-1 g/kg/dose; repeat as needed; maximum dose: six g/kg/day

Albumisol® *see* Albumin Human *on this page*

Albustix® [OTC] *see* Diagnostic Test for Protein in Urine *on page 108*

Albuterol (al byoo' ter ole)
Brand Names Proventil®; Ventolin®
Synonyms Salbutamol
Use Used as a bronchodilator in reversible airway obstruction due to asthma or COPD
Pregnancy Risk Factor C
Usual Dosage

Adult and Children: > 12 years:
Oral: 2-4 mg 3-4 times daily
Metered dose inhaler: Two inhalations every 4-6 hours (90 μg/spray)
Nebulizer: 2.5 mg 3-4 times daily (2.5 mg=0.5 mL of the 0.5% inhalation solution) in 2.5 mL of normal saline

Children: 6-11 years of age:
Oral: 2 mg 3-4 times/day
Nebulizer: 2.5 mg (0.5 mL of 0.5% solution) in 2 mL normal saline every 4-6 hours; not recommended in children < 12 years of age

Children: 2-6 years:
Oral: 0.1 mg/kg three times/day (not to exceed 6 mg/day); dose may be gradually increased to 0.2 mg/kg (0.5 mL/kg) three times daily (not to exceed 12 mg daily)
Nebulizer: 0.01-0.03 mL/kg (maximum 1 mL) in 2 mL normal saline every 6-8 hours

Alcaine® *see* Proparacaine Hydrochloride *on page 302*

Alclometasone Dipropionate (al kloe met' a sone)
Brand Names Aclovate®
Use Inflammation of corticosteroid-responsive dermatosis
Pregnancy Risk Factor C
Usual Dosage Apply 2-3 times daily

Alcohol and Dextrose (al' koe hol)
Use Increasing caloric intake and replenishing fluids
Usual Dosage
Adult: I.V.: 1-2 L of 5% solution over 24 hours
Children: I.V.: 40 mL/kg/24 hours

Alcohol, Ethyl
Brand Names Lavacol® [OTC]
Synonyms Ethanol
Use Topical anti-infective; pharmaceutical aid
Pregnancy Risk Factor D/X

Alconefrin® Nasal Solution [OTC] *see* Phenylephrine Hydrochloride *on page 282*

Aldactazide® *see* Hydrochlorothiazide and Spironolactone *on page 172*

Aldactone® *see* Spironolactone *on page 332*

Aldoclor® *see* Chlorothiazide and Methyldopa *on page 72*

Aldomet® *see* Methyldopa *on page 230*

Aldoril® *see* Methyldopa and Hydrochlorothiazide *on page 230*

Alfenta® *see* Alfentanil Hydrochloride *on this page*

Alfentanil Hydrochloride (al fen' ta nill)
Brand Names Alfenta®
Use As analgesic adjunct given in incremental doses in maintenance of anesthesia with barbiturate or NO_2 or a primary anesthetic agent for the induction of anesthesia in patients undergoing general surgery in which endotracheal intubation and mechanical ventilation are required
Restrictions C-II
Pregnancy Risk Factor C
(Continued)

11

Alfentanil Hydrochloride *(Continued)*

Alfentanil

Indication	Approximate Duration of Anesthesia (min)	Induction Period (Initial Dose) (μg/kg)	Maintenance Period (Increments/ Infusion)	Total Dose (μg/kg)	Effects
Incremental injection	≤ 30	8–20	3–5 μg/kg or 0.5–1 μg/kg/min	8–40	Spontaneously breathing or assisted ventilation when required.
	30–60	20–50	5–15 μg/kg	Up to 75	Assisted or controlled ventilation required. Attenuation of response to laryngoscopy and intubation.
Continuous infusion	> 45	50–75	0.5–3.0 μg/kg/min average infusion rate 1–1.5 μg/kg/min	Dependent on duration of procedure	Assisted or controlled ventilation required. Some attenuation of response to intubation and incision, with intraoperative stability.
Anesthetic induction	> 45	130–245	0.5–1.5 μg/kg/min or general anesthetic	Dependent on duration of procedure	Assisted or controlled ventilation required. Administer slowly (over three minutes). Concentration of inhalation agents reduced by 30–50% for initial hour.

Usual Dosage No pediatric dosage data available in children < 12 years of age. See table.

ALG
Brand Names ALG Minnesota
Restrictions Investigational drug
Usual Dosage Skin testing for hypersensitivity should be performed prior to administration. Dosage: 10-30 mg/kg/day administered as a 1% solution (10 mg/mL) in 0.9% sodium chloride over 4-6 hours, through a 5 micron filter

ALG Minnesota *see* ALG *on this page*

Alimenazine Tartrate *see* Trimeprazine Tartrate *on page 363*

Alkeran® *see* Melphalan *on page 217*

Allantoin and Coal Tar *(a lan' toyn)*
Brand Names Tegrin® [OTC]
Synonyms Coal Tar and Allantoin
Use Symptomatic relief of psoriasis
Usual Dosage Adult: Apply 2-4 four times daily

Allbee® With C [OTC] *see* Vitamin B Complex With Vitamin C *on page 377*

Aller-Chlor® [OTC] *see* Chlorpheniramine Maleate *on page 74*

Allerest® 12 Hours Nasal Solution [OTC] *see* Oxymetazoline Hydrochloride *on page 265*

Allerest® Eye Drops [OTC] *see* Naphazoline Hydrochloride *on page 246*

Allergenic Extracts
Use Relief of allergic symptoms due to specifically identified materials by means of a graduated schedule of doses; diagnosis of specific allergies
Pregnancy Risk Factor C
Usual Dosage Inject subcutaneously usually every 3-14 days

Allopurinol (al oh pure' i nole)
Brand Names Lopurin™; Zurinol®; Zyloprim®
Use Prevention of attack of gouty arthritis and nephropathy; also used to treat secondary hyperuricemia which may occur during treatment of tumors or leukemia, and to prevent recurrent calcium oxalate calculi
Pregnancy Risk Factor C
Usual Dosage Adjust dosage in renal impairment

Adult:
Gout: 200-300 mg/day (mild), 400-600 mg/day (severe)
Myeloproliferative neoplastic disorders: 200-800 mg/day for 2-3 days (doses > 300 mg should be divided and given twice a day)

Children: 10 mg/kg/day in divided doses every eight hours
6-10 years: 300 mg/day in three doses every eight hours
< 6 years: 150 mg/day in three doses every eight hours

Aloe Vera (al' oh)
Brand Names Dermaide®
Use Soothing moisturizer for dry itchy skin, minor burns and sunburn, minor cuts, scrapes and mild skin irritations
Usual Dosage Adult: Apply 2-4 times daily

Alophen Pills® [OTC] *see* Phenolphthalein *on page 280*

Alpha Keri® [OTC] *see* Bath Oil, Antipruritic *on page 37*

Alphatrex® *see* Betamethasone *on page 43*

Alpidine® *see* Apraclonidine Hydrochloride *on page 28*

Alprazolam (al pray' zoe lam)
Brand Names Xanax®
Use Treatment of anxiety and as an adjunct in the treatment of depression; also may be used in the management of panic attacks
Restrictions C-IV
Pregnancy Risk Factor D
Usual Dosage Adult: Oral: 0.25-0.5 mg 2-3 times daily, up to 4 mg/day

Alprostadil (al pross' ta dil)

Brand Names Prostin VR Pediatric®

Synonyms PGE₁; Prostaglandin E₁

Use Temporary maintenance of patency of ductus arteriosus in neonates with ductal-dependent congenital cyanotic or acyanotic heart disease until surgery can be performed

Usual Dosage I.V., Intra-arterial, Intra-aortic: 0.05-0.1 μg/kg/minute with therapeutic response, rate is reduced to lowest effective dosage level; with unsatisfactory dose, rate is increased gradually to 0.2 μg/kg/minute to 0.4 μg/kg/minute

PGE_1 is usually given at an infusion rate of 0.1 μg/kg/minute, but it is often possible to reduce the dosage to one half or even one tenth without losing the therapeutic effect. The mixing schedule is shown in the following table.

Add 1 Ampule (500 μg) to:	Concentration (μg/mL)	Infusion Rate	
		mL/min/kg Needed to Infuse 0.1 μg/kg/min	mL/kg/24 h
250 mL	2	0.05	72
100 mL*	5	0.02	28.8
50 mL	10	0.01	14.4
25 mL	20	0.005	7.2

AL-R® [OTC] *see* Chlorpheniramine Maleate *on page 74*

Alteplase (al' te place)

Brand Names Activase®

Synonyms Tissue Plasminogen Activator, Recombinant; t-PA

Use Management of acute myocardial infarction for the lysis of thrombi in coronary arteries

Pregnancy Risk Factor C

Usual Dosage 60 mg over three hour period

ALternaGEL® [OTC] *see* Aluminum Hydroxide *on next page*

Alu-Cap® [OTC] *see* Aluminum Hydroxide *on next page*

Aluminum Acetate

Brand Names Acid Mantle®; Domeboro®

Synonyms Burow's Solution

Use Astringent wet dressing for relief of inflammatory conditions of the skin

Pregnancy Risk Factor C

Usual Dosage Apply every 15-30 minutes for 4-8 hours

Aluminum Carbonate (a loo' mi num)

Brand Names Basaljel® [OTC]

Use Hyperacidity; hyperphosphatemia

Usual Dosage Adult: Oral:

Antacid: 2 tablets/capsules or 10 mL of suspension every 2 hours, up to 12 times daily

Hyperphosphatemia: 2 tablets/capsules or 12 mL of suspension with meals

Aluminum Chloride

Brand Names Drysol™

Use As an astringent in the management of hyperhidrosis

Usual Dosage Adult: Topical: Apply at bedtime

Aluminum Hydroxide

Brand Names ALternaGEL® [OTC]; Alu-Cap® [OTC]; Alu-Tab® [OTC]; Amphojel® [OTC]; Dialume® [OTC]; Nephrox Suspension [OTC]

Use Hyperacidity; hyperphosphatemia

Usual Dosage Oral:

Adult: 500-1800 mg, 3-6 times daily, between meals and at bedtime

Children: Hyperphosphatemia: 50-150 mg/kg/24 hours in divided doses every 4-6 hours

Aluminum Hydroxide and Magnesium Hydroxide

Brand Names Maalox® [OTC]; Maalox® Therapeutic Concentrate [OTC]

Synonyms Magnesium Hydroxide and Aluminum Hydroxide

Use Antacid, hyperphosphatemia in renal failure

Pregnancy Risk Factor C

Usual Dosage 5-10 mL or 1-2 tablets 4-6 times daily, between meals and at bedtime; may be used every hour for severe symptoms

Aluminum Hydroxide, Magnesium Hydroxide and Simethicone

Brand Names Di-Gel® [OTC]; Gelusil® [OTC]; Maalox® Plus [OTC]; Mylanta® [OTC]; Mylanta®-II [OTC]

Use Temporary relief of hyperacidity

Pregnancy Risk Factor C

Aluminum Hydroxide, Magnesium Trisilicate, Sodium Bicarbonate and Alginic Acid

Brand Names Gaviscon® Foamtabs [OTC]

Use Temporary relief of hyperacidity

Pregnancy Risk Factor C

Usual Dosage Adult: Oral: Chew 2-4 tablets four times daily

Aluminum Phosphate

Brand Names Phosphaljel® [OTC]

Use Reduce fecal excretion of phosphates

Usual Dosage Adult: Oral: 15 mL-30 mL every 2 hours between meals

Alupent® *see* Metaproterenol Sulfate *on page 223*

Alu-Tab® [OTC] *see* Aluminum Hydroxide *on previous page*

Amantadine Hydrochloride (a man' ta deen)
Brand Names Symadine®; Symmetrel®
Use Symptomatic initial and adjunct treatment of parkinsonism; also used in prophylaxis and treatment of influenza A viral infection
Pregnancy Risk Factor C
Usual Dosage

Adult:
Parkinson's disease: 100 mg twice daily
Influenza A viral infection: 100 mg twice daily

Children: 4.4-8.8 mg/kg/day up to 150 mg/d in 2-3 divided doses

Ambenonium Chloride (am be noe' nee um)
Brand Names Mytelase®
Use Treatment of myasthenia gravis
Pregnancy Risk Factor C
Usual Dosage Adult: Oral: 5-25 mg 3 or 4 times daily

Ambenyl® *see* Bromodiphenhydramine and Codeine *on page 47*

Amcinonide (am sin' oh nide)
Brand Names Cyclocort®
Use Relief of the inflammatory and pruritic manifestations of corticosteroid-responsive dermatoses
Pregnancy Risk Factor C
Usual Dosage Apply in a thin film 2-4 times daily

Amcort® *see* Triamcinolone *on page 359*

Amdinocillin (am dee' noe sill in)
Brand Names Coactin®
Use Treatment of complicated and uncomplicated urinary tract infections to susceptible organisms
Pregnancy Risk Factor B
Usual Dosage Adult: I.M., I.V.: 10 mg/kg every 4-6 hours

Americaine® [OTC] *see* Benzocaine *on page 40*

Amesec® [OTC] *see* Aminophylline, Amobarbital and Ephedrine *on page 19*

A-methaPred® *see* Methylprednisolone *on page 231*

Amethocaine Hydrochloride *see* Tetracaine Hydrochloride *on page 346*

Amethopterin *see* Methotrexate *on page 227*

Amfepramone *see* Diethylpropion Hydrochloride *on page 112*

Amicar® *see* Aminocaproic Acid *on page 18*

Amidate® *see* Etomidate *on page 142*

Amikacin Sulfate (am i kay' sin)
Brand Names Amikin®
Use Useful in treatment of gram-negative bacillary infections due to staphylococci where penicillins or other less toxic drugs are contraindicated
Pregnancy Risk Factor D
Usual Dosage I.M., I.V.:

Adult: 15 mg/kg/day in divided doses every 8-12 hours

Children: 15 mg/kg/day in divided doses every 8-12 hours

Neonate: 10 mg/kg initially, then 7.5 mg/kg every 12 hours

Amikin® *see* Amikacin Sulfate *on this page*

Amiloride and Hydrochlorothiazide
Brand Names Moduretic®
Synonyms Hydrochlorothiazide and Amiloride
Use Antikaluretic diuretic, antihypertensive
Pregnancy Risk Factor B
Usual Dosage Adult: Oral: Start with one tablet daily, then may be increased to two tablets daily in needed; usually given in a single dose

Amiloride Hydrochloride (a mill' oh ride)
Brand Names Midamor®
Use To counteract potassium loss induced by other diuretics in congestive heart failure or hypertension
Pregnancy Risk Factor B
Usual Dosage

Adult: 5-10 mg/day (up to 20 mg)

Children: Although safety and efficacy has not been established by the FDA in children, a dosage of 0.625 mg/kg/day has been used in children weighing 6-20 kg

Aminacrine Hydrochloride (am in ak' rin)
Synonyms 9-Aminoacridine Hydrochloride
Use Topical anti-infective

Amin-Aid® [OTC] *see* Nutritional Formula, Enteral/Oral *on page 258*

2-Amino-6-mercaptopurine *see* Thioguanine *on page 352*

Amino Acid Injection
Brand Names Aminosyn®; HepatAmine®
Use In parenteral nutrition to prevent nitrogen loss or treat negative nitrogen balance when alimentary cannot be used, GI absorption is impaired, bowel rest is needed and metabolic requirements for protein are substantially increased
Pregnancy Risk Factor C
(Continued)

17

Amino Acid Injection *(Continued)*

Usual Dosage Adult: I.V.:

Peripheral: 1-1.7 g/kg/day
Central: 500 mL with dextrose solution over 8 hour period

Aminoacridine

Use Bacteriostatic agent

9-Aminoacridine Hydrochloride *see* Aminacrine Hydrochloride *on previous page*

Aminocaproic Acid *(a mee noe ka proe' ik)*

Brand Names Amicar®

Use Treatment of excessive bleeding

Pregnancy Risk Factor C

Usual Dosage In the management of acute bleeding syndromes, oral dosage regimens are the same as the I.V. dosage regimens in adults and children

Adult:

Oral: For the treatment of acute bleeding syndromes due to elevated fibrinolytic activity, give 5 g during first hour, followed by 1-1.25 g/hour for about eight hours or until bleeding stops

I.V.: Give 4-5 g in 250 mL of diluent during first hour followed by continuous infusion at the rate of 1-1.25 g/hour in 50 mL of diluent, continue for eight hours or until bleeding stops

Children: Oral, I.V.: 100 mg/kg or 3 g/m² during the first hour, followed by continuous infusion at the rate of 33.3 mg/kg/hour or 1 g/m²/hour; total dosage should not exceed 18 g/m²/24 hours

Amino-Cerv™ Vaginal Cream *see* Urea *on page 369*

Aminoglutethimide *(a mee noe gloo teth' i mide)*

Brand Names Cytadren®

Use Suppression of adrenal function in selected patients with Cushing's syndrome; also used successfully in postmenopausal patients with advanced breast carcinoma and in patients with metastatic prostate carcinoma

Pregnancy Risk Factor D

Usual Dosage 250 mg every six hours may be increased to a total of 2 g/day

Aminohippurate Sodium *(a mee noe hip' yoor ate)*

Use Diagnostic aid for renal plasma flow

Usual Dosage I.V.: 6-10 mg/kg loading dose, followed by 10-24 mg/min continuous infusion

Aminophyllin™ *see* Aminophylline *on this page*

Aminophylline *(am in off' i lin)*

Brand Names Aminophyllin™; Amoline®; Phyllocontin®; Somophyllin®; Somophyllin®-DF; Truphylline®

Synonyms Theophylline Ethylenediamine

Use As a bronchodilator in reversible airway obstruction due to asthma or COPD

Pregnancy Risk Factor C

Usual Dosage

Apnea: (Aminophylline concentration 2 mg/mL):
Loading dose: 5 mg/kg; dilute dose in one hour I.V. fluid via syringe pump over one hour
Maintenance: 2 mg/kg every 8-12 hours or 1-3 mg/kg/dose every 8-12 hours; administer I.V. push 1 mL/minute (2 mg/minute)

Wheezing: 4-6 mg/kg every six hours; theophylline levels should be drawn every 4-6 hours initially - longer intervals are OK when infant is stable

Treatment of acute bronchospasm in older patients: (> 6 months of age): Loading dose (in patients not currently receiving theophylline): 6 mg/kg (based on aminophylline) given I.V. over 20-30 minutes; 4.7 mg/kg (based on theophylline) given I.V. over 20-30 minutes; administration rate should not exceed 20 mg (1 mL)/minute (theophylline) or 25 mg (1 mL)/minute (aminophylline)

Approximate maintenance dosage for treatment of acute bronchospasm (first 12 hours):
Children: 6 months - 9 years of age: 1.2 mg/kg/hour (aminophylline); 0.95 mg/kg/hour (theophylline)
9-16 years and young adult smokers: 1 mg/kg/hour (aminophylline); 0.79 mg/kg/hour (theophylline)
Adult (healthy, nonsmoking): 0.7 mg/kg/hour (aminophylline); 0.55 mg/kg/hour (theophylline)
Older patients and patients with cor pulmonale: 0.6 mg/kg/hour (aminophylline); 0.47 mg/kg/hour (theophylline)
Patients with CHF or liver failure: 0.5 mg/kg/hour (aminophylline); 0.39 mg/kg/hour (theophylline)
Dosage should be adjusted according to serum level during the second 12-hour period

Aminophylline, Amobarbital and Ephedrine

Brand Names Amesec® [OTC]

Use Symptomatic relief of asthma

Pregnancy Risk Factor C

Usual Dosage Adult: Oral: One capsule every 6 hours

Aminosalicylate Sodium *see* Para-aminosalicylate Sodium
on page 268

Aminosalicylic Acid (a mee noe sal i sill' ik)

Brand Names Pamisyl®

Synonyms PAS

Use Treatment of tuberculosis with combination drugs

Usual Dosage Oral:
Adult: 14-16 g/day in 2 or 3 divided doses
Children: 275-420 mg/day in 3 or 4 divided doses

5-Aminosalicylic Acid *see* Mesalamine *on page 220*

Aminosyn® *see* Amino Acid Injection *on page 17*

Amiodarone Hydrochloride (a mee' oh da rone)
Brand Names Cordarone®
Use Used only in the management and prophylaxis of life-threatening ventricular arrhythmias unresponsive to conventional therapy with less toxic agents
Pregnancy Risk Factor C
Usual Dosage 800-1600 mg/day in 1-2 doses for 1-3 weeks, then 600-800 mg/day in 1-2 doses for one month, then 400 mg/day maintenance dose

Amipaque® *see* Metrizamide *on page 234*

Amitriptyline and Chlordiazepoxide
Brand Names Limbitrol®
Synonyms Chlordiazepoxide and Amitriptyline
Use Treatment of moderate to severe anxiety and/or agitation and depression
Restrictions C-IV
Pregnancy Risk Factor D
Usual Dosage Initial dose 3-4 tablets in divided doses, this may be increased to six tablets daily as required; some patients respond to smaller doses and can be maintained on two tablets

Amitriptyline and Perphenazine
Brand Names Etrafon®; Triavil®
Synonyms Perphenazine and Amitriptyline
Use Treatment of patients with moderate to severe anxiety and depression
Pregnancy Risk Factor D
Usual Dosage One tablet 2-4 times daily

Amitriptyline Hydrochloride (a mee trip' ti leen)
Brand Names Elavil®; Endep®; Enovil®
Use Used in the treatment of various forms of depression, often in conjunction with psychotherapy
Pregnancy Risk Factor D
Usual Dosage

Children: For pain management: Oral: Initial: 0.1 mg/kg at bedtime, may advance as tolerated over 2-3 weeks to 0.5-2 mg/kg at bedtime

Adult:
Oral: 30-100 mg/day single bedtime dose or divided doses; dose may be gradually increased up to 300 mg/day
I.M.: 20-30 mg four times daily

Ammonia Spirit, Aromatic (a moe' nee a)
Use Respiratory and circulatory stimulant
Pregnancy Risk Factor C
Usual Dosage Used as "smelling salts" to treat or prevent fainting

Ammonium Chloride

Use Diuretic or systemic and urinary acidifying agent and treatment of hypochloremic states

Pregnancy Risk Factor B

Usual Dosage

Oral: 1 g three times daily for no longer than six days

I.V.: 100-200 mEq for 500-1000 mL NaCl 0.9% injection, give 5 mL/minutes in adults, monitor dosage by repeated serum bicarbonate determinations

Amobarbital (am oh bar' bi tal)

Brand Names Amytal®

Use Oral: Hypnotic in short-term treatment of insomnia, to reduce anxiety and provide sedation preoperatively. I.M. or I.V.: Used to control status epilepticus or acute seizure episodes. Also used in catatonic, negativistic, or manic reactions.

Restrictions C-II

Pregnancy Risk Factor D

Usual Dosage

Insomnia: Oral: 100-200 mg at bedtime

Preanesthetic: 200 mg 1-2 hours before surgery

I.M.: 65-500 mg

I.V.: 65-500 mg

Amobarbital and Secobarbital

Brand Names Tuinal®

Synonyms Secobarbital and Amobarbital

Use Short-term treatment of insomnia

Restrictions C-II

Pregnancy Risk Factor D

Usual Dosage Adult: Oral: One or two capsules at bedtime

Amoline® see Aminophylline on page 18

Amonidrin® [OTC] see Guaifenesin on page 162

Amoxapine (a mox' a peen)

Brand Names Asendin®

Use Treatment of neurotic and endogenous depression and mixed symptoms of anxiety and depression

Pregnancy Risk Factor C

Usual Dosage 200-300 mg/day - initially 25 mg 2-3 times a day, if tolerated, dosage may be increased to 100 mg 2-3 times daily; once an effective dose has been reached the drug may be given in a single bedtime

Amoxicillin (a mox i sill' in)

Brand Names A-Cillin®; Amoxil®; Larotid®; Polymox®; Trimox®; Wymox®

Synonyms Amoxycillin; p-Hydroxyampicillin

Use Infections caused by susceptible organisms involving the respiratory tract, otitis media, sinusitis, skin, and urinary tract

(Continued)

Amoxicillin *(Continued)*

Pregnancy Risk Factor B
Usual Dosage Oral:

Adult:
250-500 mg every eight hours
Gonorrhea: 3 g plus probenecid 1 g in a single dose

Children:
> 20 kg: 250-500 mg every eight hours
6-20 kg: 20 mg/kg in divided doses every eight hours
Gonorrhea: ≥ 2 years: 50 mg/kg plus probenecid 25 mg/kg in a single dose; do not use this regimen in children < two years of age; probenecid is contraindicated in this age group

Amoxicillin and Clavulanate Potassium *see* Amoxicillin and Clavulanic Acid *on this page*

Amoxicillin and Clavulanic Acid

Brand Names Augmentin®
Synonyms Amoxicillin and Clavulanate Potassium
Use Infections caused by susceptible organisms involving the lower respiratory tract, otitis media, sinusitis, skin and skin structure, and urinary tract
Pregnancy Risk Factor B
Usual Dosage Oral:

Adult: 250-500 mg every eight hours

Children: < 40 kg: 20-40 mg/kg/day in divided doses every eight hours

Amoxil® *see* Amoxicillin *on previous page*

Amoxycillin *see* Amoxicillin *on previous page*

Amphetamine Sulfate *(am fet' a meen)*

Synonyms Racemic Amphetamine Sulfate
Use Narcolepsy; exogenous obesity; abnormal behavioral syndrome in children (minimal brain dysfunction)
Restrictions C-II
Pregnancy Risk Factor D
Usual Dosage

Narcolepsy:
Adult: Oral: 5-60 mg/day in divided doses
Children: > 12 years of age: 10 mg/day, increase by 10 mg at weekly intervals; 6-12 years of age: 5 mg/day, increase by 5 mg at weekly intervals

Minimal brain dysfunction: Children: Oral:
> 6 years: 5 mg/day, increase by 5 mg at weekly intervals
3-5 years of age: 2.5 mg/day, increase by 2.5 mg at weekly intervals

Short-term adjunct to exogenous obesity: Adult and Children: > 12 years: 10 mg or 15 mg long-acting capsule daily, up to 30 mg/day; or 5-30 mg/day in divided doses

Amphojel® [OTC] *see* Aluminum Hydroxide *on page 15*

Amphotericin B (am foe ter' i sin)

Brand Names Fungizone®

Use Treatment of severe systemic infections and meningitis caused by susceptible fungi

Restrictions 1:10 dilution

Pregnancy Risk Factor B

Usual Dosage

Adult: I.V.:

Test dose: 1 mg in 250 mL dextrose 5% over 2-4 hours

Initial: 0.25 mg/kg administered over six hours; dose should be gradually increased over one week to a dose of 0.5 mg/kg/day; dosage may range up to 1 mg/kg/day or 1.5 mg/kg on alternate days; do not exceed 1.5 mg/kg/day

Adult: I.T.: Initial: 0.025 mg diluted with 10-20 mL of CSF and administered by barbotage; dose is administered 2-3 times a week; dosage may be gradually increased to a maximum of 0.5-1 mg

Children: I.V.:

Test dose: 0.1 mg/kg/day, up to a maximum of 1 mg/dose

Initial: 0.25 mg/kg/day; increase to 1 mg/kg/day by increments of 0.125-0.25 mg/kg/day or every other day

Maximum dose: 1.5 mg/kg/day

Alternate day dose: 1.5 mg/kg/day on alternate days

Children: Topical. Apply 2-4 times daily

Ampicillin (am pi sill' in)

Brand Names Amplin®; Omnipen®; Penamp®; Pfizerpen® A; Polycillin®; Principen®; Totacillin®

Use Treatment of susceptible bacterial infections

Pregnancy Risk Factor B

Usual Dosage

Adult:

Oral: 250-500 mg every six hours

I.M., I.V.: 8-12 g/day in divided doses every 3-4 hours

Children:

Oral: > 20 kg: 250-500 mg every six hours; < 20 kg: 50-100 mg/kg in divided doses every 6-8 hours

I.M., I.V.: > 40 kg: 8-12 g in divided doses every 3-4 hours; < 40 kg: 25-50 mg/kg/day in divided doses every 6-8 hours, up to 100-200 mg/kg/day

Ampicillin and Sulbactam

Brand Names Unasyn®

Synonyms Sulbactam and Ampicillin

Use Treatment of susceptible bacterial infections

Pregnancy Risk Factor B

Usual Dosage 1.5-3 g every six hours

Amplin® *see* Ampicillin *on previous page*

AMPT *see* Metyrosine *on page 235*

Amrinone Lactate (am' ri none)
Brand Names Inocor®
Use Treatment of low cardiac output states (sepsis, congestive heart failure); adjunctive therapy of pulmonary hypertension
Pregnancy Risk Factor C
Usual Dosage Note: Dose should not exceed 10 mg/kg/24 hours

Adult: 0.75 mg/kg I.V. bolus over 2-3 minutes followed by maintenance infusion of 5-10 µg/kg/minute

Children: 0.75 mg/kg I.V. bolus over 2-3 minutes followed by maintenance infusion 5-10 µg/kg/minute; I.V. bolus may need to be repeated in 30 minutes

Neonate: Should receive lower maintenance infusion 3-5 µg/kg/minute

Amstat® *see* Tranexamic Acid *on page 358*

Amvisc® *see* Sodium Hyaluronate *on page 328*

Amyl Nitrite (am' il)
Use Coronary vasodilator in angina pectoris
Pregnancy Risk Factor C
Usual Dosage Adult: Inhalation: 0.18-0.3 mL, as needed

Amytal® *see* Amobarbital *on page 21*

Anabolin® *see* Nandrolone *on page 246*

Anacin® [OTC] *see* Aspirin *on page 30*

Anacin-3® [OTC] *see* Acetaminophen *on page 4*

Anadrol® *see* Oxymetholone *on page 265*

Anafranil® *see* Clomipramine *on page 83*

Ana-Kit® *see* Insect Sting Kit *on page 185*

Analgesic Balm *see* Rubs and Liniments *on page 319*

Anaprox® *see* Naproxen *on page 246*

Anaspaz® *see* Hyoscyamine Sulfate *on page 180*

Ancef® *see* Cefazolin Sodium *on page 63*

Ancobon® *see* Flucytosine *on page 149*

Andralone-D® *see* Nandrolone *on page 246*

Andro® *see* Testosterone *on page 345*

Andro-Cyp® *see* Testosterone *on page 345*

Android® *see* Methyltestosterone *on page 232*

Android-F® *see* Fluoxymesterone *on page 152*

Andro-L.A.® *see* Testosterone *on page 345*

Androlan® *see* Testosterone *on page 345*

Androlone® *see* Nandrolone *on page 246*

Andronaq® *see* Testosterone *on page 345*

Andronaq®-L.A. *see* Testosterone *on page 345*

Andronate® *see* Testosterone *on page 345*

Andropository® *see* Testosterone *on page 345*

Andryl® *see* Testosterone *on page 345*

Anectine® Chloride *see* Succinylcholine Chloride *on page 334*

Anectine® Flo-Pack® *see* Succinylcholine Chloride *on page 334*

Anergan® *see* Promethazine Hydrochloride *on page 301*

Anestacon® *see* Lidocaine Hydrochloride *on page 204*

Anestatal® *see* Thiamylal Sodium *on page 351*

Aneurine Hydrochloride *see* Thiamine Hydrochloride *on page 351*

Angio-Conray® *see* Iothalamate Sodium *on page 190*

Anhydron® *see* Cyclothiazide *on page 94*

Anisotropine Methylbromide (an iss oh troe' peen)
Brand Names Valpin® 50
Use Adjunctive treatment of peptic ulcer
Pregnancy Risk Factor C
Usual Dosage Adult: Oral: 50 mg three times a day

Anisoylated Plasminogen Streptokinase Activatory Complex
see Anistreplase *on this page*

Anistreplase
Brand Names Eminase®
Synonyms Anisoylated Plasminogen Streptokinase Activatory Complex; APSAC
Use Management of acute myocardial infarction (AMI) in adults; lysis of thrombi obstructing coronary arteries, reduction of infarct size; and reduction of mortality associated with AMI
Pregnancy Risk Factor C
Usual Dosage Adult: I.V.: 30 units injected over 2-5 minutes as soon as possible after onset of symptoms

Anocol® *see* Chloramphenicol *on page 69*

Ansaid® *see* Flurbiprofen Sodium *on page 153*

Anspor® *see* Cephradine *on page 67*

Answer® [OTC] *see* Diagnostic Test for Pregnancy *on page 108*

Answer® 2 [OTC] *see* Diagnostic Test for Pregnancy *on page 108*

Answer® Plus [OTC] *see* Diagnostic Test for Pregnancy *on page 108*

Antabuse® *see* Disulfiram *on page 120*

Antepar® *see* Piperazine Citrate *on page 286*

Anthra-Derm® *see* Anthralin *on this page*

Anthralin (an' thra lin)
Brand Names Anthra-Derm®; Drithocreme®; Lasan®
Use Treatment of psoriasis
Pregnancy Risk Factor C
Usual Dosage Adult: Topical: Apply in a thin film at bedtime

Antidiuretic Hormone *see* Vasopressin *on page 373*

Antihemophilic Factor, Human (an tee hee moe fill' ik)
Brand Names Hemofil® M; Humate-P®; Kōate®-HS; Kōate®-HT; Monoclate®; Profilate® HP; Prolifate® SD
Synonyms AHF; Factor VIII
Use Management of hemophilia A
Pregnancy Risk Factor C
Usual Dosage Individualize dosage. Hospitalized patients: 20-50 units/g/dose; may be higher for special circumstances. Dose can be given every 12-24 hours and more frequently in special circumstances.

Antilirium® *see* Physostigmine Salicylate *on page 284*

Antiminth® *see* Pyrantel Pamoate *on page 308*

Antipyrine and Benzocaine (an tee pye' reen)
Brand Names Auralgan®
Synonyms Benzocaine and Antipyrine
Use Acute otitis media and facilitates ear wax removal
Usual Dosage Fill ear canal; moisten cotton pledget, place in external ear, repeat every 1-2 hours until pain and congestion is relieved. For ear wax removal instill drops 3-4 times daily.

Antirabies Serum, Equine Origin (an tee ray' beez)
Synonyms ARS
Use Rabies prophylaxis
Pregnancy Risk Factor C
Usual Dosage 1000 IU/55 pounds in a single dose, infiltrate up to 50% of dose around the wound

Antithymocyte Immunoglobulin *see* Lymphocyte Immune Globulin *on page 208*

Antivenin, Black Widow Spider (Equine)
Synonyms Black Widow Spider Species Antivenin *Latrodectus mactans*
Use Treat patients with symptoms of black widow spider bites
Pregnancy Risk Factor C
Usual Dosage

Adult and Children: I.M.: 2.5 mL

Children or Adult (severe): < 12 years of age: I.V.: 2.5 mL in 10-50 mL over 15 minutes

Antivenin (Crotalidae) Polyvalent (kroe tal' ih day)
Synonyms Crotaline Antivenin, Polyvalent; North and South American Antisnake-bite Serum; Snake (Pit Vipers) Antivenin
Use For neutralization of the venoms of North and South America Crotalids: rattlesnake, copperhead, cottonmouth, tropical moccasins, Fer-de-lance, bushmaster
Pregnancy Risk Factor C
Usual Dosage Initial intradermal sensitivity test. The entire initial dose of antivenin should be administered as soon as possible to be most effective (within 4 hours after the bite).

Adult and Children: I.V.: Minimal envenomation: 20-40 mL; moderate envenomation: 50-90 mL; severe envenomation: 100-150 mL
Additional doses of antivenin is based on clinical response to the initial dose. If swelling continues to progress, symptoms increase in severity or hypotension, decrease if hematocrit appear, an additional 10-50 mL should be administered.
For I.V. Infusion: 1:1 to 1:10 dilution of reconstituted antivenin in normal saline or D₅W should be prepared.

Antivenin (*Micrurus fulvius*)
Synonyms North American Coral Snake Antivenin
Use Neutralize the venom of Eastern coral snake and Texas coral snake but not neutralize venom of Arizona or Sonoran coral snake
Pregnancy Risk Factor C
Usual Dosage I.V.: 3-5 vials by slow injection

Antivert® *see* Meclizine Hydrochloride *on page 215*

Antrizine® *see* Meclizine Hydrochloride *on page 215*

Anturane® *see* Sulfinpyrazone *on page 338*

Anxanil® *see* Hydroxyzine *on page 178*

APAP *see* Acetaminophen *on page 4*

Apatate® [OTC] *see* Vitamin B Complex *on page 377*

Aphrodyne™ *see* Yohimbine Hydrochloride *on page 381*

A.P.L.® *see* Chorionic Gonadotropin *on page 78*

Aplisol® *see* Tuberculin *on page 367*

Aplitest® *see* Tuberculin *on page 367*

Apomorphine Hydrochloride (a poe mor' feen)
Use To produce emesis in acute oral overdoses or poisoning
(Continued)

Apomorphine Hydrochloride *(Continued)*

Pregnancy Risk Factor C

Usual Dosage I.M., S.C.:

Adult: 2-10 mg followed by oral administration of water or evaporated milk; dose not to be repeated

Children: 0.07-0.1 mg/kg or 3 mg/m^2 followed by oral administration of water; dose not to be repeated

APPG *see* Penicillin G Procaine, Aqueous *on page 273*

Apraclonidine Hydrochloride (a pra kloe' ni deen)

Brand Names Alpidine®; Iopidine®

Use Prevention and treatment of postsurgical intraocular pressure elevation

Usual Dosage One drop in operative eye one hour prior to laser surgery, second drop in eye upon completion of procedure

Apresazide® *see* Hydralazine and Hydrochlorothiazide *on page 171*

Apresoline® *see* Hydralazine Hydrochloride *on page 171*

APSAC *see* Anistreplase *on page 25*

Aquacare® [OTC] *see* Urea *on page 369*

AquaMEPHYTON® *see* Phytonadione *on page 285*

Aquaphyllin® *see* Theophylline *on page 348*

Aquasol A® [OTC] *see* Vitamin A *on page 376*

Aquasol® E [OTC] *see* Vitamin E *on page 378*

Aquatensen® *see* Methyclothiazide *on page 229*

Aquazide-H® *see* Hydrochlorothiazide *on page 172*

Aqueous Procaine Penicillin G *see* Penicillin G Procaine, Aqueous *on page 273*

Aqueous Testosterone *see* Testosterone *on page 345*

Ara-A *see* Vidarabine *on page 375*

Ara-C *see* Cytarabine Hydrochloride *on page 95*

Aralen® Phosphate *see* Chloroquine Phosphate *on page 71*

Aralen® Phosphate With Primaquine Phosphate *see* Chloroquine and Primaquine *on page 70*

Aramine® *see* Metaraminol Bitartrate *on page 223*

Arfonad® *see* Trimethaphan Camsylate *on page 363*

Argesic®-SA *see* Salsalate *on page 320*

Arginine Hydrochloride (ar' ji neen)

Brand Names R-Gene®; R-Gene® 10

Use Pituitary function test (growth hormone); management of extreme metabolic alkalosis

Usual Dosage

Adult and Children: Metabolic alkalosis: Dosage (in grams) is estimated by multiplying the desired decrease in plasma bicarbonate concentrate (mEq/L) by the patient's weight (kg) and dividing this by 9.6

Adult: I.V.: 30 g administered at a constant rate over 30 minutes

Children: I.V.: 500 mg/kg/dose administered over 30 minutes

Argyrol® S.S. 20% [OTC] see Silver Protein, Mild on page 324

Aristocort® Forte see Triamcinolone on page 359

Aristocort® Intralesional Suspension see Triamcinolone on page 359

Aristocort® Tablet see Triamcinolone on page 359

Aristospan® see Triamcinolone on page 359

Arlidin® see Nylidrin Hydrochloride on page 258

Arm-a-Med® Isoetharine see Isoetharine on page 191

Armour® Thyroid see Thyroid on page 354

ARS see Antirabies Serum, Equine Origin on page 26

Artane® see Trihexyphenidyl Hydrochloride on page 362

Artha-G® see Salsalate on page 320

Artificial Tears

Brand Names Tearisol® [OTC]
Use Ophthalmic lubricant
Pregnancy Risk Factor C
Usual Dosage Use as needed to relieve symptoms

ASA see Aspirin on next page

A.S.A. [OTC] see Aspirin on next page

5-ASA see Mesalamine on page 220

Ascorbic Acid (a skor' bik)

Brand Names Ascorbicap® [OTC]; Cecon® [OTC]; Cee-1000® T.D. [OTC]; Cetane® [OTC]; Cevalin® [OTC]; Ce-Vi-Sol® [OTC]; Cevita® [OTC]; C-Span® [OTC]; Flavorcee® [OTC]; Vita-C® [OTC]
Synonyms Vitamin C [OTC]
Use Prevention and treatment of scurvy and to acidify the urine; large doses may decrease the severity of "colds"; dietary supplementation
Pregnancy Risk Factor C
Usual Dosage Oral:

Adult:
Scurvy: 100-250 mg 1-2 times daily
Urinary acidification: 4-12 g/day in 3-4 divided doses
Dietary supplement: 50-60 mg/day
Prevention and treatment of cold: 1-3 g/day

(Continued)

29

Ascorbic Acid *(Continued)*

Children:
Scurvy: 100-300 mg/day in divided doses
Urinary acidification: 500 mg every 6-8 hours
Dietary supplement: 35-45 mg

Ascorbic Acid and Ferrous Sulfate *see* Ferrous Sulfate and Ascorbic Acid *on page 146*

Ascorbicap® [OTC] *see* Ascorbic Acid *on previous page*

Ascriptin® [OTC] *see* Aspirin *on this page*

Asendin® *see* Amoxapine *on page 21*

Asmalix® *see* Theophylline *on page 348*

ASN-ase *see* Asparaginase *on this page*

Asparaginase *(a spare' a gi nase)*
Brand Names Colaspase; Elspar®; Kidrolase®
Synonyms A-ase; ASN-ase; Colaspase
Use Treatment of acute lymphocytic leukemia
Pregnancy Risk Factor C
Usual Dosage Perform desensitization before the first treatment. Dose must be individualized based upon clinical response and tolerance of the patient.

Aspergillus - Allergenic Extract
Use Diagnosis of specific allergies; hypersensitization treatment
Usual Dosage Normally given S.C. every 3-14 days

Aspergum® [OTC] *see* Aspirin *on this page*

Aspirin *(as' pir in)*
Brand Names Anacin® [OTC]; A.S.A. [OTC]; Ascriptin® [OTC]; Aspergum® [OTC]; Bayer® Aspirin [OTC]; Bufferin® [OTC]; Easprin®; Ecotrin® [OTC]; Empirin® [OTC]; Measurin® [OTC]; Synalgos® [OTC]; ZORprin®
Synonyms Acetylsalicylic Acid; ASA
Use Treatment of mild to moderate pain, inflammation and fever; may be used as a prophylaxis of myocardial infarction and transient ischemic episodes
Pregnancy Risk Factor D
Usual Dosage

Adult and Children: > 11 years of age:
Analgesics and antipyretics: Oral and rectal: 325-650 mg every 4-6 hours up to 4 g/day
Anti-inflammatory: Oral: 2.4-5.4 g/day in divided doses
Ischemic episodes: Oral: 1.3 g daily in 2-4 divided doses
Myocardial infarction: Oral: 325 mg/day

Children:
Analgesia and antipyretics: Oral and rectal, 2-11 years: 65 mg/kg/day in 4-6 divided doses; total rectal dose should not exceed 2.5 g/m^2
Anti-inflammatory: ≤ 25 kg: 60-90 mg/kg/day (maximum 3.6 g/day); > 25 kg: 2.4-3.6 g/day

Antirheumatic: Oral: 100 mg/kg/day in divided doses every four hours

Aspirin and Codeine
Brand Names Empirin® With Codeine
Synonyms Codeine and Aspirin
Use Relief of mild to moderate pain
Restrictions C-III
Pregnancy Risk Factor D
Usual Dosage 1-2 tablets every 4-6 hours as needed for pain

Aspirin and Meprobamate
Brand Names Equagesic®
Synonyms Meprobamate and Aspirin
Use As an adjunct to treatment of skeletal muscular disease in patients exhibiting tension and/or anxiety
Restrictions C-IV
Pregnancy Risk Factor D
Usual Dosage One tablet 3-4 times daily

Astemizole (a stem' mi zole)
Brand Names Hismanal®
Use Perennial and seasonal allergic rhinitis and other allergic symptoms including urticaria
Pregnancy Risk Factor C
Usual Dosage Adult and Children: > 12 years of age: Oral: 10-30 mg/day; give 30 mg on first day, 20 mg on second day, then 10 mg/day in a single dose

AsthmaHaler® see Epinephrine on page 131

Astramorph™ PF see Morphine Sulfate on page 240

Atabrine® see Quinacrine Hydrochloride on page 311

Atarax® see Hydroxyzine on page 178

Atenolol (a ten' oh lole)
Brand Names Tenormin®
Use Treatment of hypertension, alone or in combination with other agents; also used in management of angina pectoris
Pregnancy Risk Factor C
Usual Dosage Oral:

Angina: 50-200 mg/day

Hypertension: 50-100 mg/day

ATG see Lymphocyte Immune Globulin on page 208

Atgam® see Lymphocyte Immune Globulin on page 208

Ativan® see Lorazepam on page 207

Atracurium Besylate (a tra kyoo' ree um)
Brand Names Tracrium®
Use To ease endotracheal intubation as an adjunct to general anesthesia and to relax skeletal muscle during surgery
(Continued)

Atracurium Besylate *(Continued)*

Pregnancy Risk Factor C
Usual Dosage I.V.:

Children 1 month - 2 years: 0.3-0.4 mg/kg initially followed by maintenance doses

Children > 2 years of age - Adult: 0.4-0.5 mg/kg then 0.08-0.1 mg/kg 20-45 minutes after initial dose to maintain neuromuscular block

Atrocholin® *see* Dehydrocholic Acid *on page 99*

Atromid-S® *see* Clofibrate *on page 83*

Atropair® *see* Atropine Sulfate *on this page*

Atropine and Diphenoxylate *see* Diphenoxylate and Atropine *on page 118*

Atropine-Care® *see* Atropine Sulfate *on this page*

Atropine Sulfate (a' troe peen)

Brand Names Atropair®; Atropine-Care®; Atropisol®; Isopto® Atropine; I-Tropine®; Ocu-Tropine®

Use Preoperative medication to inhibit salivation and secretions; treatment of sinus bradycardia; management of peptic ulcer; treat exercise-induced bronchospasm; antidote for organophosphate pesticide poisoning; used to produce mydriasis and cycloplegia for examination of the retina and optic disk and accurate measurement of refractive errors; uveitis

Pregnancy Risk Factor C
Usual Dosage

Adult:
Preanesthetic: I.M., S.C.: 0.4-0.6 mg 30-60 minutes preop
Bradycardia: I.V.: 0.5-1 mg every five minutes
Ophthalmic, 1% solution: 1-2 drops one hour before exam

Children:
Preanesthetic: I.M., S.C.: 30-40 kg: 0.4 mg 30-60 minutes preop; 18-30 kg: 0.3 mg 30-60 minutes preop; 11 18 kg: 0.2 mg 30-60 minutes preop; 8-11 kg: 0.15 mg 30-60 minutes preop; 3-7 kg: 0.1 mg 30-60 minutes preop
Bradycardia: I.V.: 0.01 mg/kg every 4-6 hours
Ophthalmic, 0.5% solution: 1-2 drops one hour before exam

Atropisol® *see* Atropine Sulfate *on this page*

Atrovent® *see* Ipratropium Bromide *on page 190*

A/T/S® *see* Erythromycin, Topical *on page 135*

Attapulgite

Brand Names Diar-Aid® [OTC]; Diasorb® [OTC]; Kaopectate® [OTC]; Rheaban® [OTC]
Use Symptomatic treatment of diarrhea

Pregnancy Risk Factor B
Usual Dosage

Adult: Oral: 1200-1500 mg after each loose bowel movement or every 2 hours

15-30 mL up to 8 times per day

Attenuvax® *see* Measles Virus Vaccine, Live, Attentuated
on page 214

Augmentin® *see* Amoxicillin and Clavulanic Acid *on page 22*

Auralgan® *see* Antipyrine and Benzocaine *on page 26*

Auranofin (au rane' oh fin)
Brand Names Ridaura®
Use Management of active stage of classic or definite rheumatoid arthritis in patients that do not respond to or tolerate other agents
Pregnancy Risk Factor C
Usual Dosage Adult: Oral: 6 mg/day; after three months may be increased to 9 mg/day; if still no responsiveness after three months at 9 mg/day, discontinue drug

Aureomycin® *see* Chlortetracyline Hydrochloride *on page 77*

Aurothioglucose (aur oh thye oh gloo' kose)
Brand Names Solganal®
Use Adjunctive treatment in adult and juvenile active rheumatoid arthritis
Pregnancy Risk Factor C
Usual Dosage I.M.:

Adult: 10 mg first week; 25 mg second and third week; then 50 mg/week until 800 mg to 1 g cumulative dose has been given - if improvement occurs without adverse reactions then give 25-50 mg every 2-3 weeks, then every 3-4 weeks indefinitely

Children: 6-12 years old: One-fourth usual adult dose, governed by body weight, not to exceed 25 mg per dose; alternately may give 1 mg/kg once weekly for 20 weeks, up to 25 mg/dose

AVC™ Cream *see* Sulfanilamide *on page 338*

AVC™ Suppository *see* Sulfanilamide *on page 338*

Aventyl® Hydrochloride *see* Nortriptyline Hydrochloride
on page 256

Avitene® *see* Microfibrillar Collagen Hemostat *on page 236*

Avlosulfon® *see* Dapsone *on page 97*

Axid® *see* Nizatidine *on page 254*

Ayr® *see* Sodium Chloride *on page 327*

Azacitidine (ay za sye' ti deen)
Synonyms AZA-CR; 5-Azacytidine; 5-AZC; Ladakamycin; NSC-102816
Use Refractory acute lymphocytic and acute myelogenous leukemia
Restrictions Investigational drug
(Continued)

Azacitidine *(Continued)*
Pregnancy Risk Factor C
Usual Dosage Adult and Children: I.V.: 200-300 mg/m^2 daily for 5-10 days, repeated at 2-3 week intervals

AZA-CR *see Azacitidine on previous page*

Azactam® *see Aztreonam on next page*

5-Azacytidine *see Azacitidine on previous page*

Azatadine and Pseudoephedrine
Brand Names Trinalin®
Synonyms Pseudoephedrine and Azatadine
Use Perennial and seasonal allergic rhinitis and other allergic symptoms including urticaria
Pregnancy Risk Factor B
Usual Dosage Adult: Oral: 1-2 mg twice daily

Azatadine Maleate *(a za' ta deen)*
Brand Names Optimine®
Use Treatment of perennial and seasonal allergic rhinitis and chronic urticaria
Pregnancy Risk Factor B
Usual Dosage Adult and Children: > 12 years: Oral: 1 mg or 2 mg twice daily

Azathioprine *(ay za thye' oh preen)*
Brand Names Imuran®
Use An adjunct with other agents in prevention of rejection of renal transplants; also used in severe rheumatoid arthritis unresponsive to other agents
Pregnancy Risk Factor D
Usual Dosage

Adult:
Renal transplantation: Oral, I.V.: 3-5 mg/kg/day to start, then 1-3 mg/kg/day maintenance
Rheumatoid arthritis: Oral: 1 mg/kg/day for 6-8 weeks; increase by 0.5 mg/kg every 4 weeks until response or up to 2.5 mg/kg/day

Children: Renal transplantation: Oral, I.V.: 3-5 mg/kg/day to start, then 1-3 mg/kg/day maintenance

5-AZC *see Azacitidine on previous page*

Azidothymidine *see Zidovudine on page 381*

Azlin® *see Azlocillin on this page*

Azlocillin *(az loe sill' in)*
Brand Names Azlin®
Use Serious infections caused by susceptible organisms, mainly those caused by *Pseudomonas aeruginosa* involving the lower respiratory tract, urinary tract, skin, bone and joints, and bacterial septicemia

Pregnancy Risk Factor B
Usual Dosage I.V.:

Adult: 3-4 g every 4-6 hours up to 24 g daily

Children: 75 mg/kg every four hours, up to 24 g daily

Azmacort™ see Triamcinolone on page 359

Azo Gantanol® see Sulfamethoxazole and Phenazopyridine on page 337

Azo Gantrisin® see Sulfisoxazole and Phenazopyridine on page 339

Azolid® see Phenylbutazone on page 281

Azo-Standard® see Phenazopyridine Hydrochloride on page 278

Azostix® [OTC] see Diagnostic Test for Blood Urea Nitrogen in Blood on page 107

AZT see Zidovudine on page 381

Aztreonam (az' tree oh nam)
Brand Names Azactam®
Use Treatment of susceptible bacterial infections, mainly gram-negative aerobic organisms
Pregnancy Risk Factor B
Usual Dosage I.M., I.V.: 0.5-2 g every 6-12 hours

Azulfidine® see Sulfasalazine on page 338

Azulfidine® EN tabo® see Sulfasalazine on page 338

BAC see Benzalkonium Chloride on page 40

Bacampicillin Hydrochloride (ba kam pi sill' in)
Brand Names Spectrobid®
Use Treatment of susceptible bacterial infections, mainly urinary tract, skin structure, upper and lower respiratory tract
Pregnancy Risk Factor B
Usual Dosage Oral:

Adult: 400-800 mg every 12 hours

Children: 25-50 mg/kg/day in divided doses every 12 hours

Bacid® [OTC] see Lactobacillus acidophilus and Lactobacillus bulgaricus on page 199

Baciguent® [OTC] see Bacitracin on this page

Bacillus Calmette-Guérin see BCG Vaccine on page 37

Bacitracin (bass i tray' sin)
Brand Names AK-Tracin®; Baciguent® [OTC]
Use Treatment of susceptible bacterial infections
Pregnancy Risk Factor C
Usual Dosage

Adult:
I.M.: 10,000-25,000 units every six hours; do not exceed 25,000 units/
(Continued)
35

Bacitracin *(Continued)*

dose or 100,000 units/day; do not administer for longer than 12 days
Topical: Apply 1-5 times daily
Ophthalmic ointment: 1/2 in ribbon every 3-4 hours until better
Drops: 1-2 drops 4-6 times daily or more often

Children: I.M.: Do not exceed these doses:
> 2.5 kg: 1000 units/kg/24 hours in 2-3 divided doses
< 2.5 kg: 900 units/kg/24 hours in 2-3 divided doses

Bacitracin and Polymyxin B

Brand Names Polysporin®
Use Treatment of superficial infections caused by susceptible organisms
Usual Dosage
Ophthalmic ointment: Apply 1/2 inch ribbon to the affected eye(s) every 3-4 hours
Topical ointment: Apply to affected area 1-3 times a day; may cover with sterile bandage if needed

Bacitracin, Neomycin and Polymyxin B

Brand Names Neosporin® Ointment [OTC]; Neosporin® Ophthalmic Ointment
Use To help prevent infection in minor cuts, scrapes and burns; short-term treatment of superficial external ocular infections caused by susceptible organisms
Pregnancy Risk Factor C
Usual Dosage Adult and Children:
Topical: Apply 1-3 times daily
Ophthalmic: Apply every 3-4 hours for 7-10 days

Bacitracin, Neomycin, Polymyxin B and Hydrocortisone

Brand Names Cortisporin® Ointment; Cortisporin® Ophthalmic Ointment
Use Prevention and treatment of susceptible superficial topical infections
Pregnancy Risk Factor C
Usual Dosage

Ophthalmic Ointment: Apply 1/2 inch ribbon to inside of lower lid every 3- 4 hours until improvement occurs

Topical: Apply sparingly 2-4 times daily

Baclofen *(bak' loe fen)*

Brand Names Lioresal®
Use Treatment of reversible spasticity associated with multiple sclerosis or spinal cord lesions
Pregnancy Risk Factor C
Usual Dosage Oral: 5 mg three times daily, may increase 5 mg/dose every three days to a maximum of 80 mg/day

Adult and Children: ≥ 8 years: Maximum 60 mg/day in three divided doses

Children: 2-7 years of age: Maximum 30-40 mg/day divided three times/day

Bactrim™ *see* Sulfamethoxazole and Trimethoprim
  on page 338

Bactrim™ DS *see* Sulfamethoxazole and Trimethoprim
  on page 338

Bactroban® *see* Mupirocin *on page 242*

Baking Soda *see* Sodium Bicarbonate *on page 326*

BAL *see* Dimercaprol *on page 116*

Balanced Salt Solution
Brand Names BSS®
Use Intraocular irrigating solution
Usual Dosage Use as needed for foreign body removal, gonioscopy and other general ophthalmic office procedures

BAL in Oil® *see* Dimercaprol *on page 116*

Balmex® Ointment [OTC] *see* Vitamin A and Vitamin D
  on page 377

Balnetar® [OTC] *see* Coal Tar, Lanolin and Mineral Oil
  on page 86

Banthine® *see* Methantheline Bromide *on page 225*

Barbita® *see* Phenobarbital *on page 279*

Barium Sulfate (ba' ree urn)
Brand Names Baro-CAT®
Use Contrast medium for radiography of the alimentary tract

Baro-CAT® *see* Barium Sulfate *on this page*

Basaljel® [OTC] *see* Aluminum Carbonate *on page 15*

Bath Oil, Antipruritic
Brand Names Alpha Keri® [OTC]
Use Treatment of dry skin
Usual Dosage To be used as needed

Bayer® Aspirin [OTC] *see* Aspirin *on page 30*

Baylocaine® *see* Lidocaine Hydrochloride *on page 204*

BCG Vaccine
Brand Names Bacillus Calmette-Guérin
Use Immunization against tuberculosis
Pregnancy Risk Factor C
Usual Dosage Intradermal:

  Adult: 0.1 mL

  Children: < 3 months of age: 0.05 mL

BCNU *see* Carmustine *on page 61*

Beclomethasone Dipropionate (be kloe meth' a sone)
Brand Names Beclovent®; Beconase®; Beconase AQ®; Vancenase®; Vancenase® AQ; Vanceril®
Use Treatment of chronic bronchial asthma
Pregnancy Risk Factor C
Usual Dosage

Adult: Two inhalations or sprays in each nostril 3-4 times daily

Children: 6-12 years of age: 1-2 inhalations or sprays in each nostril 3-4 times daily

Beclovent® see Beclomethasone Dipropionate on this page

Beconase® see Beclomethasone Dipropionate on this page

Beconase AQ® see Beclomethasone Dipropionate on this page

Becotin® [OTC] see Vitamin B Complex on page 377

Beef NPH Iletin® II see Insulin, Isophane Suspension on page 185

Beef Regular Iletin® II see Insulin, Regular on page 186

Beepen-VK® see Penicillin V Potassium on page 274

Beesix® see Pyridoxine Hydrochloride on page 309

Belladonna (bell a don' a)
Use To decrease gastrointestinal activity in functional bowel disorders and to delay gastric emptying as well as decrease gastric secretion
Pregnancy Risk Factor C
Usual Dosage Adult: Oral:
Extract: 10.8-21.6 mg three to four times daily
Tincture: 0.3-1 mL three to four times daily

Belladonna and Butabarbital
Brand Names Butibel®
Synonyms Butabarbital and Belladonna
Use Relief of moderate to severe pain associated with ureteral spasm
Pregnancy Risk Factor C
Usual Dosage One suppository as needed 1-2 times daily

Belladonna and Opium
Brand Names B&O Supprettes®
Synonyms Opium and Belladonna
Use For relief of moderate to severe pain associated with rectal or bladder tenesmus that may occur in postoperative states and neoplastic situations; pain associated with ureteral spasms not responsive to nonnarcotic analgesics and to space intervals between injections of opiates
Restrictions C-II
Pregnancy Risk Factor C
Usual Dosage Adult: Rectal: One suppository once or twice daily, up to four doses daily

Belladonna, Phenobarbital and Ergotamine Tartrate

Brand Names Bellergal-S®

Use Management and treatment of menopausal disorders, gastrointestinal disorders and recurrent throbbing headache

Pregnancy Risk Factor D

Usual Dosage One tablet each morning and evening

Belladonna, Phenobarbital and Pepsin

Brand Names Donnazyme®

Use Relief of symptoms associated with nervous indigestion and other functional gastrointestinal disorders in the absence of organic pathology

Pregnancy Risk Factor C

Usual Dosage Adult: Oral: Two tablets after each meal

Bellergal-S® *see* Belladonna, Phenobarbital and Ergotamine Tartrate *on this page*

Benadryl® [OTC] *see* Diphenhydramine Hydrochloride *on page 117*

Ben-Aqua® [OTC] *see* Benzoyl Peroxide *on page 41*

Bendroflumethiazide (ben droe floo meth eye' a zide)

Brand Names Naturetin®

Use Management of mild to moderate hypertension, edema associated with congestive heart failure, pregnancy, or nephrotic syndrome; reportedly does not alter serum electrolyte concentrations appreciably at recommended doses

Pregnancy Risk Factor B

Usual Dosage Oral:

Adult: 2.5-20 mg daily or twice a day in divided doses

Children: Initially 0.1-0.4 mg/kg in one or two doses; maintenance dosage is 0.05-0.1 mg/kg daily in one or two doses

Benemid® *see* Probenecid *on page 297*

Benoxyl® *see* Benzoyl Peroxide *on page 41*

Bentiromide (ben teer' oh mide)

Brand Names Chymer®

Synonyms BTPABA

Use Screening test for pancreatic exocrine insufficiency

Pregnancy Risk Factor B

Usual Dosage Oral:

Adult and Children: > 12 years of age: Administer following an overnight fast and morning void, single 500 mg dose and follow with eight ounces of water

Children: < 12 years: 14 mg/kg followed with eight ounces of water

Bentyl® Hydrochloride *see* Dicyclomine Hydrochloride *on page 111*

Benylin® Cough Syrup [OTC] *see* Diphenhydramine Hydrochloride *on page 117*

Benzac W® *see* Benzoyl Peroxide *on next page*

Benzalkonium Chloride (benz al koe' nee um)
Brand Names Zephiran® [OTC]
Synonyms BAC
Use Bacteriostatic in low concentrations, bacteriostatic in high concentrations; may be used for application to skin and mucous membranes or for the sterilization of inanimate articles, such as surgical instruments
Pregnancy Risk Factor C
Usual Dosage Thoroughly rinse anionic detergents and soaps from the skin or other areas prior to use of solutions because they reduce the antibacterial activity of BAC; to protect metal instruments stored in BAC solution, add crushed Anti-Rust Tablets, four tablets per quart, to antiseptic solution, change solution at least once a week; not to be for storage of aluminum or zinc instruments, instruments with lenses fastened by cement, lacquered catheters or some synthetic rubber goods

Benzathine Benzylpenicillin *see* Penicillin G Benzathine, Oral *on page 272*

Benzathine Benzylpenicillin *see* Penicillin G Benzathine, Parenteral *on page 272*

Benzathine Penicillin G *see* Penicillin G Benzathine, Oral *on page 272*

Benzathine Penicillin G *see* Penicillin G Benzathine, Parenteral *on page 272*

Benzazoline Hydrochloride *see* Tolazoline Hydrochloride *on page 357*

Benzene Hexachloride *see* Lindane *on page 204*

Benzhexol Hydrochloride *see* Trihexyphenidyl Hydrochloride *on page 362*

Benzocaine (ben' zoe kane)
Brand Names Americaine® [OTC]; BiCOZENE® [OTC]; Chiggertox® [OTC]; Dermoplast® [OTC]; Foille Plus® [OTC]; Hurricaine®; Rhulicaine® [OTC]; Solarcaine® [OTC]; Unguentine® [OTC]
Synonyms Ethyl Aminobenzoate
Use Temporary relief of pain associated with local anesthetic for pruritic dermatosis, pruritus, minor burns, acute congestive and serious otitis media, swimmer's ear, otitis externa, toothache, minor sore throat pain, canker sores, hemorrhoids, rectal fissures, anesthetic lubricant for passage of catheters and endoscopic tubes
Pregnancy Risk Factor C
Usual Dosage
Gel: Apply a small amount on affected area
Otic: Fill ear canal; insert moistened cotton pledget; repeat 3-4 times/day or repeat once every 1-2 hours as needed otalgia for 2 days
Spray: To affected area as needed

Benzocaine and Antipyrine *see* Antipyrine and Benzocaine *on page 26*

Benzocaine and Cetylpyridinium Chloride *see* Cetylpyridinium Chloride and Benzocaine *on page 67*

Benzocaine, Butyl Aminobenzoate, Tetracaine and Benzalkonium Chloride

Brand Names Cetacaine®

Synonyms Tetracaine Hydrochloride, Benzocaine Butyl Aminobenzoate and Benzalkonium Chloride

Use Topical anesthetic to control pain or gagging

Pregnancy Risk Factor C

Usual Dosage Apply to affected area for approximately one second or less

Benzocaine, Gelatin, Pectin and Sodium Carboxymethylcellulose

Brand Names Orabase® With Benzocaine [OTC]

Use Topical anesthetic and emollient for oral lesions

Pregnancy Risk Factor C

Usual Dosage Apply 2-4 times daily

Benzoic Acid and Salicylic Acid (ben zoe' ik)

Brand Names Whitfield's Ointment [OTC]

Synonyms Salicylic Acid and Benzoic Acid

Use Treatment of athlete's foot and ringworm of the scalp

Usual Dosage Apply 1-4 times daily

Benzoin Tincture (ben' zoin)

Use A protective application for irritations of the skin; sometimes used in boiling water as steam inhalants for their expectorant and soothing action

Usual Dosage Apply once or twice daily

Benzonatate (ben zoe' na tate)

Brand Names Tessalon® Perles

Use Symptomatic relief of nonproductive cough

Pregnancy Risk Factor C

Usual Dosage Oral:

Adult and Children: > 10 years of age: 100 mg three times a day up to 600 mg/day

Children: < 10 years: 8 mg/kg in 3-6 divided doses

Benzoyl Peroxide (ben' zoe ill)

Brand Names Ben-Aqua® [OTC]; Benoxyl®; Benzac W®; Clear By Design® [OTC]; Clearsil® [OTC]; Desquam-X®; Dry and Clear® [OTC]; Loroxide® [OTC]; Oxy-5® [OTC]; PanOxyl® [OTC]; PanOxyl®-AQ; Persa-Gel®; pHisoAc BP® [OTC]; Vanoxide® [OTC]; Xerac BP® [OTC]; Zeroxin®

(Continued)

41

Benzoyl Peroxide *(Continued)*

Use Adjunctive treatment of mild to moderate acne vulgaris and acne rosacea

Pregnancy Risk Factor C

Usual Dosage Apply once or twice daily

Benzphetamine Hydrochloride

Brand Names Didrex®

Use Short term adjunct in exogenous obesity

Restrictions C-III

Pregnancy Risk Factor X

Usual Dosage Adult: Oral: 25-50 mg 2-3 times day, preferably twice daily, midmorning and midafternoon

Benzquinamide Hydrochloride (benz kwin' a mide)

Brand Names Emete-Con®

Use Antiemetic associated with anesthesia and surgery

Pregnancy Risk Factor C

Usual Dosage Not recommended for use in < 12 years of age; safety and efficacy has not been established

I.M.: 50 mg (0.5-1 mg/kg) may be repeated in one hour, then 3-4 hours as needed

I.V.: 25 mg (0.2-0.4 mg/kg)

Benztropine Mesylate (benz' troe peen)

Brand Names Cogentin®

Use Adjunctive treatment of Parkinson's disease; also used in treatment of drug-induced extrapyramidal effects and acute dystonic reactions

Pregnancy Risk Factor C

Usual Dosage

Drug induced: Extrapyramidal reaction: Oral, I.M., I.V.:
Adult: 1-4 mg/dose 1-2 times/day

Parkinsonism: Oral: 0.5-6 mg/day in 1-2 divided doses; if one dose is greater, give at bedtime
Children: 0.02-0.05 mg/kg/dose 1-2 times/day

Benzylpenicillin Potassium *see* Penicillin G, Parenteral
on page 273

Benzylpenicillin Sodium *see* Penicillin G, Parenteral
on page 273

Benzylpenicilloyl-polylysine

Brand Names Pre-Pen®

Use As an adjunct in assessing the risk of administering penicillin (penicillin or benzylpenicillin) in adults with a history of clinical penicillin hypersensitivity

Usual Dosage Use scratch technique with a 20 gauge needle to make 3-5 mm scratch on epidermis, apply a small drop of solution to scratch, rub in gently with applicator or toothpick. A positive reaction consists of a pale wheal surrounding the scratch site which develops within 10 minutes and ranges from 5-15 mm or more in diameter.

Beta-2® *see* Isoetharine *on page 191*

Beta Carotene (kare' oh teen)
Brand Names Solatene®
Use To protect against and to reduce severity of photosensitivity reaction in patients with erythropoietic protoporphyria
Pregnancy Risk Factor C
Usual Dosage Oral:

Adult: 30-300 mg/day

Children: < 14 years of age: 30-150 mg/day

Betachron® *see* Propranolol Hydrochloride *on page 304*

Betadine® [OTC] *see* Povidone-Iodine *on page 292*

Betagan® Liquifilm® *see* Levobunolol Hydrochloride *on page 201*

Betalin®S *see* Thiamine Hydrochloride *on page 351*

Betamethasone (bay ta meth' a sone)
Brand Names Alphatrex®; Betatrex®; Beta-Val®; B-S-P®; Celestone®; Celestone® Soluspan®; Diprolene®; Diprosone®; Maxivate®; Selestoject®; Uticort®; Valisone®
Use Glucocorticoid
Pregnancy Risk Factor C
Usual Dosage
I.M.: Up to 9 mg/day
Oral: 0.6-7.2 mg/day
Topical: Apply thin film 2-3 times daily

Betamethasone Dipropionate and Clotrimazole
Brand Names Lotrisone®
Use Topical treatment of various dermal fungal infections
Pregnancy Risk Factor C
Usual Dosage Apply twice daily

Betapen®-VK *see* Penicillin V Potassium *on page 274*

Betatrex® *see* Betamethasone *on this page*

Beta-Val® *see* Betamethasone *on this page*

Betaxolol Hydrochloride (be tax' oh lol)
Brand Names Betoptic®
Use Treatment of chronic open-angle glaucoma, ocular hypertension
Pregnancy Risk Factor C
Usual Dosage One drop twice daily

Betazole Hydrochloride
Brand Names Histalog™
Use Test gastric secretory capabilities
Usual Dosage 50 mg

Bethanechol Chloride (be than' e kole)

Brand Names Duvoid®; Urabeth®; Urecholine®

Use Nonobstructive urinary retention and retention due to neurogenic bladder

Pregnancy Risk Factor C

Usual Dosage

Adult:
Oral: 10-50 mg 2-4 times daily
S.C.: 2.5-5 mg 3-4 times daily, up to 7.5-10 mg every four hours for neurogenic bladder

Children: Oral:
Abdominal distention or urinary retention: 0.6 mg/kg/day 3-4 times/day
Gastroesophageal reflux: 0.1-0.2 mg/kg/dose given 30 minutes to 1 hour before each meal to a maximum of four times/day

Children: S.C.: 0.15-0.2 mg/kg/day 3-4 times/day

Betoptic® *see* Betaxolol Hydrochloride *on previous page*

Biamine® *see* Thiamine Hydrochloride *on page 351*

Biavax®ₗₗ *see* Rubella and Mumps Vaccines, Combined *on page 318*

Bicillin® *see* Penicillin G Benzathine, Parenteral *on page 272*

Bicillin® C-R *see* Penicillin G Benzathine and Procaine Combined *on page 272*

Bicillin® C-R 900/300 *see* Penicillin G Benzathine and Procaine Combined *on page 272*

Bicillin® L-A *see* Penicillin G Benzathine, Parenteral *on page 272*

Bicitra® *see* Sodium Citrate and Citric Acid *on page 327*

BiCNU® *see* Carmustine *on page 61*

BiCOZENE® [OTC] *see* Benzocaine *on page 40*

Bile Salts, Pancreatin and Pepsin

Brand Names Entozyme®

Use Relief of steatorrhea, pyrosis, flatulence and belching associated with incomplete digestion of food due to enzyme deficiency

Pregnancy Risk Factor C

Usual Dosage Adult: Oral: Two tablets with each meal, 1-2 tablets with each snack

Bili-Labstix® [OTC] *see* Diagnostic Test for Acetone, Bilirubin, Blood, Glucose, pH and Protein in Urine *on page 106*

Bilopaque® *see* Tyropanoate Sodium *on page 368*

Biltricide® *see* Praziquantel *on page 293*

Bio-Gan® *see* Trimethobenzamide Hydrochloride *on page 364*

Biozyme-C® *see* Collagenase *on page 88*

Biperiden Hydrochloride (bye per' i den)

Brand Names Akineton®

Use Treatment of all forms of Parkinsonism including drug induced type (extrapyramidal symptoms)

Pregnancy Risk Factor C

Usual Dosage Adult:

Parkinsonism: Oral: 2 mg 3-4 times daily

Extrapyramidal:
Oral: 2-6 mg 2-3 times daily
I.M., I.V.: 2 mg every 30 minutes up to four doses or 8 mg/daily

Biphenabid see Probucol on page 297

Bisacodyl (bis a koe' dill)

Brand Names Clysodrast®; Dulcolax® [OTC]; Fleet® Bisacodyl Prep [OTC]

Use Treatment of constipation

Pregnancy Risk Factor C

Usual Dosage

Adult:
Oral: 5-15 mg as single dose (up to 30 mg when complete evacuation of bowel is required)
Rectal enema: 1.5-4.5 mg (1 3 packets)
Rectal suppository: 10 mg as single dose

Children:
Oral: > 3 years of age: 5-10 mg or 0.3 mg/kg
Rectal suppository: > 2 years: 10 mg; < 2 years: 5 mg

Bishydroxycoumarin see Dicumarol on page 111

Bismuth

Brand Names Devrom® [OTC]; Pepto-Bismol® [OTC]

Synonyms Bismuth Subgallate; Bismuth Subsalicylate

Use Symptomatic treatment of mild, nonspecific diarrhea

Pregnancy Risk Factor C/D

Usual Dosage Nonspecific diarrhea: Subsalicylate:

Adult: Two tablets or 30 mL every 30 minutes to one hour as needed

Children:
9-12 years of age: One tablet or 15 mL every 30 minutes to one hour as needed
6-9 years: 2/3 tablet or 10 mL every 30 minutes to one hour as needed
3-6 years: 1/3 tablet of 5 mL every 30 minutes to one hour as needed

Adult: Subgallate: Oral: 1-2 tablets three times a day with meals

Bismuth Subgallate see Bismuth on this page

Bismuth Subsalicylate see Bismuth on this page

Bistropamide see Tropicamide on page 367

Bitolterol Mesylate (bye tole' ter ole)
    Brand Names Tornalate®
    Use To prevent and treat bronchial asthma and bronchospasm
    Pregnancy Risk Factor C
    Usual Dosage Adult and Children: > 12 years:

    Bronchospasm: Two inhalations at an interval of at least 1-3 minutes, followed by a third inhalation if needed

    Prevention of bronchospasm: Two inhalations every eight hours

Black and White Cocktail see Cascara Sagrada Fluid Extract and Milk of Magnesia on page 61

Black Draught® [OTC] see Senna on page 322

Black Widow Spider Species Antivenin *Latrodectus mactans* see Antivenin, Black Widow Spider (Equine) on page 27

Blenoxane® see Bleomycin Sulfate on this page

Bleomycin Sulfate (blee oh mye' sin)
    Brand Names Blenoxane®
    Synonyms BLM
    Use Palliative treatment of squamous cell carcinomas, testicular carcinoma and the following lymphomas: Hodgkin's, lymphosarcoma and reticulum cell sarcoma
    Pregnancy Risk Factor D
    Usual Dosage I.M., I.V., S.C.: 0.25-0.50 units/kg once or twice weekly; dosage may vary depending upon protocol

Bleph®-10 see Sodium Sulfacetamide on page 330

Blephamide® see Sodium Sulfacetamide and Prednisolone Acetate on page 330

Blistex® see Camphor and Menthol on page 55

BLM see Bleomycin Sulfate on this page

Blocadren® see Timolol Maleate on page 355

Bonine® [OTC] see Meclizine Hydrochloride on page 215

Boric Acid (bor' ik)
    Brand Names Borofax® [OTC]
    Use Mild antiseptic used for inflamed eyelids
    Usual Dosage Apply to lower eyelid once or twice daily

Boric Acid, Menthol and Camphor see Rubs and Liniments on page 319

Borofax® [OTC] see Boric Acid on this page

B&O Supprettes® see Belladonna and Opium on page 38

Breatheasy® see Epinephrine on page 131

Breokinase® see Urokinase on page 370

Breonesin® [OTC] see Guaifenesin on page 162

Brethaire® *see* Terbutaline Sulfate *on page 343*

Brethine® *see* Terbutaline Sulfate *on page 343*

Bretylium Tosylate (bre til' ee um)
Brand Names Bretylol®
Use Ventricular tachycardia and fibrillation; also used in the treatment of other serious ventricular arrhythmias resistant to lidocaine
Usual Dosage

Adult: Immediately life-threatening ventricular arrhythmias; ventricular fibrillation; unstable ventricular tachycardia
Initial dose: I.V.: 5 mg/kg (undiluted) over one minute; if ventricular fibrillation persists, give 10 mg/kg (undiluted) over one minute and repeat as necessary (usually at 15-30 minute intervals) up to a total dose of 30 ng/kg

Adult: Other life-threatening ventricular arrhythmias:
Initial dose: I.M., I.V.: 5-10 mg/kg, may repeat every 1-2 hours; if arrhythmias persist, give I.V. dose (diluted) over 10-30 minutes
Maintenance dose: I.M.: 5-10 ng/kg every 6-8 hours; I.V.: 5-10 ng/kg every six hours; I.V. infusion: 1-2 mg/minute (little experience with doses > 40 mg/kg/day)

Children (safety and efficacy not established):
I.M.: 2-5 mg/kg as a single dose
I.V.: 5 mg/kg (initial dose); repeat with 10 mg/kg if ventricular fibrillation persists

Bretylol® *see* Bretylium Tosylate *on this page*

Brevibloc® *see* Esmolol Hydrochloride *on page 135*

Brevital® Sodium *see* Methohexital Sodium *on page 227*

Bricanyl® *see* Terbutaline Sulfate *on page 343*

Bromarest® [OTC] *see* Brompheniramine Maleate
on next page

Brombay® [OTC] *see* Brompheniramine Maleate *on next page*

Bromocriptine Mesylate (broe moe krip' teen)
Brand Names Parlodel®
Use Treatment of parkinsonism in patients unresponsive or allergic to levodopa; also used in conditions associated with hyperprolactinemia and to suppress lactation
Pregnancy Risk Factor C
Usual Dosage Oral:

Parkinsonism: 1.25 mg twice daily, increased by 2.5 mg/day in 2-4 week intervals (usual dose range is 30-90 mg/day in three divided doses)

Hyperprolactinemia and postpartum lactation: 2.5 mg 2-3 times daily

Bromodiphenhydramine and Codeine
(brome oh dye fen hye' dra meen)
Brand Names Ambenyl®
Synonyms Codeine and Bromodiphenhydramine
Use Relief of upper respiratory symptoms and cough associated with allergies or common cold
(Continued)

47

Bromodiphenhydramine and Codeine *(Continued)*

Restrictions C-V
Pregnancy Risk Factor C
Usual Dosage 5-10 mL every 4-6 hours

Bromophen® [OTC] *see* Brompheniramine Maleate
on this page

Brompheniramine and Phenylpropanolamine

Brand Names Dimetapp® [OTC]
Synonyms Phenylpropanolamine and Brompheniramine
Use Temporary relief of nasal congestion, running nose, sneezing, and itchy, watery eyes
Pregnancy Risk Factor B
Usual Dosage
Adult and Children > 12 years: Oral: 10 mL or one regular tablet every 4 hours or one Extentab® every 12 hours
Children 6-12 years: Oral: 5 mL or one-half tablet every 4 hours
Children 2-6 years: 2.5 mL every 4 hours

Brompheniramine Maleate *(brome fen ir' a meen)*

Brand Names Bromarest® [OTC]; Brombay® [OTC]; Bromophen® [OTC]; Brotane® [OTC]; Chlorphed® [OTC]; Codimal-A®; Cophene-B®; Dehist®; Diamine T.D.® [OTC]; Dimetane® [OTC]; Histaject®; Nasahist B®; ND-Stat®; Oraminic® II; Sinusol-B®; Veltane®
Synonyms Parabromdylamine
Use Perennial and seasonal allergic rhinitis and other allergic symptoms including urticaria
Pregnancy Risk Factor B
Usual Dosage Oral:

Adult: 4 mg every 4-6 hours or 8 mg of sustained release form every 8-12 hours or 12 mg of sustained release every 12 hours; maximum 24 g/day

Children:
6-12 years: 2-4 mg every 6-8 hours; maximum 12-16 mg/day
< 6 years of age: 0.125 mg/kg/dose given every six hours; maximum 6-8 mg/day

Brompheniramine, Phenylpropanolamine and Codeine

Brand Names Dimetane®-DC
Use For relief of coughs and upper respiratory symptoms, including nasal congestion, associated with allergy or the common cold
Restrictions C-V
Pregnancy Risk Factor C
Usual Dosage
Adult and Children: > 12 years: 10 mL every 4 hours
Children 6-12 years: 5 mL every 4 hours
Children 2-6 years: 2.5 mL every 4 hours

Bronitin® *see* Epinephrine *on page 131*

Bronkaid® Mist *see* Epinephrine *on page 131*

Bronkephrine® *see* Ethylnorepinephrine Hydrochloride *on page 141*

Bronkodyl® *see* Theophylline *on page 348*

Bronkometer® *see* Isoetharine *on page 191*

Bronkosol® *see* Isoetharine *on page 191*

Brotane® [OTC] *see* Brompheniramine Maleate *on previous page*

Bryrel® *see* Piperazine Citrate *on page 286*

B-S-P® *see* Betamethasone *on page 43*

BSS® *see* Balanced Salt Solution *on page 37*

BTPABA *see* Bentiromide *on page 39*

Bucladin®-S Softab® *see* Buclizine Hydrochloride *on this page*

Buclizine Hydrochloride (byoo' kli zeen)
Brand Names Bucladin®-S Softab®; Vibazine®
Use Prevention and treatment of motion sickness; symptomatic treatment of vertigo
Pregnancy Risk Factor X
Usual Dosage Adult: Oral:
Motion sickness (prophylaxis): 50 mg thirty minutes prior to traveling; may repeat 50 mg after 4-6 hours
Vertigo: 50 mg twice daily, up to 150 mg/day

Bufferin® [OTC] *see* Aspirin *on page 30*

Bumetanide (byoo met' a nide)
Brand Names Bumex®
Use Used in the management of edema secondary to congestive heart failure or hepatic or renal disease; may also be used alone or in combination with antihypertensives in the treatment of hypertension
Pregnancy Risk Factor C
Usual Dosage Oral, I.M., I.V.: 0.5-2 mg/day (up to 10 mg/day); larger may be needed in renal insufficiency

Bumex® *see* Bumetanide *on this page*

Bupivacaine Hydrochloride (byoo piv' a kane)
Brand Names Marcaine®; Sensorcaine®
Use Local anesthetic (injectable) for peripheral nerve block, infiltration, sympathetic block, caudal or epidural block, retrobulbar block
Pregnancy Risk Factor C
Usual Dosage Dose varies with procedure, depth of anesthesia, vascularity of tissues, duration of anesthesia and condition of patient
Adult (with or without epinephrine):
Caudal block: 15-30 mL of 0.25 or 0.5%
Epidural block (other than caudal block): 10-20 mL of 0.25 or 0.5%
Peripheral nerve block: 5 mL dose of 0.25 or 0.5% (12.5-25 mg); up to a maximum of 400 mg/day
Sympathetic nerve block: 20-50 mL of 0.25% (no epinephrine) solution

Buprenex® *see* Buprenorphine Hydrochloride *on this page*

Buprenorphine Hydrochloride (byoo pre nor' feen)
Brand Names Buprenex®
Use Management of moderate to severe pain
Restrictions C-V
Pregnancy Risk Factor C
Usual Dosage Adult: I.M., slow I.V.: 0.3-0.6 mg every six hours as needed

Bupropion (byoo proe' pee on)
Brand Names Wellbutrin®
Use Treatment of depression
Pregnancy Risk Factor B
Usual Dosage Adult: Oral: 100 mg three times a day; begin at 100 mg twice a day

Burow's Solution *see* Aluminum Acetate *on page 14*

BuSpar® *see* Buspirone Hydrochloride *on this page*

Buspirone Hydrochloride (byoo spye' rone)
Brand Names BuSpar®
Use Management of anxiety
Pregnancy Risk Factor B
Usual Dosage 15 mg/day (5 mg, three times daily)

Busulfan (byoo sul' fan)
Brand Names Myleran®
Use Chronic myelogenous leukemia and bone marrow disorders
Pregnancy Risk Factor D
Usual Dosage

Adult:
Oral: 4-8 mg/day (may be as high as 12 mg/day)
Unapproved uses: Polycythemia vera: 2-5 mg/day; thrombocytosis: 4-6 mg/day
Maintenance doses: Controversial, range from 1-4 mg/day to 2 mg/week

Children: Oral: 0.06-0.12 mg/kg/day or 1.8-4.6 mg/m^2/day; titrate dosage to maintain leukocyte count about 20,000/mm^3 (dosages > 4 mg/day are especially likely to reduce the leukocyte count)

Butabarbital and Belladonna *see* Belladonna and Butabarbital *on page 38*

Butabarbital Sodium (byoo ta bar' bi tal)
Brand Names Butalan®; Buticaps®; Butisol Sodium®
Use Sedative, hypnotic
Restrictions C-III

Pregnancy Risk Factor D
Usual Dosage Oral:

Adult:
Sedative: 15-30 mg 3-4 times daily
Hypnotic: 50-100 mg
Preop: 50-100 mg 1-1.5 hours before surgery

Children:
Sedative: 6 mg/kg/day in three divided doses
Hypnotic: Not established for children, based on age and weight
Preop: 2-6 mg/kg/dose; maximum 100 mg

Butalan® *see* Butabarbital Sodium *on previous page*

Butalbital and Codeine Compound
Brand Names Fiorinal® With Codeine
Synonyms Codeine Compound and Butalbital
Use Mild to moderate pain when sedation is needed
Restrictions C-III
Pregnancy Risk Factor D
Usual Dosage 1-2 capsules every 4-6 hours as needed for pain

Butalbital Compound
Brand Names Fioricet®; Fiorinal®
Use Relief of the symptomatic complex of tension or muscle contraction headache
Restrictions C-III
Pregnancy Risk Factor D
Usual Dosage Adult: Oral: 1-2 tablets or capsules every four hours; not to exceed six per day

Butazolidin® *see* Phenylbutazone *on page 281*

Butibel® *see* Belladonna and Butabarbital *on page 38*

Buticaps® *see* Butabarbital Sodium *on previous page*

Butisol Sodium® *see* Butabarbital Sodium *on previous page*

Butoconazoie Nitrate (byoo toe koe' na zole)
Brand Names Femstat®
Use Local treatment of vulvovaginal candidiasis
Pregnancy Risk Factor C
Usual Dosage

Nonpregnant: One applicatorful (225 g) intravaginally at bedtime every three days

Pregnant: Use only during second or third trimesters

Butorphanol Tartrate (byoo tor' fa nole)
Brand Names Stadol®
Use Management of moderate to severe pain
Pregnancy Risk Factor C
(Continued)

Butorphanol Tartrate *(Continued)*

Usual Dosage Adult:
    I.M.: 1-4 mg every 3-4 hours as needed
    I.V.: 0.5-2 mg every 3-4 hours as needed

C8-CCK *see* Sincalide *on page 325*

Cafergot® *see* Ergotamine *on page 133*

Cafergot® PB *see* Ergotamine *on page 133*

Caffeine and Sodium Benzoate (kaf' een)

Synonyms Sodium Benzoate and Caffeine
Use Emergency stimulant in acute circulatory failure; as a diuretic; and to relieve spinal puncture headache
Pregnancy Risk Factor C
Usual Dosage

Adult: I.M., I.V.: 500 mg, maximum single dose 1 g

Children: I.M., I.V., S.C.: 8 mg/kg every four hours as needed

Caffeine, Citrated

Use Central nervous system stimulant; can be used in treatment of poisoning, acute circulatory failure
Pregnancy Risk Factor C
Usual Dosage I.M., I.V.:

Adult: 500 mg with range of 200-500 mg

Children: 8 mg/kg every four hours as needed

Calamine Lotion (kal' a meen)

Use Employed chiefly as an astringent and protectant for soothing conditions such as poison ivy or sunburn
Usual Dosage Apply 1-4 times daily as needed

Calan® *see* Verapamil Hydrochloride *on page 374*

Calcifediol (kal si fe dye' ole)

Brand Names Calderol®
Synonyms 25-HCC; 25-Hydroxyvitamin D_3
Use Treatment and management of metabolic bone disease associated with chronic renal failure
Pregnancy Risk Factor C
Usual Dosage Oral: Initially 300-350 μg/week given on a daily or alternate day schedule

Calciferol™ *see* Ergocalciferol *on page 132*

Calcimar® *see* Calcitonin *on this page*

Calciparine® *see* Heparin *on page 167*

Calcitonin (kal si toe' nin)

Brand Names Calcimar®; Cibacalcin®
Synonyms Calcitonin (Human); Calcitonin (Salmon)
Use Treatment of Paget's disease of bone and as adjunctive therapy for hypercalcemia; also used in postmenopausal osteoporosis

Pregnancy Risk Factor C

Usual Dosage Adult: Paget's disease: I.M., S.C.: 0.5 mg per day or 0.5 mg 2-3 times weekly

Calcitonin (Human) *see* Calcitonin *on previous page*

Calcitonin (Salmon) *see* Calcitonin *on previous page*

Calcitriol (kal si trye' ole)

Brand Names Rocaltrol®

Synonyms 1,25 dihydroxycholecalciferol

Use Management of hypocalcemia in patients on chronic renal dialysis; reduce elevated parathyroid hormone levels

Pregnancy Risk Factor C

Usual Dosage Individualize dosage

Calcium Carbonate

Brand Names Os-Cal® 250 [OTC]; Os-Cal® 500 [OTC]; Tums® [OTC]

Use As an adjunct in prevention of postmenopausal osteoporosis, treatment and prevention of calcium depletion

Pregnancy Risk Factor C

Usual Dosage Oral:

Adult: 1-2 g/day (doses in g of elemental calcium)

Children: 45-65 mg/kg/day

Calcium Carbonate and Simethicone

Brand Names Titralac® Plus Liquid [OTC]

Synonyms Simethicone and Calcium Carbonate

Use Relief of acid indigestion, heartburn, peptic esophagitis, hiatal hernia and gas

Pregnancy Risk Factor C

Usual Dosage 0.5-2 g 4-6 times a day

Calcium Chloride

Brand Names Cal Plus®

Use Emergency treatment of hypoglycemia; treatment of hypermagnesemia; cardiac disturbances of hyperkalemia; cardiac resuscitation when epinephrine fails to improve myocardial contractions

Pregnancy Risk Factor C

Usual Dosage Adult:

Cardiac Resuscitation: Intraventricular: 200-800 mg directly into cardiac ventricle

Hypocalcemia: I.V.: 500 mg - 1 g at 1-3 day intervals

Calcium Citrate

Brand Names Citracal® [OTC]

Use As an adjunct in prevention of postmenopausal osteoporosis, treatment and prevention of calcium depletion

Pregnancy Risk Factor C

(Continued)

Calcium Citrate *(Continued)*

Usual Dosage Oral:

Adult: 1-2 g/day (doses in g of elemental calcium)

Children: 45-65 mg/kg/day

Calcium Disodium Versenate® *see* Edetate Calcium Disodium *on page 127*

Calcium EDTA *see* Edetate Calcium Disodium *on page 127*

Calcium Glubionate (gloo bye' oh nate)

Brand Names Neo-Calglucon® [OTC]

Use As an adjunct in prevention of postmenopausal osteoporosis, treatment and prevention of calcium depletion

Pregnancy Risk Factor C

Usual Dosage Oral:

Adult: 1-2 g/day (doses in g of elemental calcium)

Children: 45-65 mg/kg/day

Calcium Gluceptate (gloo sep' tate)

Use Emergency treatment of hypoglycemia; treatment of hypermagnesemia; cardiac disturbances of hyperkalemia; cardiac resuscitation when epinephrine fails to improve myocardial contractions

Pregnancy Risk Factor C

Usual Dosage Adult:

Cardiac Resuscitation: Intraventricular: 200-800 mg directly into cardiac ventricle

Hypocalcemia: I.V.: 500 mg - 1 g at 1-3 day intervals

Calcium Gluconate (gloo' koe nate)

Use Emergency treatment of hypoglycemia; treatment of hypermagnesemia; cardiac disturbances of hyperkalemia; cardiac resuscitation when epinephrine fails to improve myocardial contractions

Pregnancy Risk Factor C

Usual Dosage Adult:

Cardiac Resuscitation: Intraventricular: 200-800 mg directly into cardiac ventricle

Hypocalcemia: I.V.: 500 mg - 1 g at 1-3 day intervals Adult:

Cardiac Resuscitation: Intraventricular: 200-800 mg directly into cardiac ventricle

Hypocalcemia: I.V.: 500 mg - 1 g at 1-3 day intervals

Calcium Lactate (lak' tate)

Use As an adjunct in prevention of postmenopausal osteoporosis, treatment and prevention of calcium depletion

Pregnancy Risk Factor C

Usual Dosage Oral:

Adult: 1-2 g/day (doses in g of elemental calcium)

Children: 45-65 mg/kg/day

Calcium Leucovorin *see* Leucovorin Calcium *on page 200*

Calcium Pantothenate *see* Pantothenic Acid *on page 268*

Calcium Phosphate, Dibasic
Use As an adjunct in prevention of postmenopausal osteoporosis, treatment and prevention of calcium depletion
Pregnancy Risk Factor C
Usual Dosage Oral:

Adult: 1-2 g/day (doses in g of elemental calcium)

Children: 45-65 mg/kg/day

Calcium Polycarbophil (pol ee kar' boe fil)
Brand Names FiberCon® [OTC]; Mitrolan® [OTC]
Use Treatment of constipation or diarrhea by restoring a more normal moisture level and providing bulk in the patient's intestinal tract
Pregnancy Risk Factor C
Usual Dosage Oral:
Adult: 1 g four times daily, up to 6 g daily
Children 6-12 years: 500 mg, 1-3 times daily, up to 3 g daily
Children 2-6 years: 500 mg, 1 or 2 times daily, up to 1.5 g daily

Calcium Undecylenate
Brand Names Caldesene® [OTC]; Cruex® [OTC]
Use Adjunctive therapy in treatment of athlete's foot and ringworm
Usual Dosage Apply as needed after cleansing and drying area

Calderol® *see* Calcifediol *on page 52*

Caldesene® [OTC] *see* Calcium Undecylenate *on this page*

Calibind® *see* Cellulose Sodium Phosphate *on page 66*

Cal Plus® *see* Calcium Chloride *on page 53*

Calusterone (kal u' ster one)
Brand Names Methosarb®
Use Palliation of metastatic breast carcinoma in which the tumor cells possess estrogen receptors
Usual Dosage Adult: Oral: 150-300 mg/day in 3 or 4 divided doses

Camphor and Menthol (kam' for)
Brand Names Blistex®
Use Lip balm
Usual Dosage Apply as needed

Camphor, Menthol and Boric Acid *see* Rubs and Liniments
on page 319

Camphor, Menthol and Phenol
Brand Names Sarna [OTC]
Use For relief of dry, itching skin
Usual Dosage Apply as needed for dry skin

Candida albicans (Monilia)
Synonyms *Monilia* Skin Test
Use A screen for detection of nonresponsiveness to antigens in immuno-compromised individuals
Usual Dosage Inject S.C. at 5-7 day intervals as indicated

Cantharidin
Brand Names Cantharone®
Use Removal of ordinary and periungual warts
Pregnancy Risk Factor C
Usual Dosage Apply directly to lesion, cover with nonporous tape, remove tape in 24 hours, reapply if necessary

Cantharone® *see* Cantharidin *on this page*

Cantil® *see* Mepenzolate Bromide *on page 218*

Capastat® Sulfate *see* Capreomycin Sulfate *on this page*

Capoten® *see* Captopril *on this page*

Capozide® *see* Captopril and Hydrochlorothiazide
on next page

Capreomycin Sulfate (kap ree oh mye' sin)
Brand Names Capastat® Sulfate
Use Used in conjunction with at least one other antituberculosis agent in the treatment of tuberculosis
Usual Dosage Adult: I.M.: 15 mg/kg/day up to 1 g/day for 60-120 days

β-Capsa I® *see* Haemophilus b Vaccine *on page 165*

Capsaicin (kap say' sin)
Brand Names Zostrix®
Use Temporary relief of pain following herpes zoster after lesions have healed
Usual Dosage Adult and Children > 2 years: Apply to area up to 3 or 4 times daily only

Captopril (kap' toe pril)
Brand Names Capoten®
Use Management of hypertension and treatment of congestive heart failure
Pregnancy Risk Factor C
Usual Dosage Oral:

Adult:
Hypertension: Initially 25 mg 2-3 times daily; may increase at 1-2 week intervals up to 50 mg three times daily; add diuretic before further dosage increases; may need to start at 12.5 mg three times/day; maximum dose 150 mg three times/day
Congestive heart failure: 6.25-25 mg three times daily (maximum 450 mg/day) in conjunction with cardiac glycoside and diuretic therapy; initial dose depends upon patient's fluid/electrolyte status

Children: 12.5 mg every 12 hours; Maintenance dose: 0.1-0.4 mg/kg/dose every 6-24 hours

Infants: 0.5-0.6 mg/kg/day every 6-12 hours

Neonates: Loading dose 0.5 mg/kg

Captopril and Hydrochlorothiazide
Brand Names Capozide®
Use Management of hypertension and treatment of congestive heart failure
Pregnancy Risk Factor C
Usual Dosage Adult: Oral:

Hypertension: Initially 25 mg 2-3 times daily; may increase at 1-2 week intervals up to 150 mg three times daily (captopril dosages)

Congestive heart failure: 6.25-25 mg three times daily (maximum 450 mg/day) (captopril dosages)

Carafate® see Sucralfate on page 335

Caramiphen and Phenylpropanolamine
Brand Names Tuss-Ornade®
Synonyms Phenylpropanolamine and Caramiphen
Use Symptomatic relief of cough and nasal congestion associated with the common cold
Usual Dosage Adult and Children: > 12 years of age: Oral: One every 12 hours

Carbachol (kar' ba kole)
Brand Names Isopto® Carbachol; Miostat®
Synonyms Carbacholine; Carbamylcholine Chloride
Use Lower intraocular pressure in the treatment of glaucoma
Pregnancy Risk Factor C
Usual Dosage 1-2 drops in eye(s) up to four times daily

Carbacholine see Carbachol on this page

Carbamazepine (kar ba maz' e peen)
Brand Names Epitrol®; Tegretol®
Use Prophylaxis of tonic-clonic mixed, and complex-partial seizures; may be used to relieve pain in trigeminal neuralgia
Pregnancy Risk Factor C
Usual Dosage Oral:

> 12 years of age: Seizure disorders: 200 mg twice daily to start, increase by 200 mg/day until therapeutic levels are achieved; usual dose is 800-1200 mg/day in divided doses every 6-8 hours; maximum dose: 1200 mg/day (some patients may require 1600-2400 mg/day) (> 16 years of age)

12-16 years: Maximum dose 1000 mg/day

(Continued)

Carbamazepine *(Continued)*

6-12 years:
Initial dose: 10 mg/kg/day; given every 12-24 hours; increase by 100 mg/day at weekly intervals depending upon response
Maintenance dose: 20-30 mg/kg/day given every 6-8 hours
Maximum dose: 1000 mg/day

< 6 years of age: Initial dose: 10 mg/kg/day given every 12-24 hours; if necessary, increase at 1-2 week intervals up to 20 mg/kg/day depending upon response and blood levels (occasionally dosages may need to exceed 20 mg/kg/day)

Carbamide *see* Urea *on page 369*

Carbamide Peroxide *(kar' ba mide)*
Brand Names Debrox® [OTC]; Gly-Oxide® [OTC]
Synonyms Urea Peroxide
Use Relief of minor inflammation of gums, oral mucosal surfaces and lips including canker sores and dental irritation; emulsify and disperse ear wax
Pregnancy Risk Factor C
Usual Dosage
Oral: Apply undiluted four times a day and at bedtime
Otic: Instill 5-10 drops twice a day up to four days

Carbamylcholine Chloride *see* Carbachol *on previous page*

Carbenicillin *(kar ben i sill' in)*
Brand Names Geocillin®; Geopen®; Pyopen®
Synonyms Carbenicillin Disodium; Carbenicillin Indanyl Sodium; Carindacillin
Use Treatment of serious infections caused by susceptible organisms and urinary tract infections
Pregnancy Risk Factor B
Usual Dosage
Adult: Oral: 1-2 tablets every six hours
Children: Oral: 30-50 mg/kg/day given every six hours; maximum dose is 2-3 grams/day

Soft tissue, septicemia, respiratory infections: I.V.:
Adult: 1.5-40 g daily in divided doses every 4-6 hours; maximum dose is 40 g/day
Children: 250-500 mg/kg in divided doses every 4-6 hours

Urinary tract infections: I.M., I.V.:
Adult: 200 mg/kg in divided doses every 4-6 hours
Children: 50-200 mg/kg in divided doses every 4-6 hours

Carbenicillin Disodium *see* Carbenicillin *on this page*

Carbenicillin Indanyl Sodium *see* Carbenicillin *on this page*

Carbidopa *(kar bi doe' pa)*
See Also Levodopa and Carbidopa
Brand Names Lodosyn®
Use In combination with levodopa in the treatment of parkinsonism
Usual Dosage Adult: Oral: 70-100 mg/day

Carbidopa and Levodopa *see* Levodopa and Carbidopa
on page 202

Carbinoxamine and Pseudoephedrine
Brand Names Rondec®
Synonyms Pseudoephedrine and Carbinoxamine
Use Symptomatic relief of seasonal and perennial allergic rhinitis and vasomotor rhinitis
Pregnancy Risk Factor C
Usual Dosage See table.

Age	Dose*	Frequency*
Rondec® oral drops 1–3 mo	$^1/_4$ dropperful ($^1/_4$ mL)	4 times/d
3–6 mo	$^1/_2$ dropperful ($^1/_2$ ml)	4 times/d
6–9 mo	$^3/_4$ dropperful ($^3/_4$ ml)	4 times/d
9–18 mo	1 dropperful (1 ml)	4 times/d
Rondec® syrup and Rondec® tablet 18 mo – 6 y	$^1/_2$ teaspoonful (2.5 mL)	4 times/d
6 y and over adults	1 teaspoonful (5 mL) or 1 tablet	4 times/d
Rondec-TR® tablet 12 y and over adults	1 tablet	2 times/d

* In mild cases or in particularly sensitive patients, less frequent or reduced doses may be adequate.

Carbinoxamine Maleate (kar bi nox' a meen)
Brand Names Clistin®; Rondec® Drops; Rondec® Filmtab®; Rondec® Syrup; Rondec-TR®
Use Perennial and seasonal allergic rhinitis and other allergic symptoms including urticaria
Pregnancy Risk Factor C
Usual Dosage Oral:

Adult: 4-8 mg 3-4 times daily

Children: 0.2-0.4 mg/kg/day

Carbinoxamine, Pseudoephedrine and Dextromethorphan
Brand Names Rondec®-DM
Use For relief of coughs and upper respiratory symptoms, including nasal congestion, associated with allergy or the common cold
Pregnancy Risk Factor C

(Continued)

Carbinoxamine, Pseudoephedrine and Dextromethorphan *(Continued)*

Usual Dosage Syrup and drops:

Adult and Children: > 6 years of age: 5 mL syrup four times/day

Children: 18 months-6 years: 2.5 mL syrup four times/day

Infant: Drops:
   1-3 months: 1/4 mL four times/day
   3-6 months: 1/2 mL four times/day
   6-9 months: 3/4 mL four times/day
   9-18 months: 1 mL four times/day

Carbocaine® *see* Mepivacaine Hydrochloride *on page 219*

Carbol-Fuchsin Solution N.F. (kar bol fook' sin)

Synonyms Castellani's Paint
Use Treatment of superficial mycotic infections
Usual Dosage Apply to affected area 2-4 times daily

Carboplatin (kar' boe pla tin)

Brand Names Paraplatin®
Use Palliative treatment of ovarian carcinoma
Pregnancy Risk Factor D
Usual Dosage I.V.: 360 mg/m^2 on day one every four weeks; dose then is adjusted on platelet count

Carboprost (kar' boe prost)

Brand Names Hemabate™
Use Termination of pregnancy
Usual Dosage I.M.: 250 µg to start, 250 µg at 1.5-3.5 hour intervals depending on uterine response; a 500 µg dose may be given if uterine response is not adequate after several 250 µg doses

Carbose D *see* Carboxymethylcellulose Sodium *on this page*

Carboxymethylcellulose Sodium

(kar box ee meth ill sell' yoo lose)
Synonyms Carbose D
Use In tablet form it is used as a hydrophilic colloid laxative; as a powder: suspending agent, tablet excipient, and viscosity-increasing agent
Usual Dosage Adult: Oral: 1.5 g 3 or 4 times daily

Cardene® *see* Nicardipine Hydrochloride *on page 251*

Cardilate® *see* Erythrityl Tetranitrate *on page 134*

Cardio-Green® *see* Indocyanine Green *on page 184*

Cardioquin® *see* Quinidine *on page 311*

Cardizem® *see* Diltiazem *on page 116*

Carindacillin *see* Carbenicillin *on page 58*

Carisoprodate *see* Carisoprodol *on next page*

Carisoprodol (kar eye soe proe' dole)
Brand Names Rela®; Sodol®; Soma®; Soprodol®; Soridol®
Synonyms Carisoprodate; Isobamate
Use Skeletal muscle relaxant
Pregnancy Risk Factor C
Usual Dosage Oral: 350 mg 3-4 times daily; take last dose at bedtime

Carmol® [OTC] *see* Urea *on page 369*

Carmol-HC® *see* Hydrocortisone and Urea *on page 175*

Carmustine (kar mus' teen)
Brand Names BiCNU®
Synonyms BCNU
Use Palliative treatment of brain tumors, multiple myeloma and Hodgkin's disease and non-Hodgkin's lymphomas
Pregnancy Risk Factor D
Usual Dosage I.V.: 150-200 mg/m^2 every six weeks as a single dose or divided into daily injections on two successive days; next dose is to be determined based on hematologic response to the previous dose

Carnation Instant Breakfast® [OTC] *see* Nutritional Formula, Enteral/Oral *on page 258*

Carnitor® *see* Levocarnitine *on page 201*

Casanthranol and Docusate *see* Docusate and Casanthranol *on page 121*

Cascara Sagrada (kas kar' a)
Use Temporary relief of constipation; sometimes used with milk of magnesia ("black and white" mixture)
Pregnancy Risk Factor C
Usual Dosage

Adult: 1 tablet; 1 mL fluid extract; 5 mL aromatic fluid extract at bedtime

Children:
   2-12 years of age: 1/2 adult dose
   < 2 years: 1/4 adult dose

Cascara Sagrada Fluid Extract and Milk of Magnesia
Synonyms Black and White Cocktail; MOM/Cascara
Use Temporary relief of constipation

Castellani's Paint *see* Carbol-Fuchsin Solution N.F. *on previous page*

Castor Oil (kas' tor)
Brand Names Neoloid® [OTC]; Purge® [OTC]
Synonyms Oleum Ricini
Use Preparation for rectal or bowel examination or surgery; rarely used to relieve constipation; also applied to skin as emollient and protectant
Pregnancy Risk Factor X

(Continued)

Castor Oil *(Continued)*
Usual Dosage Oral:
Adult: 15-60 mL
Children:
6-12 years of age: 5-15 mL
< 6 years: 1.25-7.5 mL
Infants: Up to 4 mL, increased dose produces no greater effect

Catapres® *see* Clonidine *on page 84*

Catarase® *see* Chymotrypsin, Alpha *on page 79*

CCNU *see* Lomustine *on page 206*

CDDP *see* Cisplatin *on page 80*

Ceclor® *see* Cefaclor *on this page*

Cecon® [OTC] *see* Ascorbic Acid *on page 29*

Cedilanid-D® *see* Deslanoside *on page 101*

Cee-1000® T.D. [OTC] *see* Ascorbic Acid *on page 29*

CeeNU® *see* Lomustine *on page 206*

Ceepryn® [OTC] *see* Cetylpyridinium Chloride *on page 67*

Cefaclor *(sef' a klor)*
Brand Names Ceclor®
Use Treatment of susceptible bacterial infection; mainly respiratory tract, skin and skin structure, bone and joint, urinary tract and gynecologic as well as septicemia; second generation cephalosporin
Pregnancy Risk Factor B
Usual Dosage Oral:

Adult: 250-500 mg every eight hours; maximum: 4 grams/day

Children: > 1 month: 20-40 mg/kg/day in divided doses every eight hours; maximum: 1 gram/day; adjust dosage according to body weight

Cefadroxil Monohydrate *(sef a drox' ill)*
Brand Names Duricef®; Ultracef®
Use Treatment of susceptible bacterial infections, including those caused by group A beta-hemolytic *Streptococcus*; first generation cephalosporin
Pregnancy Risk Factor B
Usual Dosage Oral:
Adult: 1-2 g/day in 1-2 divided doses

Children: 15 mg/kg twice daily

Cefadyl® *see* Cephapirin Sodium *on page 66*

Cefamandole Nafate *(sef a man' dole)*
Brand Names Mandol®
Use Treatment of susceptible bacterial infection; mainly respiratory tract, skin and skin structure, bone and joint, urinary tract and gynecologic as well as septicemia; second generation cephalosporin

Pregnancy Risk Factor B
Usual Dosage I.M., I.V.:

Adult: 500-1000 mg every 4-8 hours

Children: 50-100 mg/kg/day in divided doses every 4-8 hours

Cefanex® *see* Cephalexin Monohydrate *on page 66*

Cefazolin Sodium (sef a' zoe lin)
Brand Names Ancef®; Kefzol®; Zolicef®
Use Treatment of susceptible bacterial infections, mainly gram-positive and some gram-negative rods; first generation cephalosporin
Pregnancy Risk Factor B
Usual Dosage I.M., I.V.:

Adult: 750-6000 mg/day (depending upon severity of infection); given every 6-8 hours

Children: > 1 month of age: 50-100 mg/kg/day given every 6-8 hours; maximum dose 4-6 grams/day

Neonates:
< 2 kg: 40 mg/kg/day given every 12 hours
> 2 kg: Age 0-7 days: 40 mg/kg/day given every 12 hours; age > 7 days: 60 mg/kg/day given every eight hours

Cefixime (sef ix' eem)
Brand Names Suprax®
Use Treatment of infections when caused by susceptible strains in uncomplicated urinary tract infections, otitis media, pharyngitis and tonsillitis, as well all as acute bronchitis and acute exacerbations of chronic bronchitis; third generation cephalosporin
Pregnancy Risk Factor B
Usual Dosage Oral:

Adult: 400 mg/day as a single dose or 200 mg twice daily

Children: 8 mg/kg/day either as a single dose or two equal doses given every 12 hours

Cefizox® *see* Ceftizoxime *on page 65*

Cefobid® *see* Cefoperazone Sodium *on this page*

Cefoperazone Sodium (sef oh per' a zone)
Brand Names Cefobid®
Use Treatment of susceptible bacterial infection; mainly respiratory tract, skin and skin structure, bone and joint, urinary tract and gynecologic as well as septicemia; third generation cephalosporin
Pregnancy Risk Factor B
Usual Dosage Adult: I.M., I.V.: 2-4 g/day in divided doses every 12 hours (up to 16 g/day)

Cefotan® *see* Cefotetan Disodium *on next page*

Cefotaxime Sodium (sef oh taks' eem)
Brand Names Claforan®
Use Treatment of susceptible bacterial infection; mainly respiratory tract, skin and skin structure, bone and joint, urinary tract and gynecologic as well as septicemia; third generation cephalosporin
Pregnancy Risk Factor B
Usual Dosage I.M., I.V.:

Adult: 1 g every 6-8 hours (up to 12 g/day)

Children: 1 month - 12 years of age (less than 50 kg): 50-180 mg/kg/day in 4-6 divided doses; > 50 kg: Use usual adult dosage

Neonates: 1-4 weeks of age: 50 mg/kg every 6-8 hours

Premature or full-term neonates: < 1 week: 50 mg/kg every 12 hours

Cefotetan Disodium (sef' oh tee tan)
Brand Names Cefotan®
Use Treatment of susceptible bacterial infection; mainly respiratory tract, skin and skin structure, bone and joint, urinary tract and gynecologic as well as septicemia; second generation cephalosporin
Pregnancy Risk Factor B
Usual Dosage Adult: I.M., I.V.: 1-6 g/day in divided doses every 12 hours, 1-2 g may be given every 24 hours for urinary tract infection

Cefoxitin Sodium (se fox' i tin)
Brand Names Mefoxin®
Use Treatment of susceptible bacterial infection; mainly respiratory tract, skin and skin structure, bone and joint, urinary tract and gynecologic as well as septicemia; second generation cephalosporin
Pregnancy Risk Factor B
Usual Dosage I.M., I.V.:

Adult: 1-2 g every 6-8 hours (I.M. injection is painful)

Children:
Mild to moderate infection: 80-100 mg/kg/day in 3-4 divided doses
Severe infection: 100-160 mg/kg/day in 4-6 divided doses
Maximum dose: 12 g/day

Ceftazidime (sef' tay zi deem)
Brand Names Fortaz®; Tazidime™
Use Treatment of documented *Pseudomonas aeruginosa* infection; pseudomonad infection resistant to ticarcillin/aminoglycoside therapy and pseudomonad infection in patient at risk of developing aminoglycoside-induced nephrotoxicity and/or ototoxicity; empiric therapy of a febrile, granulocytopenic patient; third generation cephalosporin
Pregnancy Risk Factor B
Usual Dosage I.M., I.V.:

Adult: 1-2 g every 8-12 hours (250-500 mg every 12 hours for urinary tract infections)

Children: 1 month-12 years: 30-50 mg/kg every eight hours; maximum dose is six grams daily (50 mg/kg dose should be reserved for immuno-compromised patients, cystic fibrosis patients, or meningitis patients)

Neonate: Four weeks: 30 mg/kg every 12 hours

Ceftin® *see* Cefuroxime *on this page*

Ceftizoxime (sef ti zox' eem)
Brand Names Cefizox®
Use Treatment of susceptible bacterial infection; mainly respiratory tract, skin and skin structure, bone and joint, urinary tract and gynecologic as well as septicemia; third generation cephalosporin
Pregnancy Risk Factor B
Usual Dosage I.M., I.V.:

Adult: 1-2 g every 8-12 hours, up to 2 g every four hours for life-threatening infections

Children: ≥ 6 months of age: 50 mg/kg every 6-8 hours to 200 mg/kg/day

Ceftriaxone Sodium (sef try ax' one)
Brand Names Rocephin®
Use Treatment of documented infection due to susceptible organisms in patients without I.V. line access; documented or suspected infection due to susceptible organisms in home care patients; treatment of documented or suspected gonococcal infection; third generation cephalosporin
Pregnancy Risk Factor B
Usual Dosage I.M., I.V.:

Adult: 1-2 g/day single dose or every 12 hours; maximum dose is 4 grams/day

Children: 50-75 mg/kg/day in divided doses every 12 hours; maximum dose is 2 g/day (100 mg/kg/day for meningitis)

Cefuroxime (se fyoor ox' eem)
Brand Names Ceftin®; Kefurox®; Zinacef®
Use A second generation cephalosporin useful in infections caused by staphylococci, group B streptococci, *H. influenzae* (type A and B), *E. coli*, *Enterobacter*, *Salmonella*, and *Klebsiella*
Pregnancy Risk Factor B
Usual Dosage

Adult:
Oral: 125-500 mg twice daily, depending on severity of infection
I.M., I.V.: 750-1500 mg every eight hours

Children:
Oral: > 12 years of age: 250 mg twice daily; < 12 years: 125 mg twice daily
I.M., I.V.: 50-100 mg/kg/day in divided doses every 6-8 hours

Celestone® *see* Betamethasone *on page 43*

Celestone® Soluspan® *see* Betamethasone *on page 43*

Cellulose, Oxidized (sell' yoo lose)
Brand Names Oxygel®; Surgicel®
Synonyms Absorbable Cotton
Use As a temporary packing for the control of capillary, venous, or small arterial hemorrhage

Cellulose Sodium Phosphate
Brand Names Calibind®

Synonyms Sodium Cellulose Phosphate

Use As an adjunct to dietary restriction to reduce renal calculi formation in absorptive hypercalciuria type I

Pregnancy Risk Factor C

Usual Dosage Adult: Oral: 5 g three times a day with meals; decrease dose to 5 g with main meal and 2.5 g with each of two other meals when urinary calcium declines to less than 150 mg/day

Celontin® *see* Methsuximide *on page 229*

Cenafed® Syrup [OTC] *see* Pseudoephedrine *on page 307*

Cenocort® *see* Triamcinolone *on page 359*

Cenocort® Forte *see* Triamcinolone *on page 359*

Cenolate® *see* Sodium Ascorbate *on page 326*

Centrax® *see* Prazepam *on page 293*

Cepacol® [OTC] *see* Cetylpyridinium Chloride *on next page*

Cepacol® Anesthetic Troches [OTC] *see* Cetylpyridinium Chloride and Benzocaine *on next page*

Cephalexin Monohydrate (sef a lex' in)
Brand Names Cefanex®; C-Lexin®; Entacef®; Keflet®; Keflex®; Keftab®

Use Treatment of susceptible bacterial infections, including those caused by group A beta-hemolytic *Streptococcus*, staphylococci, *Klebsiella pneumoniae*, *E. coli*, *Proteus mirabilis*, and *Shigella*; first generation cephalosporin

Pregnancy Risk Factor B

Usual Dosage Oral:

Adult: 250-500 mg every six hours

Children: 25-50 mg/kg/day in divided doses every six hours; severe infections: 50-100 mg/kg/day in divided doses every six hours

Cephalothin Sodium (sef a' loe thin)
Brand Names Keflin®

Use Treatment of susceptible bacterial infections, including those caused by group A beta-hemolytic *Streptococcus*; first generation cephalosporin

Pregnancy Risk Factor B

Usual Dosage

Adult: I.M., I.V.: 500 g - 1 g every 4-6 hours

Children: I.V.: 14-27 mg/kg every 4 hours; 20-40 mg/kg every six hours

Cephapirin Sodium (sef a pye' rin)
Brand Names Cefadyl®

Use Treatment of infections when caused by susceptible strains in serious respiratory, genitourinary, gastrointestinal, skin and soft-tissue, bone and joint infections; septicemia; endocarditis; first generation cephalosporin

Pregnancy Risk Factor B
Usual Dosage I.M., I.V.:

Adult: 500 mg every 4-6 hours up to 12 g per day

Children: 10-20 mg/kg every 6 hours

Cephradine (sef' ra deen)
Brand Names Anspor®; Ro-Ceph®; Velosef®
Use Treatment of susceptible bacterial infections, including those caused by group A beta-hemolytic *Streptococcus*; first generation cephalosporin
Pregnancy Risk Factor B
Usual Dosage

Adult:
Oral: 250-500 mg every six hours or 500 mg - 1 g every 12 hours up to 4 g/day
I.M., I.V.: 2-4 g/day in four equally divided doses up to 8 g/day

Children:
Oral: ≥ 9 months of age: 25-50 mg/kg/day in equally divided doses every 6-12 hours up to 4 g/day
I.M., I.V.: > 1 year of age: 50-100 mg/kg/day in equally divided doses every six hours up to 8 g/day

Cephulac® *see* Lactulose *on page 199*

Cerespan® *see* Papaverine Hydrochloride *on page 200*

Cerubidine® *see* Daunorubicin Hydrochloride *on page 98*

Cerumenex® *see* Triethanolamine Polypeptide Oleate-Condensate *on page 361*

C.E.S. *see* Estrogen, Conjugated *on page 136*

Cesamet® *see* Nabilone *on page 243*

Cetacaine® *see* Benzocaine, Butyl Aminobenzoate, Tetracaine and Benzalkonium Chloride *on page 41*

Cetane® [OTC] *see* Ascorbic Acid *on page 29*

Cetapred® *see* Sodium Sulfacetamide and Prednisolone Acetate *on page 330*

Cetylpyridinium Chloride (see' til peer i di' nee um)
Brand Names Ceepryn® [OTC]; Cepacol® [OTC]
Use Temporary relief of sore throat
Usual Dosage Use as needed for sore throat

Cetylpyridinium Chloride and Benzocaine
Brand Names Cepacol® Anesthetic Troches [OTC]
Synonyms Benzocaine and Cetylpyridinium Chloride
Use Symptomatic relief of sore throat
Usual Dosage Use as needed for sore throat

Cevalin® [OTC] *see* Ascorbic Acid *on page 29*

Ce-Vi-Sol® [OTC] *see* Ascorbic Acid *on page 29*

Cevita® [OTC] *see* Ascorbic Acid *on page 29*

Charcoaid® [OTC] *see* Charcoal *on this page*

Charcoal

Brand Names Actidose-Aqua® [OTC]; Actidose® With Sorbitol [OTC]; Adsorba® 300 C [OTC]; Charcoaid® [OTC]; Charcocaps® [OTC]; Insta-Char® [OTC]; Liqui-Char® [OTC]; SuperChar® [OTC]

Synonyms Activated Carbon; Adsorbent Charcoal, Activated Charcoal; Liquid Antidote; Medicinal Charcoal

Use Emergency treatment in poisoning by drugs and chemicals; repetitive doses gastric dialysis in uremia to adsorb various waste products

Pregnancy Risk Factor C

Usual Dosage

Acute poisoning: Adult and Children: Oral: 30-100 g in at least 6-8 ounces of water; in general dose is 1 g/kg or approximately 5-10 times estimated weight of ingested poison

Gastric Dialysis: 20-40 g every six hours for 1-2 days

Charcocaps® [OTC] *see* Charcoal *on this page*

Chemstrip bG® [OTC] *see* Diagnostic Test for Glucose in Blood *on page 107*

Chemstrip® K [OTC] *see* Diagnostic Test for Acetone in Urine *on page 106*

Chemstrip uG® [OTC] *see* Diagnostic Test for Glucose in Urine *on page 107*

Chiggertox® [OTC] *see* Benzocaine *on page 40*

Chlo-Amine® [OTC] *see* Chlorpheniramine Maleate *on page 74*

Chloracol® *see* Chloramphenicol *on next page*

Chloral *see* Chloral Hydrate *on this page*

Chloral Hydrate

Brand Names Noctec®; Somnos®

Synonyms Chloral; Hydrated Chloral; Trichloroacetaldehyde Monohydrate

Use Short-term sedative and hypnotic (< 2 weeks)

Restrictions C-IV

Pregnancy Risk Factor C

Usual Dosage Oral, rectal:

Adult:
Sedation, anxiety: 250 mg three times daily
Insomnia: 500-1000 mg at bedtime

Children:
Sedation, anxiety: 25 mg/kg/day in divided doses every eight hours
Hypnotic: 50 mg/kg/dose
Prior to EEG: 20-25 mg/kg

Chlorambucil (klor am' byoo sil)
Brand Names Leukeran®
Use Management of chronic lymphocytic leukemia, malignant lymphoma, and Hodgkin's disease
Pregnancy Risk Factor D
Usual Dosage Oral:

Adult: 0.1-0.2 mg/kg/day for 3-6 weeks, then adjust dose on basis of blood counts

Children: 0.1-0.2 mg/kg/day or 4.5 mg/m^2/day

Chloramphenicol (klor am fen' i kole)
Brand Names AK-Chlor®; Anocol®; Chloracol®; Chlorofair®; Chloromyce-tin®; Chloroptic®; Econochlor®; I-Chlor®; Ocu-Chlor®; Ophthochlor®; Spectro-Chlor®
Use Treatment of susceptible bacterial infections, mainly gram-negative, when less toxic agents cannot be used
Pregnancy Risk Factor C
Usual Dosage

Adult and Children:
Oral, I.V.: 50 mg/kg/day in divided doses every six hours
Ophthalmic: Apply 1-2 drops or small amount of ointment every 3-6 hours
Otic: 2-3 drops 2-3 times daily

Newborn: Oral, I.V.: 25 mg/kg every 12 hours

Chloramphenicol and Prednisolone
Brand Names Chloroptic-P®
Use Topical anti-infective and corticosteroid for treatment of ocular infections
Usual Dosage Instill one or two drops in eye(s) 2-4 times daily

Chlordiazepoxide (klor dye az e pox' ide)
Brand Names Libritabs®; Librium®
Use Management of anxiety and as a preoperative sedative, symptoms of alcohol withdrawal
Restrictions C-IV
Pregnancy Risk Factor D
Usual Dosage

Adult:
Anxiety: Oral: 5-10 mg 3-4 times daily
Preoperative sedation: Oral: 5-10 mg 3-4 times daily, one day preop; I.M.: 50-100 mg one hour preop
Alcohol withdrawal symptoms: Oral: 50-100 mg, repeated until agitation is controlled, up to 300 mg/day; I.V.: 50-100 mg to start, dose may be repeated in 2-4 hours

Children: Anxiety: Oral: 5 mg 2-4 times daily, up to 10 mg three times daily > 6 years

Chlordiazepoxide and Amitriptyline *see* Amitriptyline and Chlordiazepoxide *on page 20*

Chlordiazepoxide and Clidinium *see* Clidinium and Chlordiazepoxide *on page 81*

Chlorhexidine Gluconate (klor hex' i deen)
Brand Names Hibiclens® [OTC]; Peridex®
Use Skin cleanser for surgical scrub, cleanser skin wounds, germicidal hand rinse, and as antibacterial dental rinse
Pregnancy Risk Factor B
Usual Dosage Oral rinse (Peridex®)

Precede use of solution by flossing and brushing teeth; completely rinse toothpaste from mouth. Swish 15 mL undiluted oral rinse around in mouth for 30 seconds, then expectorate. Caution patient not to swallow the medicine. Avoid eating for 2-3 hours after treatment. (The cap on bottle of oral rinse is a measure for 15 mL.)

Staining of oral surfaces (mucosa, teeth, dorsum of tongue) may be visible as soon as one week after therapy begins and is more pronounced when there is a heavy accumulation of unremoved plaque and when teeth fillings have rough surfaces. Stain does not have a clinically adverse effect but because removal may not be possible, patient with frontal restoration should be advised of the potential permanency of the stain.

When used as a treatment of gingivitis, the regimen begins with oral prophylaxis. Patient treats mouth with 15 mL chlorhexidine; swish for 30 seconds, then expectorate. This is repeated twice daily (morning and evening). Patient should have a re-evaluation followed by a dental prophylaxis every six months.

Inform patient that reduced taste perception during treatment is reversible with discontinuation of chlorhexidine.

Chloroethane *see* Ethyl Chloride *on page 141*

Chlorofair® *see* Chloramphenicol *on previous page*

Chloromycetin® *see* Chloramphenicol *on previous page*

Chloroprocaine Hydrochloride (klor oh proe' kane)
Brand Names Nesacaine®
Use For infiltration anesthesia and for peripheral and epidural anesthesia
Pregnancy Risk Factor C
Usual Dosage Dosage varies with anesthetic procedure, the area to be anesthetized, the vascularity of the tissues, depth of anesthesia required, degree of muscle relaxation required, and duration of anesthesia

Chloroptic® *see* Chloramphenicol *on previous page*

Chloroptic-P® *see* Chloramphenicol and Prednisolone *on previous page*

Chloroquine and Primaquine
Brand Names Aralen® Phosphate With Primaquine Phosphate
Synonyms Primaquine and Chloroquine
Use Prophylaxis of malaria, regardless of species, in all areas where the disease is endemic.

Pregnancy Risk Factor C
Usual Dosage

Adult: Start at least one day before entering the endemic area; take one tablet weekly on the same day each week; continue for eight weeks after leaving the endemic area

Children: For suggested dosage (based on body weight), see table:

Weight		Chloroquine Base (mg)	Primaquine Base (mg)	Dose* (mL)
lb	**kg**			
10–15	4.5–6.8	20	3	2.5
16–25	7.3–11.4	40	6	5
26–35	11.8–15.9	60	9	7.5
36–45	16.4–20.5	80	12	10
46–55	20.9–25	100	15	12.5
56–100	25.4–45.4	150	22.5	$^1/_2$ tablet
100+	> 45.4	300	45	1 tablet

* Dose based on liquid containing approximately 40 mg of chloroquine base and 6 mg primaquine base per 5 mL, prepared from chloroquine phosphate with primaquine phosphate tablets.

Chloroquine Phosphate (klor' oh kwin)

Brand Names Aralen® Phosphate

Use Suppression prophylaxis and treatment of acute attacks of malaria; suppressive treatment of malaria; extraintestinal amebiasis; rheumatoid arthritis

Acute attack:

Dose	Time	Dosage (in mg of base)	
		Adults	**Children**
Initial dose	Day 1	600 mg	10 mg/kg
2nd dose	6 h later	300 mg	5 mg/kg
3rd dose	Day 2	300 mg	5 mg/kg
4th dose	Day 3	300 mg	5 mg/kg

Age	Chloroquine PO$_4$	Chloroquine Base Equivalent
< 1 y	62 mg	37.5 mg
1–3 y	125 mg	75 mg
4–6 y	165 mg	100 mg
7–10 y	250 mg	150 mg
11–16 y	375 mg	225 mg

(Continued)

Pregnancy Risk Factor C
Usual Dosage

Suppression:

Adult: 300 mg (base) weekly, on the same day each week. Begin two weeks prior to exposure; continue for 6-8 weeks after leaving endemic area. If suppressive therapy is not begun prior to exposure, double the initial loading dose (adults - 600 mg base; children - 10 mg base/kg) and give in two divided doses, six hours apart.

Children: Administer 5 mg base/kg weekly or titrate dosage. See table.

Extraintestinal amebiasis: Oral:

Adult: 600 mg base/day for two days followed by 300 mg base daily for at least 2-3 weeks

Children: 10 mg/kg once daily for 2-3 weeks (up to 300 mg base/day)

Rheumatoid arthritis: Adult: 150 mg base once daily with evening meal

Chlorothiazide (klor oh thye' a zide)

Brand Names Diuril®

Use Management of mild to moderate hypertension, edema associated with congestive heart failure, pregnancy, or nephrotic syndrome

Pregnancy Risk Factor B

Usual Dosage Oral:

Adult: 250-500 mg per dose four times/day; maximum dose is 2 grams/day

Children:

> 6 months: 20 mg/kg/day in two divided doses every 12 hours

< 6 months: 20-30 mg/kg/day in two divided doses every 12 hours

Chlorothiazide and Methyldopa

Brand Names Aldoclor®

Synonyms Methyldopa and Chlorothiazide

Use Treatment of hypertension

Pregnancy Risk Factor C

Usual Dosage One tablet 2-3 times daily for first 48 hours, then adjust

Chlorothiazide and Reserpine

Brand Names Diupres-250®; Diupres-500®

Synonyms Reserpine and Chlorothiazide

Use Management of hypertension

Pregnancy Risk Factor C

Usual Dosage 1-2 tablets once or twice daily

Chlorotrianisene (klor oh trye an' i seen)

Brand Names TACE®

Use Treat inoperable prostatic cancer; management of atrophic vaginitis, female hypogonadism, vasomotor symptoms of menopause; prevention of postpartum breast engorgement (no longer recommended because increased risk of thrombophlebitis)

Pregnancy Risk Factor X
Usual Dosage Oral:

Prostatic cancer: Adult: 12-25 mg/day

Atrophic Vaginitis: Adult: 12-25 mg/day in 28-day cycles (21 days on and seven days off)

Female Hypogonadism: Adult: 12-25 mg for 21 days followed by I.M. progesterone 100 mg or five days of oral progestin; next course may begin on days of induced uterine bleeding

Menopause: Adult: 12-25 mg for 30 days

Postpartum breast engorgement: Adult: 12 mg four times a day for seven days or 72 mg twice a day for two days

Chlorpactin® WCS-90 *see* Oxychlorosene Sodium
on page 264

Chlorphed® [OTC] *see* Brompheniramine Maleate
on page 48

Chlorphed®-LA Nasal Solution [OTC] *see* Oxymetazoline
Hydrochloride *on page 265*

Chlorphenesin Carbamate (klor fen' e sin)
Brand Names Maolate®
Use Adjunctive treatment of discomfort in short-term, acute, painful musculoskeletal conditions
Pregnancy Risk Factor C
Usual Dosage Adult: Oral: 800 mg three times a day, then adjusted to lowest effective dosage, usually 400 mg four times a day for up to a maximum of two months

Chlorpheniramine and Phenylephrine
Brand Names Novahistine® Elixir [OTC]; Ru-Tuss® Liquid
Synonyms Phenylephrine and Chlorpheniramine
Use Temporary relief of nasal congestion and eustachian tube congestion as well as runny nose, sneezing, itching of nose or throat, itchy and watery eyes
Pregnancy Risk Factor C
Usual Dosage Oral:

Adult: 10 mL every four hours

Children:
6-12 years of age: 5 mL every four hours
2-5 years: 2.5 mL every four hours

Chlorpheniramine and Phenylpropanolamine
Brand Names Ornade® Spansule®; Triaminic® Cold Syrup [OTC]
Synonyms Phenylpropanolamine and Chlorpheniramine
Use Symptomatic relief of nasal congestion, runny nose, sneezing, itchy nose or throat, and itchy or watery eyes due to the common cold or allergic rhinitis
(Continued)

73

Chlorpheniramine and Phenylpropanolamine
(Continued)
Pregnancy Risk Factor B
Usual Dosage

Adult and Children: > 12 years: One capsule every 12 hours; 5-10 mL every 3-4 hours

Children: < 12 years: 5 mL every 3-4 hours

Chlorpheniramine and Pseudoephedrine
Brand Names Deconamine® SR; Novafed® A

Synonyms Pseudoephedrine and Chlorpheniramine

Use Relief of nasal congestion associated with the common cold, hay fever, and other allergies, sinusitis, eustachian tube blockage, and vasomotor and allergic rhinitis

Pregnancy Risk Factor B
Usual Dosage

Capsule: One capsule every 12 hours
Tablet: One tablet 3-4 times daily

Chlorpheniramine, Codeine and Guaifenesin
Brand Names Tussar® SF

Use Relief of severe coughs due to respiratory conditions caused by common cold, bronchitis, and influenza

Usual Dosage 5 mL three to four times daily up to 40 mL in a 24 hour period

Chlorpheniramine, Ephedrine, Phenylephrine and Carbetapentane
Brand Names Rynatuss® Pediatric Suspension

Use Symptomatic relief of cough

Pregnancy Risk Factor C
Usual Dosage Children:

> 6 years: 5-10 mL every 12 hours
2-6 years: 2.5-5 mL every 12 hours
< 2 years: Titrate dose individually

Chlorpheniramine Maleate (klor fen ir' a meen)
Brand Names Aller-Chlor® [OTC]; AL-R® [OTC]; Chlo-Amine® [OTC]; Chlorpro® [OTC]; Chlor-Trimeton® [OTC]; Kloromin® [OTC]; Teldrin® [OTC]

Use Perennial and seasonal allergic rhinitis and other allergic symptoms including urticaria

Pregnancy Risk Factor B
Usual Dosage Oral:

Adult: 4 mg every 4-6 hours or 8-12 mg of sustained release formulation every 8-12 hours, not to exceed 24 mg/day

Children:
6-12 years: 2 mg every 4-6 hours or 8 mg of sustained release formulation once daily, not to exceed 12 mg/day
2-6 years: 1 mg every 4-6 hours

Chlorpheniramine, Phenylephrine and Phenyltoloxamine

Brand Names Comhist®; Comhist® LA

Use Symptomatic relief of rhinitis and nasal congestion due to colds or allergy

Pregnancy Risk Factor C

Usual Dosage One capsule every 8-12 hours; 1-2 tablets three times a day

Chlorpheniramine, Phenylpropanolamine and Dextromethorphan

Brand Names Triaminicol® Multi-Symptom Cold Syrup [OTC]

Use Provides relief of runny nose, sneezing, suppresses cough, promotes nasal and sinus drainage.

Pregnancy Risk Factor C

Usual Dosage

Adult: 10 mL every four hours

Children: 6-12 years of age: 5 mL every four hours

Chlorpheniramine, Phenyltoloxamine, Phenylpropanolamine and Phenylephrine

Brand Names Naldecon®; Tri-Phen-Chlor®

Use Symptomatic treatment of nasal and eustachian tube congestion associated with sinusitis and acute upper respiratory infection; symptomatic relief of perennial and allergic rhinitis

Pregnancy Risk Factor C

Usual Dosage Oral:

Adult and Children > 12 years: 5 mL (syrup) or one tablet every 3-4 hours

Children 6-12 years: 2.5 mL (syrup) or 10 mL (pediatric syrup) or one-half tablet every 3-4 hours

Children 1-6 years: 5 mL (pediatric syrup) or 1 mL (pediatric drops) every 3-4 hours

Children 6-12 months: 2.5 mL (pediatric syrup) or 1/2 mL (pediatric drops) every 3-4 hours

Children 3-6 months: 1/4 mL (pediatric drops) every 3-4 hours

Chlorpheniramine, Pseudoephedrine and Codeine

Brand Names Histadyl® E.C.; Novahistine® DH

Use Temporary relief of cough associated with minor throat or bronchial irritation or nasal congestion due to common cold, allergic rhinitis, or sinusitis

Restrictions C-V

Pregnancy Risk Factor C

Usual Dosage Oral:

Adult: 10 mL every 4-6 hours, up to four doses in 24-hour period

Children:

50-90 lbs: 2.5-5 mL every 4-6 hours, up to four doses in 24-hour period

25-50 lbs: 1.25-2.50 mL every 4-6 hours, up to four doses in 24-hour period

(Continued)

Chlorpheniramine, Pyrilamine and Phenylephrine
Brand Names Rynatan® Pediatric Suspension
Use Symptomatic relief of nasal congestion associated with upper respiratory tract condition
Pregnancy Risk Factor C
Usual Dosage Children:
> > 6 years of age: 5-10 mL every 12 hours
> 2-6 years of age: 2.5-5 mL every 12 hours
> < 2 years of age: Titrate dose individually

Chlorpro® [OTC] *see* Chlorpheniramine Maleate *on page 74*

Chlorpromazine Hydrochloride (klor proe' ma zeen)
Brand Names Thorazine®
Use Treatment of psychoses, nausea, vomiting, and intractable hiccups
Pregnancy Risk Factor C
Usual Dosage

Adult:
Psychosis: Oral: 30-800 mg/day in 1-4 divided doses, usual dose is 200 mg/day; dosage may be gradually increased twice weekly by 20-50 mg until symptoms are controlled; some patients may require 1-2 g/day; I.M.: 25 mg initially, may increase to a maximum of 400 mg every 4-6 hours

Nausea and vomiting: Oral: 10-25 mg every 4-6 hours; rectal: 50-100 mg every 6-8 hours; I.M.: 25-50 mg every 3-4 hours

Intractable hiccups: Oral: 25-50 mg 3-4 times daily; I.M.: 25-80 mg 3-4 times daily, if no response to oral; I.V.: 25-80 mg by slow infusion

Children:
Psychosis: Oral: > 6 months of age: 0.55 mg/kg every 4-6 hours; rectal: > 6 months: 1.1 mg/kg every 6-8 hours; I.M.: > 6 months: 0.55 mg/kg every 4-6 hours; maximum I.M. dosage in children < 22.7 kg and < 5 years of age is 40 mg/daily

Nausea and vomiting: Oral: > 6 months: 0.55 mg/kg every 4-6 hours; rectal: 1.1 mg/kg every 6-8 hours; I.M.: 0.55 mg/kg every 6-8 hours; maximum I.M. dosage in children 22.7-45.5 kg and 5-12 years of age should not exceed 75 mg daily

Chlorpropamide (klor proe' pa mide)
Brand Names Diabinese®
Use To control blood sugar in adult onset, noninsulin-dependent diabetes (type II)
Pregnancy Risk Factor D
Usual Dosage Adult: Oral: 500 mg in 1-2 divided doses; initial dose in elderly patients should be 100 mg

Chlorprothixene (klor proe thix' een)
Brand Names Taractan®
Use Management of psychotic disorders
Pregnancy Risk Factor C
Usual Dosage

Adult:

Oral: 25-50 mg 3-4 times daily, to be increased as needed; doses exceeding 600 mg/day are rarely required

I.M.: 25-50 mg up to 3-4 times daily

Children: > 6 years: Oral: 10-25 mg 3-4 times daily

Chlortetracycline Hydrochloride (klor te tra sye' kleen)
Brand Names Aureomycin®; Fermycin® Soluble
Use Treatment of superficial infections of the skin due to susceptible organisms, also infection prophylaxis in minor skin abrasions
Pregnancy Risk Factor D
Usual Dosage Apply 1-5 times daily, cover with sterile bandage if needed

Chlorthalidone (klor thal' i done)
Brand Names Hygroton®
Use Management of mild to moderate hypertension, used alone or in combination with other agents; treatment of edema associated with congestive heart failure, nephrotic syndrome, or pregnancy
Pregnancy Risk Factor B
Usual Dosage Oral:

Adult: 25-100 mg/day or 100 mg three times weekly

Children: 2 mg/kg three times weekly

Chlor-Trimeton® [OTC] see Chlorpheniramine Maleate
on page 74

Chlorzoxazone (klor zox' a zone)
Brand Names Paraflex®; Parafon Forte™ DSC; Strifon® Forte DSC
Use Symptomatic treatment of muscle spasm and pain associated with acute musculoskeletal conditions
Pregnancy Risk Factor C
Usual Dosage Oral:

Adult: 250-500 mg 3-4 times a day up to 750 mg 3-4 times daily

Children: 20 mg/kg/day or 600 mg/m^2 in 3-4 divided doses

Cholac® see Lactulose on page 199

Choledyl® see Oxtriphylline on page 263

Cholera Vaccine (kol' er a)
Use Primary immunization for cholera prophylaxis
Pregnancy Risk Factor C
Usual Dosage I.M., S.C.:

Adult and Children: > 10 years of age: 0.5 mL in two doses one week to one month or more apart

(Continued)

Cholera Vaccine *(Continued)*

Children:
5-10 years of age: 0.3 mL with same dosage schedule
6 months - 4 years of age: 0.2 mL with same dosage schedule

Cholestyramine Resin (koe less' tir a meen)
Brand Names Quemid®; Questran®
Use As an adjunct in the management of primary hypercholesterolemia; to relieve pruritus associated with elevated levels of bile acids
Pregnancy Risk Factor C
Usual Dosage Adult: Oral: 3-4 g 3-4 times daily

Choline Magnesium Salicylate (koe' leen)
Brand Names Trilisate®
Use Management of osteoarthritis, rheumatoid arthritis, and other arthritides
Pregnancy Risk Factor C
Usual Dosage Adult: Oral: 500 mg-1.5 g 2-3 times daily

Choline Theophyllinate *see* Oxtriphylline *on page 263*

Cholografin® Meglumine *see* Iodipamide Meglumine *on page 188*

Choloxin® *see* Dextrothyroxine Sodium *on page 106*

Chondroitin Sulfate-Sodium Hyaluronate
Brand Names Viscoat®
Synonyms Sodium Hyaluronate-Chrondroitin Sulfate
Use Surgical aid in anterior segment procedures, protects corneal endothelium and coats intraocular lens thus protecting it
Usual Dosage Carefully introduce into anterior chamber after thoroughly cleaning the chamber with a balanced salt solution

Chorex® *see* Chorionic Gonadotropin *on this page*

Chorionic Gonadotropin (go nad' oh troe pin)
Brand Names A.P.L.®; Chorex®; Choron®; Corgonject®; Follutein®; Glukor®; Gonic®; Pregnyl®; Profasi® HP
Synonyms hCG
Use To induce ovulation and pregnancy; treatment of hypogonadotropic hypogonadism
Pregnancy Risk Factor X
Usual Dosage I.M. only:

Prepubertal cryptorchidism: 4000 USP units, three times weekly for three weeks; 5000 USP units every second day for four injections

Hypogonadotropic hypogonadism: 500-1000 USP units three times a week for three weeks, followed by the same dose twice a week for three weeks

Induction of ovulation: 5000-10,000 USP units one day following the last dose of menotropins

Choron® *see* Chorionic Gonadotropin *on previous page*

Chroma-Pak® *see* Trace Metals *on page 358*

Chromium *see* Trace Metals *on page 358*

Chronulac® *see* Lactulose *on page 199*

Chymer® *see* Bentiromide *on page 39*

Chymodiactin® *see* Chymopapain *on this page*

Chymopapain (kye' moe pa pane)
Brand Names Chymodiactin®; Discase®
Use Alternative to surgery in patients with herniated lumbar intervertebral disks
Pregnancy Risk Factor C
Usual Dosage 2000-4000 units/disk with a maximum cumulative dose not to exceed 8000 units for patients with multiple disk herniations

Chymotrypsin, Alpha (kye moe trip' sin)
Brand Names Catarase®; Zolyse®
Use Enzymatic zonulysis for intracapsular lens extraction in cataract surgery
Pregnancy Risk Factor C
Usual Dosage Irrigate area with 1-2 mL containing 150 units

Cibacalcin® *see* Calcitonin *on page 52*

Cibalith-S® *see* Lithium *on page 205*

Ciclopirox Olamine (sye kloe peer' ox)
Brand Names Loprox®
Use Treatment of tinea pedis, tinea cruris, tinea corporis, cutaneous candidiasis, tinea versicolor
Pregnancy Risk Factor B
Usual Dosage Adult and Children: > 10 years of age: Apply twice a day, gently massage into affected areas

Cilloral® *see* Penicillin G, Parenteral *on page 273*

Cimetidine (sye met' i deen)
Brand Names Tagamet®
Use Short-term treatment of active duodenal ulcers and benign gastric ulcers; long-term prophylaxis of duodenal ulcer and gastric hypersecretory states
Pregnancy Risk Factor B
Usual Dosage Adult: (Not recommended for children under 16 years of age; if potential benefits outweigh the risks, can use a dosage of 20-40 mg/kg/day)

Short-term treatment of active ulcers:
   Oral: 300 mg four times a day or 800 mg at bedtime or 400 mg twice daily for up to eight weeks

(Continued)

Cimetidine *(Continued)*
I.M., I.V.: 300 mg every six hours

Duodenal ulcer prophylaxis: Oral: 400-800 mg at bedtime

Gastric hypersecretory conditions: Oral, I.M., I.V.: 300-600 mg every six hours

Cinobac® *see* Cinoxacin *on this page*

Cinonide® *see* Triamcinolone *on page 359*

Cinoxacin (sin ox' a sin)
Brand Names Cinobac®
Use Urinary tract infections
Pregnancy Risk Factor B
Usual Dosage Adult and Children: > 12 years: 1 g daily in 2-4 doses

Cin-Quin® *see* Quinidine *on page 311*

Cipro™ *see* Ciprofloxacin Hydrochloride *on this page*

Ciprofloxacin Hydrochloride (sip roe flox' a sin)
Brand Names Cipro™
Use For treatment of susceptible bacterial infections, mainly lower respiratory tract, skin and skin structure, bone and joint, urinary tract and infectious diarrhea
Pregnancy Risk Factor C
Usual Dosage 250-750 mg every 12 hours, depending on severity of infection and susceptibility

Cisplatin (sis' pla tin)
Brand Names Platinol®; Platinol®-AQ
Synonyms CDDP
Use Management of metastatic testicular or ovarian carcinoma, advanced bladder cancer, head or neck cancer, cervical cancer, lung cancer, or other tumors, used alone or with other agents
Pregnancy Risk Factor D
Usual Dosage Adult: I.V.: 20 mg/m^2 daily for five days or 50-100 mg/m^2 single dose; repeat every three weeks

13-*cis*-Retinoic Acid *see* Isotretinoin *on page 194*

Citracal® [OTC] *see* Calcium Citrate *on page 53*

Citrate of Magnesia *see* Magnesium Citrate *on page 210*

Citric acid and d-gluconic acid irrigant *see* Citric Acid Bladder Mixture *on this page*

Citric Acid Bladder Mixture (si' trik)
Brand Names Renacidin®
Synonyms Citric acid and d-gluconic acid irrigant; Hemiacidrin
Use Preparing solutions for irrigating indwelling urethral catheters; to dissolve or prevent formation of calcifications

Usual Dosage 30-60 mL of 10% (sterile) solution 2-3 times a day by means of a rubber syringe

Citroma® [OTC] *see* Magnesium Citrate *on page 210*

Citrotein® [OTC] *see* Nutritional Formula, Enteral/Oral *on page 258*

Citrovorum Factor *see* Leucovorin Calcium *on page 200*

Citrucel® [OTC] *see* Methylcellulose *on page 230*

CI-719 *see* Gemfibrozil *on page 156*

Claforan® *see* Cefotaxime Sodium *on page 64*

Clearblue® [OTC] *see* Diagnostic Test for Pregnancy *on page 108*

Clear By Design® [OTC] *see* Benzoyl Peroxide *on page 41*

Clear Eyes® [OTC] *see* Naphazoline Hydrochloride *on page 246*

Clearplan® [OTC] *see* Diagnostic Test for Ovulation *on page 107*

Clearsil® [OTC] *see* Benzoyl Peroxide *on page 41*

Clemastine Fumarate (klem' as teen)
Brand Names Tavist®
Use Perennial and seasonal allergic rhinitis and other allergic symptoms including urticaria
Pregnancy Risk Factor C
Usual Dosage Oral:

Adult: 1.34 mg twice daily to 2.68 three times a day; do not exceed 8.04 mg/day

Children:
> 12 years: 1.34 mg twice daily to 2.68 three times a day; do not exceed 8.04 mg/day
< 12 years: 0.67-1.34 mg every 8-12 hours as needed

Cleocin HCl® *see* Clindamycin *on next page*

Cleocin Pediatric® *see* Clindamycin *on next page*

Cleocin Phosphate® *see* Clindamycin *on next page*

Cleocin T® *see* Clindamycin *on next page*

C-Lexin® *see* Cephalexin Monohydrate *on page 66*

Clidinium and Chlordiazepoxide (kli di' nee um)
Brand Names Librax®
Synonyms Chlordiazepoxide and Clidinium
Use Adjunct treatment of peptic ulcer, treatment of irritable bowel syndrome
Pregnancy Risk Factor D
Usual Dosage 1-2 capsules 3-4 times daily, before meals or food and at bedtime

Clindamycin (klin da mye' sin)

Brand Names Cleocin HCl®; Cleocin Pediatric®; Cleocin Phosphate®; Cleocin T®

Use Useful agent against aerobic and anaerobic streptococci (except enterococci), most staphylococci, *Bacteroides* sp. and *Actinomyces israelii*; used topically in treatment of severe acne

Pregnancy Risk Factor C

Usual Dosage

Adult and Children: Topical: Apply twice daily

Adult:

Oral: 150-450 mg every six hours

I.M., I.V.: 300-600 mg every 6-8 hours up to 2.7 g/day (up to 4.8 g daily in life-threatening infections); single I.M. doses should not exceed 600 mg

Children:

Oral: 8-25 mg/kg/day in divided doses every 6-8 hours; or, children < 10 kg: minimum oral dose is 37.5 mg three times/day

I.M., I.V.: > one month of age: 15-40 mg/kg in divided doses every 6-8 hours

Neonate: < 1 month of age: I.M., I.V.: 15-20 mg/kg/day in divided doses every 6-8 hours

Clinistix® [OTC] *see* Diagnostic Test for Glucose in Urine *on page 107*

Clinitest® [OTC] *see* Diagnostic Test for Glucose in Urine *on page 107*

Clinoril® *see* Sulindac *on page 340*

Clioquinol *see* Iodochlorhydroxyquin *on page 189*

Clistin® *see* Carbinoxamine Maleate *on page 59*

Clobetasol Dipropionate (kloe bay' ta sol)

Brand Names Temovate®

Use Short-term relief of inflammation of moderate to severe corticosteroid-responsive dermatosis

Pregnancy Risk Factor C

Usual Dosage Apply twice a day for up to two weeks with no more than 50 g/week

Clocortolone Pivalate (kloe kor' toe lone)

Brand Names Cloderm®

Use Inflammation of corticosteroid-responsive dermatoses

Pregnancy Risk Factor C

Usual Dosage Apply sparingly and gently rub into affected area from 1-4 times daily

Clocream® [OTC] *see* Vitamin A and Vitamin D *on page 377*

Cloderm® *see* Clocortolone Pivalate *on this page*

Clofazimine (kloe fa' zi meen)
Brand Names Lamprene®
Use Treatment of dapsone-resistant leprosy; multibacillary dapsone-sensitive leprosy; erythema nodosum leprosum; *Mycobacterium avium* - intracellular infections
Pregnancy Risk Factor C
Usual Dosage Adult: Oral:

Dapsone-resistant leprosy: 100 mg/day in combination with one or more antileprosy drugs for three years; then alone 100 mg/day

Dapsone-sensitive multibacillary leprosy: Triple drug therapy for at least two years and continue until negative skin smears are obtained, then institute single drug therapy with appropriate agent

Erythema nodosum leprosum: 100-300 mg up to 90 days then taper dose to 100 mg/day when possible

Clofibrate (kloe fye' brate)
Brand Names Atromid-S®
Use As an adjunct to dietary therapy in the management of hyperlipidemias associated with high triglyceride levels
Pregnancy Risk Factor C
Usual Dosage Adult: Oral: 500 mg four times a day

Clomid® see Clomiphene Citrate *on this page*

Clomiphene Citrate (kloe' mi feen)
Brand Names Clomid®; Milophene®; Serophene®
Use Treatment of ovulatory failure in patients desiring pregnancy
Pregnancy Risk Factor C
Usual Dosage Oral: 50 mg/day for five days (first course). Start the regimen on or about the fifth day of cycle. If ovulation occurs do not increase dosage; if not, increase next course to 100 mg/day for five days.

Clomipramine (kloe mi' pra meen)
Brand Names Anafranil®
Use Treatment of obsessions and compulsions
Pregnancy Risk Factor C
Usual Dosage

Adult: Oral: 25 mg daily initially and gradually increase, as tolerated to 100 mg daily the first two weeks, may then be increased to a total of 250 mg/day

Children: Oral: 25 mg daily initially and gradually increase, as tolerated to a maximum of 3 mg/kg or 100 mg, whichever is greater

Clonazepam (kloe na' ze pam)
Brand Names Klonopin™
Use Prophylaxis of petit mal, petit mal variant, akinetic, and myoclonic seizures
Restrictions C-IV
Pregnancy Risk Factor C
(Continued)

Clonazepam *(Continued)*

Usual Dosage Oral:

Adult: Initial daily dose not to exceed 1.5 mg given in three divided doses; may increase by 0.5-1 mg every third day until therapeutic levels are achieved, not to exceed 20 mg/day maintenance dose

Children: < 10 years or 30 kg: Initial daily dose 0.01-0.03 mg/kg (up to 0.05 mg/kg) given in 2-3 divided doses; increase by no more than 0.5 mg every third day until therapeutic levels are achieved; not to exceed 0.2 mg/kg daily dose

Clonidine (kloe' ni deen)

Brand Names Catapres®

Use Management of mild to moderate hypertension; either used alone or in combination with other antihypertensives

Pregnancy Risk Factor C

Usual Dosage Adult:

Oral: Initial dose 0.1 mg twice daily, dosage may be increased by 0.1-0.2 daily or every few days until the desired response is seen; usual maintenance dose is 0.2-1.2 mg/day in 2-3 divided doses

Topical: Applied once a week as transdermal delivery system; initiate therapy with 0.1 mg/24 hours applied once every seven days; adjust dosage based on response

Clonidine and Chlorthalidone

Brand Names Combipres®

Use Management of mild to moderate hypertension

Pregnancy Risk Factor C

Usual Dosage One tablet once or twice daily

Clopra® *see* Metoclopramide *on page 233*

Clorazepate Dipotassium (klor az' e pate)

Brand Names Tranxene® T-Tab™

Use Treatment of anxiety and management of alcohol withdrawal; may also be used as an anticonvulsant in management of simple partial seizures

Restrictions C-IV

Pregnancy Risk Factor D

Usual Dosage

Adult: Oral:

Anxiety: 7.5-15 mg 2-4 times daily, or given as single dose of 22.5 mg at bedtime

Alcohol withdrawal: 30 mg initially, then 15 mg 2-4 times daily on first day, then gradually decreased over subsequent days

Anticonvulsant: 7.5 mg three times a day, can increase by no more than 7.5 mg/day at weekly intervals, up to 90 mg

Children: 9-12 years: Anticonvulsant: 7.5 mg twice daily; increase dose by no more than 7.5 mg/day at weekly intervals, up to 60 mg/day

Clotrimazole (kloe trim' a zole)

Brand Names Gyne-Lotrimin®; Lotrimin®; Mycelex®

Use Treatment of susceptible fungi infections, including oropharyngeal, candidiasis, dermatophytoses, superficial mycoses, and cutaneous candidiasis, as well as vulvovaginal candidiasis

Pregnancy Risk Factor B
Usual Dosage

> Adult: Vaginal: 100 mg every day for seven days, 200 mg every day for three days, 500 mg single dose or 5 g of 1% vaginal cream daily for 7-14 days

> Adult and Children: > 3 years:
> Oral: 10 mg troche dissolved slowly five times daily
> Topical: Apply twice daily

Cloxacillin Sodium (klox a sill' in)
Brand Names Cloxapen®; Tegopen®
Use Treatment of susceptible bacterial infections, notably penicillinase-producing staphylococci causing respiratory tract, skin and skin structure, bone and joint, urinary tract infections, endocarditis, septicemia, and meningitis
Pregnancy Risk Factor B
Usual Dosage Oral, I.V.:

> Adult and Children: > 20 kg: 250-500 mg every six hours

> Children: > 1 month and < 20 kg: 50-100 mg/kg/day in divided doses every six hours

Cloxapen® see Cloxacillin Sodium on this page

Clozapine (kloe' za peen)
Brand Names Clozaril®
Use Management of schizophrenic patients
Pregnancy Risk Factor B
Usual Dosage Adult: Oral: 25 mg once or twice daily initially and increased, as tolerated to a target dose of 300-450 mg/day, but may require doses as high as 600-900 mg/day

Clozaril® see Clozapine on this page

Clysodrast® see Bisacodyl on page 45

Coactin® see Amdinocillin on page 16

Coal Tar
Brand Names Fototar® [OTC]; Pentrax® [OTC]; Polytar® [OTC]; T/Gel® [OTC]; Zetar® [OTC]
Synonyms L.C.D.
Use Used topically for controlling dandruff, seborrheic dermatitis or psoriasis
Usual Dosage Shampoo: Apply topically to the scalp as a shampoo; apply to wet hair and massage vigorously into the scalp twice weekly

Coal Tar and Allantoin see Allantoin and Coal Tar
on page 12

Coal Tar and Salicylic Acid
Brand Names X-seb® T [OTC]
Use Seborrheal dermatitis; dandruff
Usual Dosage Use as shampoo twice weekly

Coal Tar, Lanolin and Mineral Oil

Brand Names Balnetar® [OTC]

Use Psoriasis; seborrheal dermatitis; atopic dermatitis; eczematoid dermatitis

Usual Dosage Add to bath water, soak for 5-20 minutes then pat dry

Cocaine Hydrochloride (koe' kane)

Use Topical anesthesia for mucous membranes

Restrictions C-II

Pregnancy Risk Factor X

Usual Dosage Dosage depends on the area to be anesthetized, tissue vascularity, technique of anesthesia, and individual patient tolerance - the lowest necessary to produce adequate anesthesia should be used

Coccidioidin Skin Test (kox i dee oh' i din)

Brand Names Spherulin®

Use Intradermal skin test in diagnosis of coccidioidomycosis; differential diagnosis of this disease from histoplasmosis, sarcoidosis and other mycotic and bacterial infections

Pregnancy Risk Factor C

Usual Dosage Adult and Children: Intradermally: 0.1 mL of 1:100 or flexor surface of forearm

Positive reaction: Induration of 5 mm or more; erythema without induration is considered negative; read the test at 24 and 48 hours, since some reactions may not be noticeable after 36 hours. A positive reaction indicates present or past infection with *Coccidioides immitis*.

Negative reaction: A negative test means the individual has not been sensitized to coccidioidin or has lost sensitivity

Codeine (koe' deen)

Synonyms Codeine Phosphate; Codeine Sulfate

Use To manage mild to moderate pain, and as an antitussive in lower doses

Restrictions C-II

Pregnancy Risk Factor C

Usual Dosage

Adult:
Analgesia: Oral, I.M., I.V., S.C.: 15-60 mg every four hours as needed
Antitussive: Oral, I.M., S.C.: 15-30 mg every 4-6 hours as needed, up to 120 mg/day

Children: ≥ 1 year of age:
Analgesia: Oral, I.M., I.V., S.C.: 0.5-1 mg/kg/dose every 4-6 hours
Antitussive: Oral, I.M., S.C., 6-11 years: 5-10 mg every 4-6 hours as needed up to 60 mg/day; oral, I.M., S.C., 2-5 years: 2.5-5 mg every 4-6 hours up to 30 mg/day or 0.25-0.5 mg/kg/dose every four hours to maximum of 30 mg/day

Codeine and Acetaminophen *see* Acetaminophen and Codeine *on page 5*

Codeine and Aspirin *see* Aspirin and Codeine *on page 31*

Codeine and Bromodiphenhydramine *see* Bromodiphenhydramine and Codeine *on page 47*

Codeine and Guaifenesin *see* Guaifenesin and Codeine *on page 162*

Codeine Compound and Butalbital *see* Butalbital and Codeine Compound *on page 51*

Codeine Phosphate *see* Codeine *on previous page*

Codeine Sulfate *see* Codeine *on previous page*

Codimal-A® *see* Brompheniramine Maleate *on page 48*

Codoxy® *see* Oxycodone Hydrochloride *on page 264*

Cogentin® *see* Benztropine Mesylate *on page 42*

Colace® [OTC] *see* Docusate *on page 121*

Colaspase *see* Asparaginase *on page 30*

Colaspase *see* Asparaginase *on page 30*

ColBENEMID® *see* Colchicine and Probenecid *on this page*

Colchicine (kol' chi seen)
Use Treat acute gouty arthritis attacks and to prevent recurrences of such attacks
Pregnancy Risk Factor C/D
Usual Dosage Adult: Acute attacks:
   Oral: 0.5-12 mg initially, then 0.5-0.6 mg every 1-2 hours or 1-1.2 mg every two hours until relief or GI side effects occur, usually 4-8 mg is required
   I.V.: 1-3 mg initially, then 0.5 mg every six hours until response, up to 4 mg

Colchicine and Probenecid
Brand Names ColBENEMID®
Synonyms Probenecid and Colchicine
Use Treatment of chronic gouty arthritis when complicated by frequent, recurrent acute attacks of gout
Pregnancy Risk Factor C/D
Usual Dosage Adult: Oral: One tablet daily for 1 week, then one tablet twice daily thereafter

Colestid® *see* Colestipol Hydrochloride *on this page*

Colestipol Hydrochloride (koe les' ti pole)
Brand Names Colestid®
Use As an adjunct in the management of primary hypercholesterolemia; to relieve pruritus associated with elevated levels of bile acids
Pregnancy Risk Factor C
Usual Dosage 15-30 g/day in divided doses 2-4 times daily

Colistimethate Sodium (koe lis ti meth' ate)
Brand Names Coly-Mycin® M Parenteral
Use Treatment of infections due to sensitive strains of certain gram-negative bacilli
   (Continued)

87

Colistimethate Sodium *(Continued)*
Pregnancy Risk Factor C
Usual Dosage Adult and Children: I.M., I.V.: 2.5-5 mg/kg/day in 2-4 divided doses

Colistin Sulfate (koe lis' tin)
Brand Names Coly-Mycin® S
Synonyms Polymyxin E
Use Treat diarrhea in infants and children caused by susceptible organisms, especially *E. coli* and *Shigella*; used to treat superficial infections of external ear canal and of mastoidectomy and fenestration cavities infections
Pregnancy Risk Factor C
Usual Dosage

Diarrhea: Children: 5-15 mg/kg/day in three divided doses given every eight hours

Ear: Adult: Four drops in ear(s) 3-4 times daily

Collagenase (kol' la je nase)
Brand Names Biozyme-C®; Santyl®
Use To promote debridement of necrotic tissue in dermal ulcers and severe burns
Usual Dosage Apply daily or every other day

Collyrium Fresh® [OTC] *see* Tetrahydrozoline Hydrochloride
on page 347

Cologel® [OTC] *see* Methylcellulose *on page 230*

Colonic Lavage Mixture
Use For bowel cleansing prior to colonoscopy and barium enema x-ray examination
Usual Dosage Drink 240 mL every 10 minutes, until 4 L are consumed

ColoScreen® [OTC] *see* Diagnostic Test for Blood in Feces
on page 107

Coly-Mycin® M Parenteral *see* Colistimethate Sodium
on previous page

Coly-Mycin® S *see* Colistin Sulfate *on this page*

Coly-Mycin® S Otic Drops *see* Hydrocortisone, Neomycin and Colistin *on page 175*

CoLyte® *see* Polyethylene Glycol-Electrolyte Solution
on page 290

Combipres® *see* Clonidine and Chlorthalidone *on page 84*

Combistix® [OTC] *see* Diagnostic Test for Glucose, pH, and Protein in Urine *on page 107*

Comfort® [OTC] *see* Naphazoline Hydrochloride *on page 246*

Comhist® *see* Chlorpheniramine, Phenylephrine and Phenyltoloxamine *on page 75*

Comhist® LA *see* Chlorpheniramine, Phenylephrine and Phenyltoloxamine *on page 75*

Compazine® *see* Prochlorperazine *on page 299*

Complex 15® *see* Emollient Cream *on page 129*

Compound F *see* Hydrocortisone *on page 174*

Compound S *see* Zidovudine *on page 381*

Conray® *see* Iothalamate Meglumine *on page 190*

Constant-T® *see* Theophylline *on page 348*

Constilac® *see* Lactulose *on page 199*

Constulose® *see* Lactulose *on page 199*

Control® [OTC] *see* Phenylpropanolamine Hydrochloride *on page 283*

Contuss® *see* Guaifenesin, Phenylpropanolamine and Phenylephrine *on page 163*

Cophene-B® *see* Brompheniramine Maleate *on page 48*

Copper *see* Trace Metals *on page 358*

Cordarone® *see* Amiodarone Hydrochloride *on page 20*

Cordran® *see* Flurandrenolide *on page 152*

Corgard® *see* Nadolol *on page 244*

Corgonject® *see* Chorionic Gonadotropin *on page 78*

Corn Oil
Brand Names Lipomul Oral [OTC]
Synonyms Maize Oil
Use As a solvent and vehicle for injections; edible oil substitute
Usual Dosage Oral:
Adult: 1 1/2 oz two to four times daily, after or between meals
Children: 1 oz one to four times daily, after or between meals

Correctol® [OTC] *see* Docusate and Phenolphthalein *on page 121*

Cortalone® *see* Prednisolone *on page 294*

Cortef® *see* Hydrocortisone *on page 174*

Corticaine® *see* Dibucaine and Hydrocortisone *on page 110*

Corticotropin (kor ti koe troe' pin)
Brand Names Acthar®; Cortrophin®; H.P. Acthar® Gel
Synonyms ACTH; Corticotropin, Repository
Use Acute exacerbations of multiple sclerosis; diagnostic aid in adreno-cortical insufficiency
Pregnancy Risk Factor C
Usual Dosage

Acute exacerbation of multiple sclerosis: I.M.: 80-120 units/day for 2-3 weeks

(Continued)

Corticotropin *(Continued)*

Diagnostic purposes:
 I.V.: 10-25 units in 500 mL 5% dextrose in water over eight hours
 I.M., S.C.: 20 units four times a day

Corticotropin, Repository *see Corticotropin on previous page*

Cortisol *see Hydrocortisone on page 174*

Cortisone Acetate *(kor' ti sone)*
Brand Names Cortone® Acetate
Use Management of adrenocortical insufficiency
Pregnancy Risk Factor C
Usual Dosage

Adult: Oral, I.M.: 25-300 mg/day

Children:
 Oral: 0.7-10 mg/kg/day or 20-30 mg/m^2/day divided in four doses
 I.M.: 0.2-1.25 mg/kg or 7-37.5 mg/m^2 1-2 times/day

Cortisporin® Cream *see Neomycin, Polymyxin and Hydrocortisone on page 248*

Cortisporin® Ointment *see Bacitracin, Neomycin, Polymyxin B and Hydrocortisone on page 36*

Cortisporin® Ophthalmic Ointment *see Bacitracin, Neomycin, Polymyxin B and Hydrocortisone on page 36*

Cortisporin® Ophthalmic Suspension *see Neomycin, Polymyxin and Hydrocortisone on page 248*

Cortisporin® Otic *see Neomycin, Polymyxin and Hydrocortisone on page 248*

Cortone® Acetate *see Cortisone Acetate on this page*

Cortran® *see Prednisone on page 295*

Cortrophin® *see Corticotropin on previous page*

Cortrosyn® *see Cosyntropin on this page*

Cosmegen® *see Dactinomycin on page 96*

Cosyntropin *(koe sin troe' pin)*
Brand Names Cortrosyn®
Use Diagnostic test to differentiate primary adrenal from secondary (pituitary) adrenocortical insufficiency
Pregnancy Risk Factor C
Usual Dosage

Adult: I.M., I.V.: 0.25 mg injected over two minutes

Children: < 2 years of age: I.V.: 0.125 mg injected over two minutes
 I.V. infusion: 0.125 mg administered over 4-8 hours at rate of approximately 0.04 mg/hour over six hours

Cotazym® *see Pancrelipase on page 267*

Cotazym-S® see Pancrelipase on page 267

Cotrim® see Sulfamethoxazole and Trimethoprim on page 338

Cotrim® DS see Sulfamethoxazole and Trimethoprim on page 338

Co-trimoxazole see Sulfamethoxazole and Trimethoprim on page 338

Coumadin® see Warfarin Sodium on page 379

Cremacoat®2 [OTC] see Guaifenesin on page 162

Creon® see Pancreatin on page 267

Criticare HN® [OTC] see Nutritional Formula, Enteral/Oral on page 258

Cromoglicic Acid see Cromolyn Sodium on this page

Cromolyn Sodium (kroe' moe lin)
Brand Names Aarane®; Intal®; Nasalcrom®; Opticrom®
Synonyms Cromoglicic Acid
Use An adjunct in the prophylaxis of allergic disorders, including rhinitis, conjunctivitis, and asthma; inhalation product may be used for prevention of exercise-induced bronchospasm
Pregnancy Risk Factor B
Usual Dosage

Adult:
Inhalation: 20 mg four times a day (Spinhaler®), two inhalations four times a day by metered spray
Nasal: One spray in each nostril 3-4 times daily
Ophthalmic: 1-2 drops 4-6 times daily

Children:
Inhalation: > 2 years: 20 mg four times a day (Spinhaler®); > 5 years: two inhalations four times a day by metered spray
Nasal: > 6 years: One spray in each nostril 3-4 times daily
Ophthalmic: > 4 years: 1-2 drops 4-6 times daily

Crotaline Antivenin, Polyvalent see Antivenin (Crotalidae) Polyvalent on page 27

Crotamiton (kroe tam' i tonn)
Brand Names Eurax®
Use Treatment of scabies and symptomatic treatment of pruritus
Pregnancy Risk Factor C
Usual Dosage

Scabicide: Adult and Children: Wash thoroughly and scrub away loose scales, then towel dry; massage drug onto skin of the entire body from the neck to the toes (with special attention to skin folds, creases, and interdigital spaces). Repeat application in 24 hours. Take a cleansing bath 48 hours after the final application.

Antipruritic: Adult and Children: Apply locally 2-3 times a day

Cruex® [OTC] *see* Calcium Undecylenate *on page 55*

Cryptenamine Tannates and Methyclothiazide *see* Methyclothiazide and Cryptenamine Tannates *on page 229*

Crystalline Penicillin *see* Penicillin G, Parenteral *on page 273*

Crystal Violet *see* Gentian Violet *on page 157*

Crysticillin® A.S. *see* Penicillin G Procaine, Aqueous *on page 273*

Crystodigin® *see* Digitoxin *on page 113*

C-Solve®2 *see* Erythromycin, Topical *on page 135*

C-Span® [OTC] *see* Ascorbic Acid *on page 29*

CS-T® [OTC] *see* Diagnostic Test for Blood in Feces *on page 107*

Culturette® 10 Minute *see* Diagnostic Test for Streptococci *on page 108*

Cuprid® *see* Trientine Hydrochloride *on page 361*

Cuprimine® *see* Penicillamine *on page 272*

Cupri-Pak® *see* Trace Metals *on page 358*

CYA *see* Cyclosporine *on page 94*

Cyanide Antidote Kit
Use Treatment of cyanide poisoning
Usual Dosage For cyanide poisoning, a 0.3 mL ampule of amyl nitrite is crushed every minute and vapor is inhaled for 15-30 seconds until an I.V. sodium nitrite infusion is available. Following administration of 300 mg I.V. sodium nitrite, inject 12.5 grams sodium thiosulfate I.V. (over approximately 10 minutes), if needed; injection of both may be repeated at 1/2 the original dose.

Cyanocobalamin (sye an oh koe bal' a min)
Brand Names Redisol®; Rubramin-PC®
Synonyms Vitamin B_{12}
Use Pernicious anemia, vitamin B_{12} deficiency, increased B_{12} requirements due to pregnancy, thyrotoxicosis, hemorrhage, malignancy, liver or kidney disease
Pregnancy Risk Factor A/C
Usual Dosage

Adult:
  Pernicious anemia: I.M., S.C.: 100 μg every day for 6-7 days
  Vitamin B_{12} deficiency: Oral: usually not recommended, maximum absorbed from a single oral dose is 2-3 μg; I.M., S.C.: 30 μg every day for 5-10 days, followed by 100-200 μg every month

Children:
  Congenital pernicious anemia (if evidence of neurologic involvement): I.M.: 1000 μg every day for at least two weeks; maintenance 50 μg per month
  Vitamin B_{12} deficiency: I.M., S.C.: 1-5 mg given in single or subcutaneous doses of 100 μg over two or more weeks

Cyclandelate (sye klan' de late)
Brand Names Cyclospasmol®
Use Adjunctive therapy in peripheral vascular disease and possibly senility
Restrictions DESI drug; not approved for HCFA reimbursement
Pregnancy Risk Factor C
Usual Dosage 400-800 mg/day in 2-4 divided doses

Cyclizine (sye' kli zeen)
Brand Names Marezine® [OTC]
Use Prevention and treatment of nausea, vomiting and vertigo associated with motion sickness; control of postoperative nausea and vomiting
Pregnancy Risk Factor B
Usual Dosage

Adult:
Oral: 50 mg taken 30 minutes before departure, may repeat in 4-6 hours if needed, up to 200 mg/day
I.M.: 50 mg every 4-6 hours as needed

Children: 6-12 years:
Oral: 25 mg up to 3 times daily
I.M.: Not recommended

Cyclobenzaprine Hydrochloride (sye kloe ben' za preen)
Brand Names Flexeril®
Use Treatment of muscle spasm associated with acute painful musculoskeletal conditions; supportive therapy in tetanus
Pregnancy Risk Factor B
Usual Dosage Adult: 10 mg three times a day

Cyclocort® see Amcinonide on page 16

Cyclogyl® see Cyclopentolate Hydrochloride on this page

Cyclomydril® see Cyclopentolate and Phenylephrine on this page

Cyclopentolate and Phenylephrine
Brand Names Cyclomydril®
Synonyms Phenylephrine and Cyclopentolate
Use Induce mydriasis greater than that produced with cyclopentolate HCl alone
Pregnancy Risk Factor C
Usual Dosage One drop every 5-10 minutes, not to exceed three instillations

Cyclopentolate Hydrochloride (sye kloe pen' toe late)
Brand Names Cyclogyl®
Use Diagnostic procedures requiring mydriasis and cycloplegia
Pregnancy Risk Factor C
Usual Dosage

Adult: One drop of 1% followed by another drop in five minutes, 2% solution in heavily pigmented iris

(Continued)

93

Cyclopentolate Hydrochloride *(Continued)*

Children: One drop of 0.5%, 1%, or 2% in eye followed by one drop in five minutes, if necessary

Cyclophosphamide (sye kloe foss' fa mide)

Brand Names Cytoxan®

Use Management of Hodgkin's disease, malignant lymphomas, multiple myeloma, leukemias, mycosis fungoides, neuroblastoma, ovarian carcinoma, breast carcinoma, and a variety of other tumors

Pregnancy Risk Factor C

Usual Dosage

Adult:
Induction: Oral: 1-5 mg/kg/day; I.V.: 40-50 mg/kg (1.5-1.8 g/m^2) in divided doses > 2-5 days
Maintenance: Oral: 1-5 mg/kg/day; I.V.: 10-15 mg/kg (350-550 mg/m^2) every 7-10 days or 3-5 mg/kg twice weekly (110-185 mg/m^2)

Children:
Induction: Oral: 2-6 mg/kg/day; I.V.: 2-6 mg/kg/day (60-250 mg/m^2)
Maintenance: Oral: 2-5 mg/kg (50-150 mg/m^2) twice weekly

Cycloserine (sye kloe ser' een)

Brand Names Seromycin® Pulvules®

Use Adjunctive treatment in pulmonary or extrapulmonary tuberculosis; treatment of acute urinary infections caused by *E. coli* or *Enterobacter* sp when more conventional therapy has failed

Pregnancy Risk Factor C

Usual Dosage Adult: Oral:

Tuberculosis: Initial 250 mg every 12 hours for 14 days, then given 500 mg - 1 g in divided doses up to 1 g/day

Urinary tract infection: 250 mg every 12 hours for 14 days

Cyclospasmol® *see* Cyclandelate *on previous page*

Cyclosporin A *see* Cyclosporine *on this page*

Cyclosporine (sye' kloe spor een)

Brand Names Sandimmune®

Synonyms CYA; Cyclosporin A

Use Immunosuppressant used with corticosteroids to prolong organ and patient survival in kidney, liver, heart, and bone marrow transplants

Pregnancy Risk Factor C

Usual Dosage Adult and Children:
Oral: 15 mg/kg/day for 1-2 weeks, then taper by 5% weekly to maintenance dose of 5-10 mg/kg/day
I.V.: 5-6 mg/kg/day initially, then change to oral

Cyclothiazide (sye kloe thye' a zide)

Brand Names Anhydron®

Use Management of mild to moderate hypertension; treatment of edema in congestive heart failure and nephrotic syndrome

Pregnancy Risk Factor B
Usual Dosage Adult: Oral: 2 mg/day; up to 2 mg 2-3 times daily

Cyklokapron® *see* Tranexamic Acid *on page 358*

Cylert® *see* Pemoline *on page 271*

Cyproheptadine Hydrochloride (si proe hep' ta deen)
Brand Names Periactin®
Use Perennial and seasonal allergic rhinitis and other allergic symptoms including urticaria
Pregnancy Risk Factor B
Usual Dosage Oral:

Adult: 12-16 mg/day every eight hours (not to exceed 0.5 mg/kg/day)

Children:
7-14 years: 4 mg every 8-12 hours (not to exceed 16 mg/day)
2-6 years: 2 mg every 8-12 hours (not to exceed 12 mg/day)

Cystografin® *see* Diatrizoate Meglumine *on page 108*

Cystospaz® *see* Hyoscyamine Sulfate *on page 180*

Cytadren® *see* Aminoglutethimide *on page 18*

Cytarabine Hydrochloride (sye tare' a been)
Brand Names Cytosar®
Synonyms Ara-C; Cytosine Arabinosine Hydrochloride
Use Adjunct in treatment of leukemias
Pregnancy Risk Factor C
Usual Dosage Adult and Children:
I.V.: 70-200 mg/m^2/day for 2-5 days
S.C.: 1.5 mg/kg single dose for maintenance
I.T.: 10-30 mg/m^2 up to three times weekly

Cytomel® *see* Liothyronine Sodium *on page 205*

Cytosar® *see* Cytarabine Hydrochloride *on this page*

Cytosine Arabinosine Hydrochloride *see* Cytarabine Hydrochloride *on this page*

Cytotec® *see* Misoprostol *on page 238*

Cytovene® *see* Ganciclovir *on page 155*

Cytoxan® *see* Cyclophosphamide *on previous page*

D-3-Mercaptovaline *see* Penicillamine *on page 272*

D$_5$1/2NS *see* Dextrose and Sodium Chloride *on page 105*

D$_5$LR *see* Dextrose in Lactated Ringer's *on page 105*

D$_5$NS *see* Dextrose and Sodium Chloride *on page 105*

D$_5$W *see* Dextrose in Water *on page 105*

D$_{10}$W *see* Dextrose in Water *on page 105*

D$_{20}$W *see* Dextrose in Water *on page 105*

D$_{50}$W see Dextrose in Water on page 105

D$_{70}$W see Dextrose in Water on page 105

Dacarbazine (da kar' ba zeen)
Brand Names DTIC-Dome®
Use Metastatic malignant melanoma and second-line therapy, in combination with other agents, in Hodgkin's disease
Pregnancy Risk Factor C
Usual Dosage I.V.:

Malignant melanoma: 2-4.5 mg/kg for 10 days, repeat in four weeks or may use 250 mg/m^2/day for five days, repeat in three weeks

Hodgkin's disease: 150 mg/m^2/day for five days, repeat every four weeks or 375 mg/m^2 on day one, repeat in 15 days

Dactinomycin (dak ti noe mye' sin)
Brand Names Cosmegen®
Synonyms Actinomycin D
Use Management, either alone or with other treatment modalities, of Wilm's tumor, rhabdomyosarcoma, Ewing's sarcoma, trophoblastic neoplasms, testicular carcinoma, and other malignancies
Pregnancy Risk Factor C
Usual Dosage Dosage for obese or edematous patients should be based upon body surface area; 400-600 μg/m^2/day for five days

Adult: I.V.: 500 μg/day for five days; repeat every 2-4 weeks

Children: I.V.: > 6 months: 15 μg/kg daily for five days; repeat every 2-4 weeks

Daisy® 2 [OTC] see Diagnostic Test for Pregnancy on page 108

Dalgan® see Dezocine on page 106

Dalmane® see Flurazepam Hydrochloride on page 152

d-Alpha Tocopherol see Vitamin E on page 378

Danazol (da' na zole)
Brand Names Danocrine®
Use Treatment of endometriosis, fibrocystic breast disease, and hereditary angioedema
Pregnancy Risk Factor X
Usual Dosage Adult: Oral:

Endometriosis: 100-400 mg twice daily

Fibrocystic breast disease: 50-200 mg twice daily for 2-6 months

Hereditary angioedema: 400-600 mg/day in 2-3 divided doses

Danocrine® see Danazol on this page

Dantrium® see Dantrolene Sodium on next page

Dantrolene Sodium (dan' troe leen)
Brand Names Dantrium®

Use Treatment of spasticity associated with spinal cord injury, stroke, cerebral palsy, or multiple sclerosis; also used as treatment of malignant hyperthermia

Pregnancy Risk Factor C

Usual Dosage

Adult:

Spasticity: Oral: 25 mg/day to start, increase by 25 mg every 4-7 days to a maximum of 100 mg 2-4 times daily

Hyperthermia: Oral: 4-8 mg/kg/day in 3-4 divided doses; I.V.: 1 mg/kg; may repeat dose up to cumulative dose of 10 mg/kg, then switch to oral dosage

Children:

Spasticity: Oral: 0.5 mg/kg twice daily, increase by 0.5 mg/kg 3-4 times daily, increase in increments of 0.5 mg/kg daily, up to 3 mg/kg 2-4 times daily; maximum dose is 400 mg/day

Hyperthermia: Oral: 4-8 mg/kg/day in 3-4 divided doses; I.V.: 1 mg/kg; may repeat dose up to cumulative dose of 10 mg/kg, then switch to oral dosage

Dapsone (dap' sone)
Brand Names Avlosulfon®

Synonyms Diaminodiphenylsulfone

Use Treatment of leprosy and dermatitis herpetiformis

Pregnancy Risk Factor C

Usual Dosage Adult: Oral:

Leprosy: 50-100 mg/day

Dermatitis herpetiformis: Start at 50 mg/day, increase to 300 mg/day, or higher to achieve full control, reduce dosage to minimum level as soon as possible

Daranide® *see* Dichlorphenamide *on page 111*

Daraprim® *see* Pyrimethamine *on page 310*

Darbid® *see* Isopropamide Iodide *on page 193*

Daricon® *see* Oxyphencyclimine Hydrochloride *on page 266*

Darvocet-N® *see* Propoxyphene and Acetaminophen *on page 304*

Darvocet-N® 100 *see* Propoxyphene and Acetaminophen *on page 304*

Darvon® *see* Propoxyphene *on page 303*

Darvon® Compound-65 Pulvules® *see* Propoxyphene and Aspirin *on page 304*

Darvon® Compound Pulvules® *see* Propoxyphene and Aspirin *on page 304*

Darvon-N® *see* Propoxyphene *on page 303*

Darvon-N® With A.S.A.® *see* Propoxyphene and Aspirin
on page 304

Darvon® With A.S.A.® Pulvules® *see* Propoxyphene and Aspirin
on page 304

Daunorubicin Hydrochloride (daw noe roo' bi sin)
Brand Names Cerubidine®
Synonyms DNR
Use In combination with other agents in the treatment of leukemias
Pregnancy Risk Factor D
Usual Dosage I.V.:

Adult: 30-60 mg/m²/day for 3-5 days, repeat dose in 3-4 weeks; total cumulative dose should not exceed 400-600 mg/m²

Children: 25-45 mg/m²; in children < 2 years of age or with a surface area < 0.5 m² → the dosage should be calculated based on weight (consult appropriate literature)

DDAVP® *see* Desmopressin Acetate *on page 101*

1-Deamino-8-D-Arginine Vasopressin *see* Desmopressin Acetate *on page 101*

Debrisan® [OTC] *see* Dextranomer *on page 104*

Debrox® [OTC] *see* Carbamide Peroxide *on page 58*

Decadron® *see* Dexamethasone *on page 102*

Decadron®-LA *see* Dexamethasone *on page 102*

Decadron® Turbinaire® *see* Dexamethasone *on page 102*

Deca-Durabolin® *see* Nandrolone *on page 246*

Decaspray® *see* Dexamethasone *on page 102*

Decholin® *see* Dehydrocholic Acid *on next page*

Declomycin® *see* Demeclocycline Hydrochloride *on next page*

Decofed® Syrup [OTC] *see* Pseudoephedrine *on page 307*

Deconamine® SR *see* Chlorpheniramine and Pseudoephedrine *on page 74*

Deferoxamine Mesylate (de fer ox' a meen)
Brand Names Desferal® Mesylate
Use Acute iron intoxication; chronic iron overload secondary to multiple transfusions; diagnostic test for iron overload; used investigationally in the treatment of aluminum accumulation in renal failure
Pregnancy Risk Factor C
Usual Dosage

Adult:
Acute iron intoxication: I.M.: 1 g stat, then 0.5 g every four hours for two doses, then 0.5 g every 4-12 hours up to 6 g/day; I.V.: same as I.M., do not exceed 15 mg/kg/hour
Chronic iron overload: I.M.: 0.5-1 g every day; S.C.: 1-2 g every day over 8-24 hours

Children: Chronic iron overload: I.M., I.V.: 50 mg/kg/dose every six hours or up to 15 mg/kg/hour by continuous I.V. infusion up to 6 g/24 hours or 2 g/dose

Degest® 2 [OTC] *see* Naphazoline Hydrochloride *on page 246*

Dehist® *see* Brompheniramine Maleate *on page 48*

Dehydrocholic Acid (dee hye droe koe' lik)
Brand Names Atrocholin®; Decholin®
Use Relief of constipation; adjunct to various biliary tract conditions
Pregnancy Risk Factor C
Usual Dosage Adult and Children: > 12 years of age: 250-500 mg 2-3 times daily after meals up to 1.5 g/day

Delatestryl® *see* Testosterone *on page 345*

Delaxin® *see* Methocarbamol *on page 227*

Delestrogen® *see* Estradiol *on page 135*

Delfen® *see* Nonoxynol 9 *on page 254*

Delsym® [OTC] *see* Dextromethorphan *on page 105*

Delta-Cortef® *see* Prednisolone *on page 294*

Deltacortisone *see* Prednisone *on page 295*

Deltadehydrocortisone *see* Prednisone *on page 295*

Deltahydrocortisone *see* Prednisolone *on page 294*

Deltanyne® *see* Dronabinol *on page 124*

Deltasone® *see* Prednisone *on page 295*

Demecarium Bromide (dem e kare' ee um)
Brand Names Humorsol®
Use Management of chronic simple glaucoma, chronic and acute angle-closure glaucoma; counter effects of cycloplegics
Pregnancy Risk Factor C
Usual Dosage 1-2 drops twice daily

Demeclocycline Hydrochloride (dem e kloe sye' kleen)
Brand Names Declomycin®
Synonyms Demethylchlortetracycline
Use Treatment of susceptible bacterial infections, both gram-negative and gram-positive; used when penicillin is contraindicated and in acute amebiasis management of chronic form of the syndrome of inappropriate antidiuretic hormone secretion
Pregnancy Risk Factor D
Usual Dosage Oral: Administer one hour before or two hours after food or milk

Adult:
150 mg four times a day or 300 mg twice daily
Gonorrhea: 600 mg stat, 300 mg every 12 hours for four days (3 g total)

Children: > 9 years: 6-12 mg/kg/24 hours given in 2-4 divided doses

Demerol® *see* Meperidine Hydrochloride *on page 218*

Demethylchlortetracycline *see* Demeclocycline Hydrochloride *on previous page*

Demser® *see* Metyrosine *on page 235*

Demulen® 1/35 *see* Ethinyl Estradiol and Ethynodiol Diacetate *on page 139*

Demulen® 1/50 *see* Ethinyl Estradiol and Ethynodiol Diacetate *on page 139*

Deodorized Opium Tincture *see* Opium, Tincture of *on page 261*

Depakene® *see* Valproic Acid and Derivatives *on page 371*

Depakote® *see* Valproic Acid and Derivatives *on page 371*

Depen® *see* Penicillamine *on page 272*

depGynogen® *see* Estradiol *on page 135*

depMedalone® *see* Methylprednisolone *on page 231*

Depo®-Estradiol *see* Estradiol *on page 135*

Depogen® *see* Estradiol *on page 135*

Depoject® *see* Methylprednisolone *on page 231*

Depo-Medrol® *see* Methylprednisolone *on page 231*

Deponit® *see* Nitroglycerin *on page 253*

Depopred® *see* Methylprednisolone *on page 231*

Depo-Provera® *see* Medroxyprogesterone Acetate *on page 216*

Depotest® *see* Testosterone *on page 345*

Depo®-Testosterone *see* Testosterone *on page 345*

Deprenyl *see* Selegiline Hydrochloride *on page 322*

Dermaide® *see* Aloe Vera *on page 13*

Dermoplast® [OTC] *see* Benzocaine *on page 40*

DES *see* Diethylstilbestrol *on page 112*

Desenex® [OTC] *see* Zinc Undecylenate *on page 382*

Desferal® Mesylate *see* Deferoxamine Mesylate *on page 98*

Desipramine Hydrochloride (dess ip' ra meen)
Brand Names Norpramin®; Pertofrane®
Use Used in the treatment of various forms of depression, often in conjunction with psychotherapy
Pregnancy Risk Factor C
Usual Dosage Oral:

Adult: 75-200 mg/day in divided doses or in a single dose; maximum dose is 300 mg

Geriatric and Adolescent: > 12 years: 25-100 mg/day, up to 150 mg

Desitin® [OTC] *see* Zinc Oxide, Cod Liver Oil and Talc
on page 382

Deslanoside (des lan' oh side)
Brand Names Cedilanid-D®
Use Rapid digitalizing effect in emergency treatment of congestive heart failure, paroxysmal atrial tachycardia, atrial fibrillation and flutter
Pregnancy Risk Factor C
Usual Dosage Stenosis:

Adult and Children: I.M., I.V.: Highly individualized

Adult: I.M., I.V.: Loading dose is 1.2-1.6 mg in two divided doses over 24 hours

Children:
> 3 years of age: 22.5 μg/kg divided into 2-3 doses every 3-4 hours
3 years - 2 weeks old: 25 μg/kg divided into 2-3 doses every 3-4 hours

Premature and full-term neonates: 22 μg divided into 2-3 doses every 3-4 hours

Desmopressin Acetate (des moe press' in)
Brand Names DDAVP®; Stimate™
Synonyms 1-Deamino-8-D-Arginine Vasopressin
Use Treatment of diabetes insipidus and controlling bleeding in certain types of hemophilia
Pregnancy Risk Factor B
Usual Dosage

Adult:
Diabetes insipidus: I.V., S.C.: 2-4 μg/day in two divided doses; intranasal: 5-40 μg 1-3 times daily
Hemophilia: I.V.: 0.3 μg/kg by slow infusion 30 minutes preop

Children:
Diabetes insipidus: 3 months - 12 years of age: Intranasal: 5-30 μg 1-2 times daily
Hemophilia: > 3 months: I.V.: 0.3 μg/kg by slow infusion 30 minutes preop

Desonide (dess' oh nide)
Brand Names Tridesilon®
Use Adjunctive therapy for inflammation in acute and chronic corticosteroid responsive dermatosis
Pregnancy Risk Factor C
Usual Dosage Apply 2-4 times daily

Desoximetasone (des ox i met' a sone)
Brand Names Topicort®; Topicort®-LP
Use Relieve inflammation and pruritic symptoms of corticosteroid-responsive dermatosis
Pregnancy Risk Factor C
Usual Dosage

Adult: Apply sparingly in a thin film twice a day

Children: Apply sparingly in a very thin film to affected area 1-2 times/day

Desoxyephedrine Hydrochloride *see* Methamphetamine Hydrochloride *on page 225*

Desoxyn® *see* Methamphetamine Hydrochloride *on page 225*

Desoxyphenobarbital *see* Primidone *on page 296*

Desoxyribonuclease and Fibrinolysin *see* Fibrinolysin and Desoxyribonuclease *on page 147*

Desquam-X® *see* Benzoyl Peroxide *on page 41*

Dessicated Thyroid *see* Thyroid *on page 354*

Desyrel® *see* Trazodone *on page 359*

Devrom® [OTC] *see* Bismuth *on page 45*

Dex-A-Diet® [OTC] *see* Phenylpropanolamine Hydrochloride *on page 283*

Dexamethasone (dex a meth' a sone)

Brand Names Decadron®; Decadron®-LA; Decadron® Turbinaire®; Decaspray®

Use Used systematically and locally for chronic inflammation, allergic hematologic, neoplastic, and autoimmune diseases; may be used in management of cerebral edema and septic shock and a diagnostic agent

Pregnancy Risk Factor C

Usual Dosage

Adult:
  Anti-inflammatory: Oral: 0.75-9 mg/day in single or 3-4 divided doses; I.M., I.V.: 0.5-24 mg/day
  Cerebral edema: I.V. 10 mg stat, 4 mg I.M. every six hours until response is maximized, then switched to oral regimen, 1-3 mg three times a day as soon as possible; taper off if appropriate
  Diagnosis for Cushing's syndrome: Oral: 1 mg at 11 PM, draw blood at 8 AM
  Inhalation: Three inhalations 3-4 times daily

Children:
  Anti-inflammatory: Oral: 83.3-333.3 µg/kg/day; I.M.: 27.76-166.65 µg/kg every 12-24 hours
  Inhalation: Two inhalations 3-4 times daily

Dexamethasone and Neomycin

Brand Names NeoDecadron®

Synonyms Neomycin and Dexamethasone

Use Treatment of steroid responsive inflammatory conditions of the palpebral and bulbar conjunctiva, lid, cornea, and anterior segment of the globe

Pregnancy Risk Factor C

Usual Dosage Apply thin coat 3-4 times a day until favorable response is observed, then reduce dose to one application per day

Dexamethasone and Tobramycin *see* Tobramycin and Dexamethasone *on page 356*

Dexamethasone, Neomycin and Polymyxin B
Brand Names Maxitrol®
Use Infectious ocular inflammations
Pregnancy Risk Factor C
Usual Dosage 1-2 drops into affected eye(s) every 3-4 hours

Dexatrim® [OTC] *see* Phenylpropanolamine Hydrochloride
on page 283

Dexbrompheniramine and Pseudoephedrine
(dex brom fen eer' a meen)
Brand Names Disophrol® [OTC]; Drixoral® [OTC]
Synonyms Pseudoephedrine and Dexbrompheniramine
Use Relief of symptoms of upper respiratory mucosal congestion in seasonal and perennial nasal allergies, acute rhinitis, rhinosinusitis and eustachian tube blockage
Pregnancy Risk Factor B
Usual Dosage Adult and Children: > 12 years of age: One tablespoonful every 12 hours, may require a tablespoonful every eight hours

Dexchlorpheniramine Maleate (dex klor fen eer' a meen)
Brand Names Polaramine®
Use Perennial and seasonal allergic rhinitis and other allergic symptoms including urticaria
Pregnancy Risk Factor B
Usual Dosage Oral:

Adult: 2 mg every 4-6 hours or 4-6 mg timed release at bedtime or 8-10 hours

Children:
6-11 years: 1 mg every 4-6 hours or 4 mg timed release at bedtime
2-5 years: 0.5 mg every 4-6 hours

Dexedrine® *see* Dextroamphetamine Sulfate *on next page*

Dexpanthenol (dex pan' the nole)
Brand Names Ilopan®; Ilopan-Choline®; Panthoderm®
Use Prophylactic use to minimize paralytic ileus, treatment of postoperative distention
Pregnancy Risk Factor C
Usual Dosage Adult: Oral: 2-3 tablets three times a day

Prevention of postoperative ileus: I.M.: 250-500 mg stat, repeat in two hours, followed by doses every six hours until danger passes

Paralyzed ileus: I.M.: 500 mg stat, repeat in two hours, followed by doses every six hours, if needed

Dextran
Brand Names Gentran®; Hyskon®; LMD®; Macrodex®; Rheomacrodex®
Synonyms Dextran 40; Dextran 70; Dextran High Molecular Weight; Dextran, Low Molecular Weight
(Continued)
103

Dextran *(Continued)*

Use Blood volume expander used in treatment of shock or impending shock when blood or blood products are not available

Pregnancy Risk Factor C

Usual Dosage I.V.:

Adult: 500-1000 mL at rate of 20-40 mL/minute

Children: Total dose should not be > 20 mL/kg during first 24 hours

Dextran 1 (dex' tran)

Brand Names Promit®

Use Prophylaxis of serious anaphylactic reactions to I.V. infusion of dextran

Pregnancy Risk Factor C

Usual Dosage I.V.:

Adult: 20 mL 1-2 minutes before I.V. infusion of dextran

Children: 0.3 mL/kg in a corresponding manner

Dextran 40 *see* Dextran *on previous page*

Dextran 70 *see* Dextran *on previous page*

Dextran High Molecular Weight *see* Dextran *on previous page*

Dextran, Low Molecular Weight *see* Dextran *on previous page*

Dextranomer (dex tran' oh mer)

Brand Names Debrisan® [OTC]

Use To clean exudative wounds

Pregnancy Risk Factor C

Usual Dosage Apply to affected area once or twice a day

Dextroamphetamine Sulfate (dex troe am fet' a meen)

Brand Names Dexedrine®

Use Narcolepsy; abnormal behavioral syndrome in children; exogenous obesity

Restrictions C-II

Pregnancy Risk Factor C

Usual Dosage

Adult:

Narcolepsy: 10 mg/day to start, may increase at 10 mg increments in weekly intervals until side effects appear

Exogenous obesity: 5-30 mg/day in divided doses of 5-10 mg, 30-60 minutes before meals

Children:

Narcolepsy: 6-12 years: 5 mg/day to start, may increase at 5 mg increments in weekly intervals until side effects appear

Abnormal behavioral syndrome: 3-5 years: 2.5 mg to start, increase by 2.5 mg/day in weekly intervals until optimal dose is obtained; 6 years and older: 6 mg once or twice daily; increase in increments of 5 mg/day at weekly intervals until optimal response is researched; up to 40 mg/day

Exogenous obesity: > 12 years: 5-30 mg/day in divided doses of 5-10 mg, 30-60 minutes before meals

Dextromethorphan (dex troe meth or' fan)

Brand Names Delsym® [OTC]

Use Symptomatic relief of coughs caused by minor viral upper respiratory tract infections or inhaled irritants; most effective for a chronic nonproductive cough

Pregnancy Risk Factor C

Usual Dosage Oral:

Adult: 10-20 mg every four hours or 30 mg every 6-8 hours; extended release oral is 60 mg twice daily

Children:

6-11 years: 5-10 mg every four hours or 15 mg every 6-8 hours; extended release is 30 mg twice daily

2-5 years: 2.5-5 mg every four hours or 7.5 mg every 6-8 hours; extended release is 50 mg twice daily

Dextromethorphan and Guaifenesin see Guaifenesin and Dextromethorphan on page 162

Dextropropoxyphene see Propoxyphene on page 303

Dextrose and Sodium Chloride (dex' trose)

Synonyms D$_5$1/2NS; D$_5$NS; Sodium Chloride and Dextrose

Use Source of calories, sodium chloride, and water for hydration

Pregnancy Risk Factor C

Dextrose and Sodium Chloride with Potassium Chloride

Synonyms Potassium Chloride, Sodium Chloride and Dextrose; Sodium Chloride, Dextrose and Potassium Chloride

Pregnancy Risk Factor C

Dextrose in Lactated Ringer's

Synonyms D$_5$LR

Pregnancy Risk Factor C

Dextrose in Water

Synonyms D$_5$W; D$_{10}$W; D$_{20}$W; D$_{50}$W; D$_{70}$W; Glucose

Pregnancy Risk Factor C

Dextrose in Water with Potassium Chloride

Synonyms Electrolytes and Dextrose

Pregnancy Risk Factor C

Dextrose, Levulose and Phosphoric Acid see Levulose, Dextrose and Phosphoric Acid on page 203

Dextrostix® [OTC] see Diagnostic Test for Glucose in Blood on page 107

Dextrothyroxine Sodium (dex troe thye rox' een)
Brand Names Choloxin®
Use Reduction of elevated serum cholesterol
Pregnancy Risk Factor C
Usual Dosage Oral:

Adult: 1-2 mg/day, up to 8 mg/day

Children: 0.1 mg/kg/day

Dey-Dose® Isoproterenol *see* Isoproterenol *on page 193*

Dey-Dose® Metaproterenol *see* Metaproterenol Sulfate
on page 223

Dey-Lute® Isoetharine *see* Isoetharine *on page 191*

Dezocine (dez' oh seen)
Brand Names Dalgan®
Use Analgesic used for pain control
Usual Dosage Adult:
I.M.: 5-20 mg initially; may be repeated every 3-6 hours as needed up
to a maximum of 120 mg/day
I.V.: 2.5-10 mg initially; may be repeated every 2-4 hours as needed

DFP *see* Isoflurophate *on page 192*

D.H.E.45® *see* Dihydroergotamine Mesylate *on page 115*

DHPG Sodium *see* Ganciclovir *on page 155*

DHT *see* Dihydrotachysterol *on page 115*

Diaβeta® *see* Glyburide *on page 159*

Diabinese® *see* Chlorpropamide *on page 76*

**Diagnostic Test for Acetone, Bilirubin, Blood, Glucose,
pH and Protein in Urine**
Brand Names Bili-Labstix® [OTC]

**Diagnostic Test for Acetone, Blood, Glucose, pH, and
Protein in Urine**
Brand Names Labstix® [OTC]

Diagnostic Test for Acetone in Urine
Brand Names Acetest® [OTC]; Chemstrip® K [OTC]; Ketostix® [OTC]

Diagnostic Test for Acid Mucopolysaccharides
Brand Names MPS® Papers [OTC]

Diagnostic Test for Bacteriuria
Brand Names Microstix-3® [OTC]; Microstix-Nitrite® [OTC]; Uricult®
[OTC]

Diagnostic Test for Bilirubin in the Urine
Brand Names Ictotest® [OTC]

Diagnostic Test for Blood, Glucose, pH, and Protein in Urine
Brand Names Hema-Combistix [OTC]

Diagnostic Test for Blood in Feces
Brand Names ColoScreen® [OTC]; CS-T® [OTC]; Early Detector® [OTC]; EZ-Detect® [OTC]; Hema-Chek® [OTC]; Hematest® [OTC]; Hemocult® II [OTC]; Hemocult® Slides
Synonyms Occult Blood Screening Test

Diagnostic Test for Blood in Urine
Brand Names Hemastix® [OTC]

Diagnostic Test for Blood Urea Nitrogen in Blood
Brand Names Azostix® [OTC]

Diagnostic Test for *Chlamydia trachomatis*
Brand Names MicroTrak®

Diagnostic Test for C-Reactive Protein
Brand Names LAtest-CRP®

Diagnostic Test for Glucose and Ketones in Urine
Brand Names Keto-Diastix® [OTC]

Diagnostic Test for Glucose and Protein in Urine
Brand Names Uristlx® [OTC]

Diagnostic Test for Glucose in Blood
Brand Names Chemstrip bG® [OTC]; Dextrostix® [OTC]; Glucostix® [OTC]; Visidex® II [OTC]

Diagnostic Test for Glucose in Urine
Brand Names Chemstrip uG® [OTC]; Clinistix® [OTC]; Clinitest® [OTC]; Diastix® [OTC]; Tes-Tape® [OTC]

Diagnostic Test for Glucose, pH, and Protein in Urine
Brand Names Combistix® [OTC]

Diagnostic Test for Mononucleosis
Brand Names Mono-Chek®; Mono-Diff®; Monospot®; Monosticon®; Mono-Sure®; Mono-Test®

Diagnostic Test for Ovulation
Brand Names Clearplan® [OTC]; First Response® Ovulation Predictor [OTC]; Fortel® Ovulation Test [OTC]; OvuSTICK® [OTC]

Diagnostic Test for Phenylketonuria
Brand Names Phenistix®

Diagnostic Test for pH in Urine
Brand Names Nitrazine® Paper [OTC]

Diagnostic Test for Pregnancy
Brand Names Advance® [OTC]; Answer® [OTC]; Answer® 2 [OTC]; Answer® Plus [OTC]; Clearblue® [OTC]; Daisy® 2 [OTC]; e.p.t.® [OTC]; e.p.t. Plus® [OTC]; Fact® [OTC]; First Response® [OTC]

Diagnostic Test for Protein in Urine
Brand Names Albustix® [OTC]

Diagnostic Test for Rheumatoid Factor
Brand Names LAtest-RF®; Rheumanosticon® Dri-Dot®

Diagnostic Test for Sickle Cell
Brand Names Sickledex™

Diagnostic Test for Streptococci
Brand Names Culturette® 10 Minute; Insta® Kit; LAtest ASO®; Rapid-Test® Strep; Respiralex®; Respirastick®; Streptonase-B®; Strepto-Sec®

Diagnostic Test for Taste Function
Brand Names Accusens T®

Diagnostic Test for Urobilinogen
Brand Names Urobilistix®

Diagnostic Test for Virus
Brand Names Abbott HTLV III EIA; MicroTrak® HSV 1/HSV 2 Culture; Rotalex® Rubacell II®

Dialose® [OTC] *see* Docusate *on page 121*

Dialose® Plus [OTC] *see* Docusate and Casanthranol *on page 121*

Dialume® [OTC] *see* Aluminum Hydroxide *on page 15*

Diamine T.D.® [OTC] *see* Brompheniramine Maleate *on page 48*

Diaminodiphenylsulfone *see* Dapsone *on page 97*

Diamox® *see* Acetazolamide *on page 5*

Diapid® *see* Lypressin *on page 209*

Diaqua® *see* Hydrochlorothiazide *on page 172*

Diar-Aid® [OTC] *see* Attapulgite *on page 32*

Diasorb® [OTC] *see* Attapulgite *on page 32*

Diastix® [OTC] *see* Diagnostic Test for Glucose in Urine *on previous page*

Diatrizoate Meglumine (dye a tri zoe' ate)
Brand Names Cystografin®
Use Retrograde cystourethrography; retrograde or ascending pyelography
Usual Dosage Varies with procedure

Diatrizoate Meglumine and Diatrizoate Sodium

Brand Names Renografin®

Synonyms Diatrizoate Sodium and Diatrizoate Meglumine

Use Radiographic examination of GI tract; angiocardiography; aortography; arteriography; cholangiography; arthrography; discography

Usual Dosage Varies with procedure

Diatrizoate Meglumine and Iodipamide Meglumine

(dye a tri zoe' ate)

Brand Names Sinografin®

Synonyms Iodipamide Meglumine and Diatrizoate Meglumine

Use Radiopaque agent to visualize the uterus

Usual Dosage Varies with procedure

Diatrizoate Sodium

Brand Names MD-50®

Use Cerebral angiography; urography; aortography; arteriography; splenoportography

Usual Dosage Varies with procedure

Diatrizoate Sodium and Diatrizoate Meglumine see Diatrizoate Meglumine and Diatrizoate Sodium on this page

Diazepam (dye az' e pam)

Brand Names Valium®

Use Management of anxiety and to provide preoperative sedation, light anesthesia, and amnesia; it can also be used in the treatment of status epilepticus and as a skeletal muscle relaxant in the treatment and management of symptoms of alcohol withdrawal

Restrictions C-IV

Pregnancy Risk Factor D

Usual Dosage

Adult:

Alcohol withdrawal: Oral: 10 mg 3-4 times daily in the first 24 hours, then decrease to 5 mg 3-4 times a day; I.M., I.V.: 10 mg initially and then 5-10 mg in 3-4 hours as needed

Anxiety and anticonvulsant: Oral: 2-10 mg 2-4 times daily; I.M., I.V.: 2-10 mg, may repeat in 3-4 hours if needed

Skeletal muscle relaxation: Oral: 2-10 mg 2-4 times daily; I.M., I.V.: 5-10 mg, may repeat in 2-4 hours

Status epilepticus: I.V.: 5-10 mg followed by up to 30 mg in 1 hour; may repeat in 2-4 hours

Pre-endoscopy: I.V.: up to 20 mg; I.M.: 5-10 mg 30 minutes before the procedure

Children:

Anxiety and anticonvulsant: Oral: > 6 months: 1-2.5 mg 3-4 times daily

Status epilepticus: I.M., I.V.: ≥ 5 years of age: 1 mg every 2-5 minutes to a total of 10 mg, repeat in 2-4 hours; 30 days to 5 years: 0.2-.5 mg every 2-5 minutes up to 5 mg

Diazoxide (dye az ox' ide)

Brand Names Hyperstat® I.V.

Use I.V. diazoxide is used for emergency lowering of blood pressure; oral diazoxide is used for management of hypoglycemia associated with leucine sensitivity, islet cell hyperplasia, nesidioblastosis, extra pancreatic malignancy, islet cell adenoma or adenomatosis

Pregnancy Risk Factor C

Usual Dosage I.V.:

Hypertensive crisis:

Adult: 1-3 mg/kg up to a maximum of 150 mg in a single injection; repeat dose in 5-15 minutes until a satisfactory reduction of blood pressure has been achieved; repeat administration at intervals of 4-24 hours; monitor the blood pressure closely

Children: 1-3 mg/kg (up to a maximum of 150 mg) every 5-15 minutes until adequate blood pressure control is achieved; repeat administration at 4-24 hour intervals

Hypoglycemia:

Adult and Children: Initial dose: 3 mg/kg/daily in three equal doses; maintenance: 3-8 mg/kg/daily in 2-3 equal doses

Newborns and Infants: Initial dose: Oral: 10 mg/kg/day in three doses every eight hours; maintenance: 3-8 mg/kg/day in 2-3 equal doses

Dibenzyline® *see* Phenoxybenzamine Hydrochloride
on page 280

Dibucaine (dye' byoo kane)

Brand Names Nupercainal® [OTC]

Use Fast, temporary relief of pain and itching due to hemorrhoids; minor burns, other minor skin conditions

Pregnancy Risk Factor C

Usual Dosage Topical: Apply gently to the affected areas; no more than 30 g for adults or 7.5 g for children should be used in any 24 hour period

Hemorrhoids: Rectal: Insert ointment into rectum using a rectal applicator; administer each morning, evening, and after each bowel movement

Dibucaine and Hydrocortisone

Brand Names Corticaine®

Synonyms Hydrocortisone and Dibucaine

Use Relief of the inflammatory and pruritic manifestations of corticosteroid-responsive dermatoses and for external anal itching

Pregnancy Risk Factor C

Usual Dosage Apply to affected areas 2-4 times daily

Dichlorodifluoromethane and Trichloromonofluoromethane

(dye klor oh dye floo or oh meth' ane)

Brand Names Fluori-Methane®

Use Management of myofascial pain, restricted motion, muscle pain; control of pain associated with injections

Usual Dosage Apply to area from approximately 12 inches away

Dichlorotetrafluoroethane and Ethyl Chloride *see* Ethyl Chloride and Dichlorotetrafluoroethane *on page 141*

Dichlorphenamide (dye klor fen' a mide)
Brand Names Daranide®
Synonyms Diclofenamide
Use Adjunct in treatment of open-angle glaucoma and perioperative treatment for angle-closure glaucoma
Pregnancy Risk Factor C
Usual Dosage Adult: Oral: 100-200 mg to start followed by 100 mg every 12 hours until desired response is obtained, then give 25-50 mg 1-3 times daily for maintenance

Diclofenac Sodium (dye kloe' fen ak)
Brand Names Voltaren®
Use Acute and chronic treatment of rheumatoid arthritis, ankylosing spondylitis, and osteoarthritis
Pregnancy Risk Factor B
Usual Dosage Adult: Oral:
  Rheumatoid arthritis: 150-200 mg/day in divided doses
  Osteoarthritis: 100-150 mg/day in divided doses
  Ankylosing spondylitis: 100-125 mg/day in divided doses

Diclofenamide *see* Dichlorphenamide *on this page*

Dicloxacillin Sodium (dye klox a sill' in)
Brand Names Dynapen®; Pathocil®; Veracillin®
Use Treatment of systemic infections caused by penicillinase-producing Staphylococci and penicillin-resistant Staphylococci
Pregnancy Risk Factor B
Usual Dosage Oral:
  Adult and Children: > 40 kg: 125-250 mg or higher every six hours
  Children: < 40 kg: 3-6 mg/kg every six hours

Dicumarol (dye koo' ma role)
Synonyms Bishydroxycoumarin
Use Prophylaxis and treatment of thromboembolic disorders
Pregnancy Risk Factor D
Usual Dosage Adult: Oral: 25-200 mg/day based on prothrombin time (PT) determinations

Dicyclomine Hydrochloride (dye sye' kloe meen)
Brand Names Bentyl® Hydrochloride; Neoquess®
Use Treatment of functional bowel and irritable bowel syndrome
Pregnancy Risk Factor C
Usual Dosage Adult:
  Oral: 160 mg per day in four equally divided doses; however, because of its side effects begin with 80 mg per day in four equally divided doses, then increase up to 160 mg
  I.M. (should not be used I.V.): 80 mg per day in four divided doses

(Continued)

Dicyclomine Hydrochloride *(Continued)*

Didrex® *see* Benzphetamine Hydrochloride *on page 42*

Didronel® *see* Etidronate Disodium *on page 142*

Dienestrol *(dye en ess' trole)*
Brand Names DV® Cream; Ortho® Dienestrol
Use Symptomatic management of atrophic vaginitis in postmenopausal women
Pregnancy Risk Factor X
Usual Dosage Adult: Vaginal: 1-2 applicators full per day for two weeks and then one-half of that dose for two weeks; maintenance dose is one applicator full 1-3 times a week for three weeks each month

Diethylpropion Hydrochloride *(dye eth il proe' pee on)*
Brand Names Tenuate®; Tepanil®
Synonyms Amfepramone
Use Short term adjunct in exogenous obesity
Restrictions C-IV
Pregnancy Risk Factor C
Usual Dosage Adult: Oral: 25 mg three times a day before meals or food or 75 mg controlled release tablet at midmorning

Diethylstilbestrol *(dye eth il stil bess' trole)*
Brand Names Diethylstilbestrol Enseals®; Stilphostrol®
Synonyms DES; Stilbestrol
Use Management of severe vasomotor symptoms of menopause, for estrogen replacement, and for palliative treatment of inoperable metastatic prostatic carcinoma
Pregnancy Risk Factor X
Usual Dosage Adult:

Hypogonadism and ovarian failure: Oral: 0.2-0.5 mg per day

Menopausal symptoms: Oral: 0.1-2 mg per day for three weeks and then off one week

Postmenopausal breast carcinoma: Oral: 15 mg per day

Prostate carcinoma: Oral: 1-3 mg per day

Prostatic cancer: I.V.: 0.5 g to start, then 1 g every 2-5 days followed by 0.25-0.5 g 1-2 times weekly as maintenance.

Diphosphate:
  Oral: 50 mg 3 times daily; increase up to 200 mg or more three times daily
  I.V.: Give 0.5 g, dissolved in 250 mL of saline or D₅W, administer slowly the first 10-15 minutes then adjust rate so that the entire amount is given in one hour

Diethylstilbestrol Enseals® *see* Diethylstilbestrol *on this page*

Diflorasone Diacetate (dye flor' a sone)

Brand Names Florone®

Use Relieve inflammation and pruritic symptoms of corticosteroid-responsive dermatosis

Pregnancy Risk Factor C

Usual Dosage Apply ointment sparingly 1-3 times a day; apply cream 2-4 times daily

Diflucan® *see* Fluconazole *on page 148*

Diflunisal (dye floo' ni sal)

Brand Names Dolobid®

Use Management of inflammatory disorders usually including rheumatoid arthritis and osteoarthritis; can be used as an analgesic for treatment of mild to moderate pain

Pregnancy Risk Factor C

Usual Dosage Adult: Oral:

Pain: 500-1000 mg initially followed by 250-500 mg every 8-12 hours

Inflammatory condition: 500-1000 mg per day in two divided doses

Di-Gel® [OTC] *see* Aluminum Hydroxide, Magnesium Hydroxide and Simethicone *on page 15*

Digibind® *see* Digoxin Immune Fab *on page 115*

Digitoxin (di ji tox' in)

Brand Names Crystodigin®; Purodigin®

Use Congestive heart failure; atrial fibrillation; atrial flutter; paroxysmal atrial tachycardia; and cardiogenic shock

Pregnancy Risk Factor C

Usual Dosage

Adult:
Rapid oral loading dose: 0.6 mg initially followed by 0.4 mg and then 0.2 mg at intervals of 4-6 hours
Slow oral loading dose: 0.2 mg twice daily for a period of four days followed by a maintenance dose
Maintenance: 0.05-0.3 mg per day
Most common dose: 0.15 mg per day

Children: The doses are very individualized; the maintenance range after neonatal period, the recommended digitalizing dose is as follows: Oral:
< 1 year: 0.045 mg/kg
1-2 years: 0.04 mg/kg
2 years: 0.03 mg/kg which is equivalent to 0.75 mg/mm^2
Maintenance: Approximately 1/10 of the digitalizing dose

Digoxin (di jox' in)

Brand Names Lanoxicaps®; Lanoxin®

Use Treatment of congestive heart failure and to slow the ventricular rate in tachyarrhythmias such as atrial fibrillation and atrial flutter
(Continued)

113

Digoxin *(Continued)*

Pregnancy Risk Factor A

Usual Dosage

Adult: The maintenance dose must be decreased in renal impairment
Oral, I.V. loading dose: 0.5-1 mg in divided doses over 24 hours; maintenance dose is then 0.125 and 0.5 mg per day

Children: Loading doses are administered in divided doses, with approximately 50% of the total dose given as the first dose; additional fractions of the loading dose (generally 25% fractions) are administered at 4- 8 hour intervals I.V. or 6-8 hour intervals orally or I.M., until an adequate therapeutic response is attained, toxic effects occur, or the total digitalizing dose has been administered. **The patient's clinical response should be carefully assessed before each additional dose is administered.** See tables.

**Usual Digitalizing and Maintenance Dosages for
Digoxin Tablets and Elixir
(normal renal function, based on lean body weight)**

Age	Digitalizing Dose (μg/kg)	Oral Maintenance Dosage (μg/kg daily)
Premature neonates	20–30	20–30% of oral loading dose*
Full–term neonates	25–35	25–35% of oral loading dose*
1–24 mo	35–60	
2–5 y	30–40	
5–10 y	20–35	
Older than 10 y	10–15	

Adapted from the American Society of Hospital Pharmacists, Inc, 1988.
* Estimated or actual digitalizing dose that provides desired clinical response.

**Usual Digitalizing and Maintenance Dosages for I.V. Digoxin
(normal renal function, based on lean body weight)**

Age	Digitalizing Dose (μg/kg)	I.V. Maintenance Dosage (μg/kg daily)
Premature neonates	15–25	20–30% of I.V. loading dose*
Full–term neonates	20–30	25–35% of I.V. loading dose*
1–24 mo	30–50	
2–5 y	25–35	
5–10 y	15–30	
Older than 10 y	8–12	

Adapted from the American Society of Hospital Pharmacists, Inc, 1988.
* Estimated or actual digitalizing dose that provides desired clinical response.

Digoxin Immune Fab

Brand Names Digibind®

Use Treatment of potentially life-threatening digoxin or digitoxin intoxication in carefully selected patients

Pregnancy Risk Factor C

Usual Dosage Determine total body load (TBL) of digoxin

TBL of digoxin (in mg) = C (in ng/mL) x 5.6 x body weight (in kg)/1000 or TBL = mg of digoxin ingested (as tablets or elixir) x 0.8; C = postdistribution digoxin concentration; calculate dose of digoxin immune Fab to neutralize digoxin in body

Dose of digoxin immune Fab (in mg) = TBL x 66.7 or dose of digoxin immune Fab (in number of 40 mg vials) = [C of digoxin (in ng/mL) x body weight (in kg)]/100

Dihydrocodeine Compound

Brand Names Synalgos®-DC

Use Management of mild to moderate pain that requires relaxation

Restrictions C-III

Pregnancy Risk Factor C

Usual Dosage Adult: 1-2 capsules every 4-6 hours as needed for pain

Dihydroergotamine Mesylate (dye hye droe or got' a meen)

Brand Names D.H.E.45®

Use Prevention of gouty arthritis; hyperuricemia; prolonged serum levels of penicillin/cephalosporin

Pregnancy Risk Factor X

Usual Dosage
I.M.: 1 mg at first sign of headache; 1 mg every six hours for two doses
I.V.: Up to 2 mg for faster effects

Dihydroergotoxine see Ergoloid Mesylates on page 133

Dihydrohydroxycodeinone see Oxycodone Hydrochloride on page 264

Dihydromorphinone see Hydromorphone Hydrochloride on page 176

Dihydrotachysterol (dye hye droe tak iss' ter ole)

Brand Names Hytakerol®

Synonyms DHT

Use Treatment of hypocalcemia associated with hypoparathyroidism; prophylaxis of hypocalcemic tetany following thyroid surgery

Pregnancy Risk Factor C

Usual Dosage Adult and Children: Oral: 0.5-2 mg daily, maintenance dose is 0.3-1.5 mg daily

1,25 dihydroxycholecalciferol see Calcitriol on page 53

Dihydroxypropyl Theophylline see Dyphylline on page 126

Diiodohydroxyquin see Iodoquinol on page 189

Diisopropyl Fluorophosphate *see* Isoflurophate *on page 192*

Dilantin® *see* Phenytoin *on page 283*

Dilatair® Ophthalmic Solution *see* Phenylephrine Hydrochloride *on page 282*

Dilaudid® *see* Hydromorphone Hydrochloride *on page 176*

Dilitrate®-SR *see* Isosorbide Dinitrate *on page 194*

Dilor® *see* Dyphylline *on page 126*

Diltiazem (dil tye' a zem)
Brand Names Cardizem®
Use Management of angina pectoris due to coronary insufficiency, hypertension
Pregnancy Risk Factor C
Usual Dosage Adult: Oral: 30-120 mg 3-4 times daily

Dimenhydrinate (dye men hye' dri nate)
Brand Names Dramamine® [OTC]
Use Treatment and prevention of nausea, vertigo, and vomiting associated with motion sickness
Pregnancy Risk Factor B
Usual Dosage

Adult: Oral, I.M., I.V.: 50-100 mg every 4-6 hours

Children:
Oral: 6-12 years: 25-50 mg every 6-8 hours; 2-5 years: 12.5-25 mg every 6-8 hours
I.M.: 1.25 mg/kg every six hours

Dimercaprol (dye mer kap' role)
Brand Names BAL in Oil®
Synonyms BAL
Use Antidote to gold arsenic and mercury poisoning
Pregnancy Risk Factor C
Usual Dosage I.M.:

Mild arsenic and gold poisoning: 2.5 mg/kg four times daily for two days, then twice daily on the third day, and once daily thereafter for 10 days

Severe arsenic and gold poisoning: 3 mg/kg every four hours for two days then four times daily on the third day, then twice daily thereafter for 10 days

Mercury poisoning: 5 mg/kg initially followed by 2.5 mg/kg 1-2 times daily for 10 days

Dimetane® [OTC] *see* Brompheniramine Maleate *on page 48*

Dimetane®-DC *see* Brompheniramine, Phenylpropanolamine and Codeine *on page 48*

Dimetapp® [OTC] *see* Brompheniramine and Phenylpropanolamine *on page 48*

Dimethoxyphenyl Penicillin Sodium *see* Methicillin Sodium
on page 226

β,β-Dimethylcysteine *see* Penicillamine *on page 272*

Dimethyl Sulfoxide
Brand Names Rimso®-50
Synonyms DMSO
Use Symptomatic relief of interstitial cystitis
Usual Dosage Instill 50 mL directly into bladder and allow to remain for 15 minutes; repeat every two weeks until maximum symptomatic relief is obtained

Dimethyl Tubocurarine Iodide *see* Metocurine Iodide
on page 233

Dinoprostone (dye noe prost' one)
Brand Names Prostin E_2®
Synonyms PGE_2; Prostaglandin E_2
Use To terminate pregnancy from 12th through 28th week of gestation; evacuate uterus in cases of missed abortion or intrauterine fetal death; manage benign hydatidiform mole
Pregnancy Risk Factor X
Usual Dosage Insert one suppository high in vagina, repeat at 3-5 hour intervals until abortion occurs up to 240 mg (maximum dose)

Dinoprost Tromethamine (dye' noe prost)
Brand Names Prostin F_2 Alpha®
Synonyms $PGF_{2\alpha}$; Prostaglandin F_2 Alpha
Use To abort second trimester pregnancy
Usual Dosage 40 mg (8 mL) via transabdominal tap, if abortion not completed in 24 hours, another 10-40 mg may be given

Dionosil Oily® *see* Propyliodone *on page 305*

Dioval® *see* Estradiol *on page 135*

Diphenhydramine Hydrochloride (dye fen hye' dra meen)
Brand Names Benadryl® [OTC]; Benylin® Cough Syrup [OTC]
Use Symptomatic relief of allergic symptoms caused by histamine release which include nasal allergies and allergic dermatosis; can be used for mild nighttime sedation; prevention of motion sickness and as an antitussive
Pregnancy Risk Factor B
Usual Dosage

Adult:
Oral: 25-50 mg every 4-6 hours
I.M., I.V.: 10-50 mg in a single dose, not to exceed 400 mg per day

Children:
Oral: > 9.1 kg: 12.5-25 mg every 4-6 hours; < 9.1 kg: 6.25-12.5 mg every 4-6 hours
I.M., I.V.: 5 mg/kg per day or 150 mg/mm² in divided doses every 6-8 hours, not to exceed 300 mg per day

Diphenoxylate and Atropine (dye fen ox' i late)
Brand Names Lomotil®
Synonyms Atropine and Diphenoxylate
Use Treatment of diarrhea
Restrictions C-V
Pregnancy Risk Factor C
Usual Dosage Oral:

Adult: Two tablets four times daily

Children:
8-12 years: 2 mg five times daily
5-8 years: 2 mg four times daily
2-5 years: 2 mg three times daily
Not recommended for children < 2 years of age

Diphenylan Sodium® see Phenytoin on page 283

Diphenylhydantoin see Phenytoin on page 283

Diphtheria and Tetanus Toxoid (dif theer' ee a)
Synonyms DT; Tetanus and Diphtheria Toxoid
Use Active immunity against diphtheria and tetanus
Usual Dosage I.M.:

Children and Infants:
6 weeks - 1 year of age: Three 0.5 mL doses at least four weeks apart;
give a reinforcing dose 6-12 months after the third injection
1-6 years: Give two 0.5 mL doses at least four weeks apart; reinforcing
dose 6-12 months after second injection; if final dose is given after
seventh birthday, use adult preparation
4-6 years (booster immunization): 0.5 mL; not necessary if all four
doses were given after fourth birthday - routinely give booster doses
at 10 year intervals with the adult preparation

Adult: > 7 years: Two primary doses of 0.5 mL each, given at an interval
of 4-6 weeks; third (reinforcing) dose of 0.5 mL 6-12 months later;
boosters every 10 years

Diphtheria and Tetanus Toxoids and Pertussis Vaccine, Adsorbed
Brand Names Tri-Immunol®
Synonyms DPT
Use Diphtheria, tetanus and whooping cough prophylaxis
Usual Dosage The primary immunization for children two months to six
years of age, ideally beginning at the age of 2-3 months or at 6-week
check-up. Administer 0.5 mL I.M. on three occasions at 4-8 week intervals with a re-enforcing dose administered one year after the third injection. The booster doses are given when the child is 4-6 years of age, 0.5
mL I.M.

Diphtheria Antitoxin
Use Passive prevention and treatment of diphtheria
Pregnancy Risk Factor D
Usual Dosage Administer I.M. or slow I.V. infusion: Dosage varies with a
range from 20,000- 120,000 units

Diphtheria CRM₁₉₇ Protein Conjugate *see Haemophilus* b Vaccine *on page 165*

Diphtheria Toxoid Conjugate *see Haemophilus* b Vaccine *on page 165*

Dipivalyl Epinephrine *see* Dipivefrin *on this page*

Dipivefrin (dye pi' ve frin)
Brand Names Propine®
Synonyms Dipivalyl Epinephrine
Use Reduce elevated intraocular pressure in chronic open-angle glaucoma
Pregnancy Risk Factor B
Usual Dosage Adult: One drop in eye every 12 hours

Diplovax® *see* Poliovirus Vaccine, Live, Trivalent *on page 289*

Diprivan® *see* Propofol *on page 303*

Diprolene® *see* Betamethasone *on page 43*

Dipropylacetic Acid *see* Valproic Acid and Derivatives *on page 371*

Diprosone® *see* Betamethasone *on page 43*

Dipyridamole (dye peer id' a mole)
Brand Names Persantine®
Use Maintain patency after surgical grafting procedures including coronary artery bypass; also used for chronic management of angina pectoris and as an additional antiplatelet agent with aspirin or an anticoagulant to prevent coronary thrombosis
Pregnancy Risk Factor C
Usual Dosage Adult: Oral: 100-400 mg per day in 2-4 divided doses

Disalcid® *see* Salsalate *on page 320*

Disalicylic Acid *see* Salsalate *on page 320*

Discase® *see* Chymopapain *on page 79*

d-Isoephedrine Hydrochloride *see* Pseudoephedrine *on page 307*

Disophrol® [OTC] *see* Dexbrompheniramine and Pseudoephedrine *on page 103*

Disopyramide Phosphate (dye soe peer' a mide)
Brand Names Norpace®
Use Suppression and prevention of unifocal and multifocal premature ventricular premature complexes, coupled ventricular tachycardia; also effective in the conversion of atrial fibrillation, atrial flutter, and paroxysmal atrial tachycardia to normal sinus rhythm and prevention of the reoccurrence of these arrhythmias after conversion by other methods
Pregnancy Risk Factor C
(Continued)

Disopyramide Phosphate *(Continued)*

Usual Dosage Oral:

Adult:
> 50 kg: 600 mg per day which breaks down to 150 mg every six hours or 300 mg every 12 hours, if used the control release dosage form;
< 50 kg: 400 mg per day or 100 mg every six hours or 200 mg every 12 hours in the control release form

Children:
12-18 years of age: is 6-15 mg/kg daily in divided doses every six hours
4-12 years: is 10-15 mg/kg daily in divided doses every six hours
1-4 years: 10-20 mg/kg daily in divided doses every six hours
< 1 year: 10-30 mg/kg daily in divided doses every six hours

Dispos-a-Med® Isoproterenol *see Isoproterenol on page 193*

Disulfiram *(dye sul' fi ram)*

Brand Names Antabuse®
Use Management of chronic alcoholics
Pregnancy Risk Factor C
Usual Dosage The maximum daily dose is 500 mg daily in a single dose for 1-2 weeks; the average maintenance dose is 250 mg daily; the range is 125-500 mg. The duration of therapy is to continue until the patient is fully recovered socially and a basis for permanent self control has been established; maintenance therapy may be required for months or even years.

Ditropan® *see Oxybutynin Chloride on page 264*

Diulo™ *see Metolazone on page 233*

Diupres-250® *see Chlorothiazide and Reserpine on page 72*

Diupres-500® *see Chlorothiazide and Reserpine on page 72*

Diuril® *see Chlorothiazide on page 72*

Diutensin® *see Methyclothiazide and Cryptenamine Tannates on page 229*

Divalproex Sodium *see Valproic Acid and Derivatives on page 371*

Dizmiss® [OTC] *see Meclizine Hydrochloride on page 215*

dl-Alpha Tocopherol *see Vitamin E on page 378*

dl-Norephedrine Hydrochloride *see Phenylpropanolamine Hydrochloride on page 283*

D-Mannitol *see Mannitol on page 212*

DMSO *see Dimethyl Sulfoxide on page 117*

DNR *see Daunorubicin Hydrochloride on page 98*

Dobutamine Hydrochloride *(doe byoo' ta meen)*

Brand Names Dobutrex®
Use Cardiac stimulant
Pregnancy Risk Factor C
Usual Dosage Adult: I.V.: 2.5-10 μg/kg minute up to 40 μg/kg/minute

To prepare for infusion:

$$\frac{6 \times \text{weight (kg)} \times \text{desired dose } (\mu g/kg/min)}{\text{I.V. infusion rate (mL/h)}} = \text{mg of drug to be added to 100 mL of I.V. fluid}$$

Dobutrex® *see* Dobutamine Hydrochloride *on previous page*

Docusate (dok' yoo sate)
Brand Names Colace® [OTC]; Dialose® [OTC]; Surfak® [OTC]
Use Stool softener in patients who should avoid straining during defecation and constipation associated with hard, dry stools
Pregnancy Risk Factor C
Usual Dosage Oral:

Adult and Children: > 12 years of age: 50-500 mg/day

Children:
6-12 years: 40-120 mg/day
3-6 years: 20-60 mg/day
< 3 years: 10-40 mg/day

Docusate and Casanthranol
Brand Names Dialose® Plus [OTC]; Peri-Colace® [OTC]
Synonyms Casanthranol and Docusate; DSS With Casanthranol
Use Treatment of constipation generally associated with lack of moisture, hardness or decreased intestinal motility
Pregnancy Risk Factor C
Usual Dosage

Adult: 1-2 capsules or 15-30 mL at bedtime or as needed

Children: 5-15 mL at bedtime or as needed; dilute in a suitable liquid for administration

Docusate and Phenolphthalein
Brand Names Correctol® [OTC]; Doxidan® [OTC]
Use Management of chronic functional constipation
Pregnancy Risk Factor C
Usual Dosage

Adult and Children: > 12 years of age: 1-2 capsules daily given at bedtime for 2-3 nights until bowel movements are normal

Children: 6-12 years of age: One capsule daily given at bedtime for 2-3 nights until bowel movements are normal

Doktors® Nasal Solution [OTC] *see* Phenylephrine Hydrochloride *on page 282*

Dolene® AP-65 *see* Propoxyphene and Acetaminophen *on page 304*

Dolobid® *see* Diflunisal *on page 113*

Dolophine® *see* Methadone Hydrochloride *on page 224*

Domeboro® *see* Aluminum Acetate *on page 14*

Donnagel® *see* Hyoscyamine, Atropine, Scopolamine, Kaolin and Pectin *on page 179*

Donnagel®-PG *see* Hyoscyamine, Atropine, Scopolamine, Kaolin, Pectin and Opium *on page 179*

Donnatal® *see* Hyoscyamine, Atropine, Scopolamine and Phenobarbital *on page 179*

Donnazyme® *see* Belladonna, Phenobarbital and Pepsin *on page 39*

Dopamine Hydrochloride (doe' pa meen)
Brand Names Intropin®
Use Emergency treatment of shock
Pregnancy Risk Factor C
Usual Dosage Adult: I.V.: 2-5 µg/kg/minute up to 50 µg/kg/minute; adjust dose by response

To prepare for infusion:

$$\frac{6 \times weight\ (kg) \times desired\ dose\ (\mu g/kg/min)}{I.V.\ infusion\ rate\ (mL/h)} = \frac{mg\ of\ drug\ to\ be\ added\ to\ 100}{mL\ of\ I.V.\ fluid}$$

Dopar® *see* Levodopa *on page 201*

Dopram® *see* Doxapram Hydrochloride *on this page*

Dorcol® [OTC] *see* Acetaminophen *on page 4*

Doriden® *see* Glutethimide *on page 159*

Dormalin® *see* Quazepam *on page 310*

Doryx® *see* Doxycycline *on next page*

Doxapram Hydrochloride (dox' a pram)
Brand Names Dopram®
Use Respiratory and CNS stimulant
Pregnancy Risk Factor C
Usual Dosage 0.5-2 mg/kg

Doxepin Hydrochloride (dox' e pin)
Brand Names Adapin®; Sinequan®
Use Antidepressant, antianxiety
Pregnancy Risk Factor C
Usual Dosage Adult: Oral: 30-150 mg/day at bedtime or 2-3 divided doses; may increase up to 300 mg/day; single dose should not exceed 150 mg

Doxidan® [OTC] *see* Docusate and Phenolphthalein *on previous page*

Doxorubicin Hydrochloride (dox oh roo' bi sin)

Brand Names Adriamycin PFS™; Adriamycin RDF™

Synonyms ADR; Hydroxydaunomycin Hydrochloride

Use Antineoplastic in treatment of various solid tumors including ovarian, breast and bladder, various lymphomas and leukemias

Pregnancy Risk Factor D

Usual Dosage I.V.:

Adult: 60-75 mg/m^2 as a single dose, repeat in three weeks or other dosage regimens like 20-30 mg/m^2/day for 2-3 days, repeat in four weeks or 20 mg/m^2 every four weeks

Investigational dose: 25-90 mg/m^2 with repeated doses per protocol; high dose regimen: 90-120 mg/m^2 every month

The lower dose regimen should be given to patients with decreased bone marrow reserve secondary to old age, prior therapy or marrow infiltration with malignant cells; use patient's ideal body weight to calculate surface area

Doxy-200® see Doxycycline on this page

Doxy-Caps® see Doxycycline on this page

Doxychel® see Doxycycline on this page

Doxycycline (dox i sye' kleen)

Brand Names Doryx®; Doxy-200®; Doxy-Caps®; Doxychel®; Doxy-Tabs®; Vibramycin®; Vibra-Tabs®

Synonyms Doxycycline Hyclate; Doxycycline Monohydrate

Use Treatment of susceptible bacterial infections of both gram-negative and gram-positive organisms

Pregnancy Risk Factor D

Usual Dosage

Adult:
Oral: 100 mg every 12-24 hours
I.V.: 100-200 mg every 24 hours

Children: Oral, I.V.: > 8 years: 2.2-4.4 mg/kg/day every 12-24 hours

Doxycycline Hyclate see Doxycycline on this page

Doxycycline Monohydrate see Doxycycline on this page

Doxy-Tabs® see Doxycycline on this page

DPA see Valproic Acid and Derivatives on page 371

D-Penicillamine see Penicillamine on page 272

DPH see Phenytoin on page 283

DPT see Diphtheria and Tetanus Toxoids and Pertussis Vaccine, Adsorbed on page 118

Dramamine® [OTC] see Dimenhydrinate on page 116

Dridase® see Oxybutynin Chloride on page 264

Drisdol® see Ergocalciferol on page 132

Dristan® Long Lasting Nasal Solution [OTC] *see*
Oxymetazoline Hydrochloride *on page 265*

Drithocreme® *see* Anthralin *on page 26*

Drixoral® [OTC] *see* Dexbrompheniramine and Pseudoephedrine
on page 103

Dronabinol (droe hab' i nol)
Brand Names Deltanyne®; Marinol®
Synonyms Tetrahydrocannabinol, THC
Use Antiemetic in patients undergoing cancer chemotherapy
Restrictions C-II
Pregnancy Risk Factor B
Usual Dosage 5 mg/m² 1-3 hours before chemotherapy, then give every
2-4 hours for a total of 4-6 doses/day; dose may be increased up to 15
mg/m² per dose if needed

Droncit® *see* Praziquantel *on page 293*

Droperidol (droe per' i dole)
Brand Names Inapsine®
Use As a tranquilizer and antiemetic in surgical and diagnostic procedures
Pregnancy Risk Factor C
Usual Dosage

Adult:
Premedication: I.M.: 2.5-10 mg 1/2-1 hour preoperatively
Adjunct to general anesthesia: I.V.: 1.25-2.5 mg
Alone in diagnostic procedures: I.M.: 2.5-10 mg 1/2-1 hour before

Children:
Premedication: I.M.: 0.088-0.165 mg/kg

Droperidol and Fentanyl
Brand Names Innovar®
Synonyms Fentanyl and Droperidol
Use To produce and maintain analgesia and sedation during diagnostic or
surgical procedures; as an adjunct to general anesthesia
Pregnancy Risk Factor C
Usual Dosage

Premedication: I.M.:
Adult: 0.5-2 mL 45-60 minutes prior to surgery
Children: 0.25 mL/20 lb body weight 45-60 minutes prior to surgery

Adjunct to General Anesthesia: I.V.:
Adult: 1 mL/20-25 lb as slow infusion until sleep occurs
Children: 0.5 mL/20 lb as slow infusion until sleep occurs

Dry and Clear® [OTC] *see* Benzoyl Peroxide *on page 41*

Drysol™ *see* Aluminum Chloride *on page 15*

DSS With Casanthranol *see* Docusate and Casanthranol
on page 121

DT *see* Diphtheria and Tetanus Toxoid *on page 118*

DTIC-Dome® *see* Dacarbazine *on page 96*

DTO *see* Opium, Tincture of *on page 261*

***d*-Tubocurarine Chloride** *see* Tubocurarine Chloride *on page 367*

Dulcolax® [OTC] *see* Bisacodyl *on page 45*

DuoDerm® *see* Hydroactive Dressing, Flexible *on page 172*

Duofilm® *see* Salicylic Acid and Lactic Acid *on page 319*

Duotrate® *see* Pentaerythritol Tetranitrate *on page 274*

Duphalac® *see* Lactulose *on page 199*

Durabolin® *see* Nandrolone *on page 246*

Duracillin® A.S. *see* Penicillin G Procaine, Aqueous *on page 273*

Dura-Estrin® *see* Estradiol *on page 135*

Duragen® *see* Estradiol *on page 135*

Duralone® *see* Methylprednisolone *on page 231*

Duralutin® *see* Hydroxyprogesterone Caproate *on page 177*

Duramorph® *see* Morphine Sulfate *on page 240*

Duranest® *see* Etidocaine Hydrochloride *on page 142*

Duraphyl™ *see* Theophylline *on page 348*

Duraquin® *see* Quinidine *on page 311*

Duratears® [OTC] *see* Ocular Lubricant *on page 259*

Duratest® *see* Testosterone *on page 345*

Durathate® *see* Testosterone *on page 345*

Durathesia® *see* Procaine Hydrochloride *on page 298*

Duration® Nasal Solution [OTC] *see* Oxymetazoline Hydrochloride *on page 265*

Duricef® *see* Cefadroxil Monohydrate *on page 62*

Duvoid® *see* Bethanechol Chloride *on page 44*

DV® Cream *see* Dienestrol *on page 112*

d-Xylose

Brand Names Xylo-Pfan®

Use For evaluating intestinal absorption and diagnosing malabsorptive states

Usual Dosage Older children should fast for eight hours prior to test; younger infants need fast only 4-6 hours; give xylose in a dose of 14.5 g/m^2 (BSA) as a 10% water solution orally or by a gastric tube (maximum 25 grams). All urine is collected for five hours and the quantity of xylose is determined colorimetrically.

Dyazide® *see* Hydrochlorothiazide and Triamterene
on page 173

Dyclone® *see* Dyclonine Hydrochloride *on this page*

Dyclonine Hydrochloride (dye' kloe neen)
Brand Names Dyclone®
Use As a local anesthetic prior to laryngoscopy, bronchoscopy, or endotracheal intubation; use topically for temporary relief of pain associated
with oral mucosa, skin, episiotomy, or anogenital lesions
Pregnancy Risk Factor C
Usual Dosage For mouth sores: 5-10 mL to oral mucosa (swab or swish
and then spit) 3-4 times/day as needed; maximum dose: 200 mg (40 mL
of 0.5% solution)/day

Dyflos *see* Isoflurophate *on page 192*

Dymelor® *see* Acetohexamide *on page 6*

Dynapen® *see* Dicloxacillin Sodium *on page 111*

Dyphylline (dye' fi lin)
Brand Names Dilor®; Lufyllin®; Neothylline®
Synonyms Dihydroxypropyl Theophylline
Use As a bronchodilator in reversible airway obstruction due to asthma or
COPD
Pregnancy Risk Factor C
Usual Dosage

Adult:
Oral: Up to 15 mg/kg four times a day, individualize dosage
I.M.: 250-500 mg, do not exceed total dosage of 15 mg/kg every six
hours

Children: I.M.: 4.4-6.6 mg/kg/day in divided doses

Dyrenium® *see* Triamterene *on page 360*

Early Detector® [OTC] *see* Diagnostic Test for Blood in Feces
on page 107

Easprin® *see* Aspirin *on page 30*

Echothiophate Iodide (ek oh thye' oh fate)
Brand Names Phospholine Iodide®
Synonyms Ecostigmine Iodide
Use Reverse toxic CNS effects caused by anticholinergic drugs; used as
miotic in treatment of glaucoma
Pregnancy Risk Factor C
Usual Dosage Instill one drop of 0.03%-0.125% solution into conjunctival
sac daily, up to one drop twice daily

Econazole Nitrate (e kone' a zole)
Brand Names Spectazole™
Use Topical treatment of tinea pedis, tinea cruris and tinea corporis, tinea
versicolor, and cutaneous candidiasis

Pregnancy Risk Factor C
Usual Dosage Tinea cruris, corporis, pedis, and cutaneous candidiasis - apply twice daily; tinea versicolor - once a day

Econochlor® *see* Chloramphenicol *on page 69*

Econopred® *see* Prednisolone *on page 294*

Econopred® Plus *see* Prednisolone *on page 294*

Ecostigmine Iodide *see* Echothiophate Iodide *on previous page*

Ecotrin® [OTC] *see* Aspirin *on page 30*

Ectasule® *see* Ephedrine Sulfate *on page 130*

E-Cypionate® *see* Estradiol *on page 135*

Edathamil Disodium *see* Edetate Disodium *on this page*

Edecrin® *see* Ethacrynic Acid *on page 138*

Edetate Calcium Disodium (ed' e tate)

Brand Names Calcium Disodium Versenate®
Synonyms Calcium EDTA
Use As an adjunct in treatment of acute and chronic lead poisoning
Pregnancy Risk Factor C
Usual Dosage

Adult: I.V., I.M.: 2-4 g/24 hours in divided doses every 12-24 hours for 5 days; may repeat course one time after at least 2 days

Children:
Asymptomatic lead poisoning: (> 55 μg/dL) or symptomatic lead poisoning without encephalopathy with level < 100 μg/dL: 1 g/m^2/day I.M./I.V. in divided doses every 8-12 hours for 3-5 days (usually 5 days); maximum 1 g/24 hours
Symptomatic lead poisoning with encephalopathy with level > 100 μg/dL: 250 mg/m^2 I.M. or intermittent I.V. infusion 4 hours after 4 mg/kg of dimercaprol, then at 4 hour intervals thereafter for 5 days (1.5 g/m^2/day); dose (1.5 g/m^2/day) can also be given as a single I.V. continuous infusion over 12-24 hours daily for 5 days; maximum 1 g/24 hours
Note: Course of therapy can be repeated in 2-3 weeks until blood lead level is normal

Edetate Disodium

Brand Names Sodium Versenate®
Synonyms Edathamil Disodium; EDTA; Sodium Edetate
Use Emergency treatment of hypercalcemia; control digitalis-induced cardiac dysrhythmias
Pregnancy Risk Factor C
Usual Dosage I.V.:

Hypercalcemia:
Adult: 50 mg/kg daily over three or more hours
Children: 40-70 mg/kg slow infusion over 3-4 hours

Dysrhythmias: Adult and Children: 15 mg/kg/hour up to 60 mg/kg/day

Edrophonium Chloride (ed roe foe' nee um)

Brand Names Enlon®; Reversol®; Tensilon®

Use Diagnosis and differentiation of myasthenia gravis, to reverse non-depolarizing neuromuscular blockers and treatment of paroxysmal atrial tachycardia

Pregnancy Risk Factor C

Usual Dosage

Adult:

Diagnosis: I.M.: 10 mg, may repeat 2 mg in 30 minutes; I.V.: 2 mg, then 8 mg if no response

Differentiation of cholinergic from myasthenic crisis: I.V.: 1 mg, may give 1 mg one minute later

Reversal of nondepolarizing neuromuscular blocking agents: I.V.: 10 mg, may repeat every 5-10 minutes up to 40 mg

Termination of paroxysmal atrial tachycardia: I.V.: 5-10 mg

Children:

Diagnosis: I.M. < 34 kg: 2 mg; > 34 kg: 5 mg

I.V.: < 34 kg: 1 mg, 1 mg every 30-45 seconds up to 5 mg; > 34 kg: 2 mg, 1 mg every 30-45 seconds up to 10 mg; if a cholinergic reaction occurs, the test should be discontinued and atropine administered I.V.

Infant: I.V.: 0.5 mg total dose; give 1/5 of the dose initially, then the remainder if no response occurs within 45 seconds

EDTA see Edetate Disodium on previous page

E.E.S.® see Erythromycin on page 134

Efedron® see Ephedrine Sulfate on page 130

Effer-Syllium® [OTC] see Psyllium on page 308

Efodine® [OTC] see Povidone-Iodine on page 292

Efudex® see Fluorouracil on page 151

EHDP see Etidronate Disodium on page 142

Elase® see Fibrinolysin and Desoxyribonuclease on page 147

Elase-Chloromycetin® see Fibrinolysin and Desoxyribonuclease on page 147

Elavil® see Amitriptyline Hydrochloride on page 20

Eldepryl® see Selegiline Hydrochloride on page 322

Electrolytes and Dextrose see Dextrose in Water with Potassium Chloride on page 105

Elemite® see Permethrin on page 277

Elixicon® see Theophylline on page 348

Elixophyllin® see Theophylline on page 348

Elixophyllin® SR see Theophylline on page 348

Elspar® see Asparaginase on page 30

Emcyt® see Estramustine Phosphate on page 136

Emete-Con® *see* Benzquinamide Hydrochloride *on page 42*

Emetine Hydrochloride (em' e teen)
Use Acute fulminating amebic dysentery; acute exacerbations of chronic amebic dysentery; amebic hepatitis and abscess
Pregnancy Risk Factor X
Usual Dosage

Adult: Deep S.C., I.M.: 1 mg/kg twice a day for 3-10 days, dosage should not exceed 65 mg/day or 650 mg in 10 days; hepatic amebiasis or abscess give for 10 days, for acute fulminating dysentery 3-5 days should be sufficient duration to control diarrhea

Children: Deep S.C.: 1 mg/kg twice a day for four days
> 8 years of age: No more than 20 mg/day
< 8 years of age: No more than 10 mg/day

Emetrol® [OTC] *see* Levulose, Dextrose and Phosphoric Acid *on page 203*

Eminase® *see* Anistreplase *on page 25*

Emollient Cream
Brand Names Complex 15®; Eucerin®; Keri®; Nivea®
Use Dry skin
Usual Dosage Apply as needed for dry skin

Emollient Lotion
Brand Names Keri® Lotion [OTC]
Use Treatment of dry skin
Usual Dosage Apply as needed for dry skin

Empirin® [OTC] *see* Aspirin *on page 30*

Empirin® With Codeine *see* Aspirin and Codeine *on page 31*

E-Mycin® *see* Erythromycin *on page 134*

E-Mycin-E® *see* Erythromycin *on page 134*

Enalapril (e nal' a pril)
Brand Names Vasotec®
Synonyms Enalaprilat
Use Management of mild to severe hypertension
Pregnancy Risk Factor C
Usual Dosage Adult: Oral: 2.5-5 mg/day then increased as required, usually 10-40 mg/day in 1-2 divided doses

Enalaprilat *see* Enalapril *on this page*

Encainide Hydrochloride (en kay' nide)
Brand Names Enkaid®
Use Ventricular arrhythmias; supraventricular arrhythmias
Pregnancy Risk Factor B
Usual Dosage Adult: Oral: 25 mg every eight hours; may increase to 35 mg every eight hours after 3-5 days if needed; increase to 50 mg every eight hours in another 3-5 days if response is not achieved

Endep® *see* Amitriptyline Hydrochloride *on page 20*

Enduron® *see* Methyclothiazide *on page 229*

Enduronyl® *see* Methyclothiazide and Deserpidine
on page 229

Enduronyl® Forte *see* Methyclothiazide and Deserpidine
on page 229

Energix® *see* Hepatitis B Vaccine *on page 168*

Enflurane (en' floo rane)
Brand Names Ethrane®
Use General induction and maintenance of anesthesia (inhalation)
Usual Dosage 0.5-3%

Enkaid® *see* Encainide Hydrochloride *on previous page*

Enlon® *see* Edrophonium Chloride *on page 128*

Enovid® *see* Mestranol and Norethynodrel *on page 222*

Enovil® *see* Amitriptyline Hydrochloride *on page 20*

Ensure® [OTC] *see* Nutritional Formula, Enteral/Oral
on page 258

Ensure Plus® [OTC] *see* Nutritional Formula, Enteral/Oral
on page 258

Entacef® *see* Cephalexin Monohydrate *on page 66*

Enterodophilus® [OTC] *see* Lactobacillus acidophilus and
Lactobacillus bulgaricus on page 199

Entex® *see* Guaifenesin, Phenylpropanolamine and Phenylephrine
on page 163

Entex® LA *see* Guaifenesin and Phenylpropanolamine
on page 163

Entolase®-HP *see* Pancrelipase *on page 267*

Entozyme® *see* Bile Salts, Pancreatin and Pepsin *on page 44*

Enulose® *see* Lactulose *on page 199*

EPEG *see* Etoposide *on page 142*

Ephedrine Sulfate (e fed' rin)
Brand Names Ectasule®; Efedron®; Ephedsol®; Vicks Vatronol®
Use Bronchial asthma; nasal congestion; acute bronchospasm
Pregnancy Risk Factor C
Usual Dosage

Adult:
Oral: 25-50 mg every 3-4 hours as needed
I.M., I.V., S.C.: 25-50 mg

Children: Oral, I.V., S.C.: 3 mg/kg/day

Ephedrine, Theophylline and Phenobarbital *see* Theophylline, Ephedrine and Phenobarbital *on page 350*

Ephedsol® *see* Ephedrine Sulfate *on previous page*

Epifrin® *see* Epinephrine *on this page*

Epinal® *see* Epinephrine *on this page*

Epinephrine (ep nef' rin)
Brand Names Adrenalin®; AsthmaHaler®; Breatheasy®; Bronitin®; Bronkaid® Mist; Epifrin®; Epinal®; EpiPen®; EpiPen® Jr; Epitrate®; Medihaler-Epi®; microNefrin®; Primatene® Mist; Sus-Phrine®; Vaponefrin®

Synonyms Adrenaline; Epinephrine Bitartrate; Epinephrine Hydrochloride; Racemic Epinephrine

Use Bronchospasms; anaphylactic reactions; cardiac arrest; management of open-angle (chronic simple) glaucoma

Pregnancy Risk Factor C

Usual Dosage

Adult:

Bronchodilator: 1-2 inhalations every 1-5 minutes; I.M., S.C.: 0.1-0.5 mg every 10-15 minutes; I.V.: 0.1-0.25 mg

Cardiac arrest: I.V., intracardiac: 0.1-1 mg every five minutes as needed; endotracheal: 1 mg

Hypersensitivity reaction: I.M., S.C.: 0.2-0.5 mg every 20 minutes to four hours

Ophthalmic: Instill 1-2 drops in eye(s) once or twice daily

Children: S.C.:

Bronchodilator: 10 µg/kg

Hypersensitivity reaction: 0.01 mg/kg every 15 minutes for two doses then every four hours as needed

Epinephrine Bitartrate *see* Epinephrine *on this page*

Epinephrine Hydrochloride *see* Epinephrine *on this page*

EpiPen® *see* Epinephrine *on this page*

EpiPen® Jr *see* Epinephrine *on this page*

Epitrate® *see* Epinephrine *on this page*

Epitrol® *see* Carbamazepine *on page 57*

EPO *see* Epoetin Alfa *on this page*

Epoetin Alfa
Brand Names Epogen®

Synonyms EPO; Erythropoietin

Use Treatment of anemia associated with chronic renal failure

Pregnancy Risk Factor C

Usual Dosage In patients on dialysis epoetin alfa usually has been administered as an I.V. bolus three times weekly. While the administration is independent of the dialysis procedure, it may be administered into the venous line at the end of the dialysis procedure to obviate the need for additional venous access. In patients with CRF not on dialysis, epoetin alfa may be given either as an I.V. or S.C. injection. See table.

Epoetin Alfa: General Therapeutic Guidelines

Starting dose	50 to 100 U/kg 3 times weekly I.V.: Dialysis patients I.V. or SC: nondialysis CRF patients
Reduce dose when	1. Target range is reached, or 2. Hematocrit increases > 4 points in any 2–week period
Increase dose if	Hematocrit does not increase by 5 to 6 points after 8 weeks of therapy, and hematocrit is below target range
Maintenance dose	Individualize. General dosage range: 25 U/kg (3 times weekly)
Target hematocrit range	30–33% (maximum 36%)

Epogen® *see* Epoetin Alfa *on previous page*

Eprolin® [OTC] *see* Vitamin E *on page 378*

Epsom Salts *see* Magnesium Sulfate *on page 211*

e.p.t.® [OTC] *see* Diagnostic Test for Pregnancy *on page 108*

EPT *see* Teniposide *on page 342*

e.p.t. Plus® [OTC] *see* Diagnostic Test for Pregnancy *on page 108*

Equagesic® *see* Aspirin and Meprobamate *on page 31*

Equanil® *see* Meprobamate *on page 220*

Eramycin® *see* Erythromycin *on page 134*

Ergocalciferol (er goe kal sif' e role)
  Brand Names Calciferol™; Drisdol®
  Synonyms Activated Ergosterol; Viosterol; Vitamin D_2
  Use Refractory rickets; hypophosphatemia; hypoparathyroidism
  Pregnancy Risk Factor C
  Usual Dosage Oral:

  Nutritional rickets and osteomalacia:
    Adult and Children: 50-125 μg daily for 6-12 weeks
    Adult with malabsorption: 250 μg to 7.5 mg
    Children with malabsorption: 250 μg to 625 μg daily
    Vitamin D deficient infants with tetanus and rickets: Administer calcium to control tetanus and 5-125 μg ergocalciferol daily until bones have healed

  Familial hypophosphatemia (vitamin D resistant rickets): Children: Initial dose is 1-2 mg daily with phosphate supplements; dosage is increased in 250-500 μg increments at 3-4 month intervals

  Vitamin D dependent rickets:
    Adult: 250 μg-1.5 mg daily

Children: 75-125 µg daily

Hypoparathyroidism:
Adult: 625 µg to 5 mg with calcium supplements
Children: 1.25-5 mg with calcium supplements

Dietary supplementation: Premature infants: 12-20 µg daily for normal bone development

Ergoloid Mesylates (er' goe loyd mess' i lates)
Brand Names Germinal®; Hydergine®; Hydergine® LC; Hydro-Ergoloid®; Niloric®; Uni-Gine®

Synonyms Dihydroergotoxine; Hydrogenated Ergot Alkaloids

Use Treatment of cerebrovascular insufficiency in primary progressive dementia, Alzheimer's dementia, and senile onset

Pregnancy Risk Factor C

Usual Dosage Adult: Oral: 1 mg three times a day up to 4.5-12 mg/day

Ergomar® see Ergotamine on this page

Ergometrine Maleate see Ergonovine Maleate on this page

Ergonovine Maleate (er goe noe' veen)
Brand Names Ergotrate® Maleate

Synonyms Ergometrine Maleate

Use Prevention and treatment of postpartum and postabortion hemorrhage caused by uterine atony or subinvolution

Pregnancy Risk Factor X

Usual Dosage Adult:
Oral: 1-2 tablets every 6-12 hours for usually 48 hours
I.M.: 0.2 mg, repeat dose in 2-4 hours as needed

Ergostat® see Ergotamine on this page

Ergotamine (er got' a meen)
Brand Names Cafergot®; Cafergot® PB; Ergomar®; Ergostat®; Wigraine®

Use To abort or prevent vascular headaches

Pregnancy Risk Factor X

Usual Dosage Adult:
Oral (Cafergot®): Two tablets at onset of attack; then one tablet every 30 minutes as needed; maximum of six tablets per attack; do not exceed 10 tablets per week

Oral (Cafergot® P-B tablets): Two tablets at first sign of an attack; follow with one tablet every 1/2 hour, if needed; maximum dose is six tablets/attack; do not exceed 10 tablets/week

Rectal (Cafergot® suppositories, Wigraine® suppositories, Cafergot® P-B suppositories): One at first sign of an attack; follow with second dose after one hour, if needed; maximum dose is 2/attack; do not exceed 5/week

Oral (Ergostat®): One tablet under tongue at first sign, then one tablet every 30 minutes, three tablets in 24 hours, five tablets per week

Ergotrate® Maleate see Ergonovine Maleate on this page

ERYC® *see* Erythromycin *on this page*

Erycette® *see* Erythromycin, Topical *on next page*

EryDerm® *see* Erythromycin, Topical *on next page*

Erymax® *see* Erythromycin, Topical *on next page*

Erypar® *see* Erythromycin *on this page*

EryPed® *see* Erythromycin *on this page*

Ery-Tab® *see* Erythromycin *on this page*

Erythrityl Tetranitrate (e ri' thri till)
Brand Names Cardilate®
Use Prophylaxis and long-term treatment of frequent or recurrent anginal pain and reduced exercise tolerance associated with angina pectoris
Pregnancy Risk Factor C
Usual Dosage Adult: Oral: 5 mg under the tongue or in the buccal pouch three times a day or 10 mg before meals or food, chewed three times a day, increasing in 2-3 days if needed

Erythrocin® *see* Erythromycin *on this page*

Erythrocin® Lactobionate-IV *see* Erythromycin *on this page*

Erythromycin (er ith roe mye' sin)
Brand Names E.E.S.®; E-Mycin®; E-Mycin-E®; Eramycin®; ERYC®; Erypar®; EryPed®; Ery-Tab®; Erythrocin®; Erythrocin® Lactobionate-IV; Ethril®; Ilosone®; Ilotycin®; Ilotycin® Gluceptate; PCE®; Pediamycin®; Robimycin®; Wintrocin®; Wyamycin® E; Wyamycin® S
Synonyms Erythromycin Base; Erythromycin Estolate; Erythromycin Ethylsuccinate; Erythromycin Gluceptate; Erythromycin Lactobionate; Erythromycin Stearate
Use Treatment of susceptible bacterial infections of the upper and lower respiratory tract and otitis media
Pregnancy Risk Factor C
Usual Dosage

Adult and Children: 15-20 mg/kg daily as a continuous I.V. infusion (every six hours in divided doses by intermittent I.V. infusion)

Adult: Oral: 250-800 every 6-8 hours

Children: Oral: 30-50 mg/kg/day in four doses every six hours; double in severe infections

Infants: 20-30 mg/kg/day in four equally divided doses

Erythromycin and Sulfisoxazole
Brand Names Pediazole®
Synonyms Sulfisoxazole and Erythromycin
Use Treatment of susceptible bacterial infections of the upper and lower respiratory tract; otitis media; and other infections in patients allergic to penicillin
Pregnancy Risk Factor C
Usual Dosage

Children: Oral: Given every 6 hours without regard to meals
> 45 kg = 10 mL

24 kg = 7.5 mL
16 kg = 5 mL
8 kg = 2.5 mL
< 8 kg = adjust dose (50 mg/kg/day erythromycin)

Erythromycin Base see Erythromycin *on previous page*

Erythromycin Estolate see Erythromycin *on previous page*

Erythromycin Ethylsuccinate see Erythromycin *on previous page*

Erythromycin Gluceptate see Erythromycin *on previous page*

Erythromycin Lactobionate see Erythromycin *on previous page*

Erythromycin Stearate see Erythromycin *on previous page*

Erythromycin, Topical
Brand Names Akne-Mycin®; A/T/S®; C-Solve®2; Erycette®; EryDerm®; Erymax®; E-Solve®2; ETS-2%®; Staticin®; T-Stat®
Use Topical treatment of acne vulgaris
Pregnancy Risk Factor B
Usual Dosage Adult and Children: Apply twice a day

Erythropoietin see Epoetin Alfa *on page 131*

Eserine Salicylate see Physostigmine Salicylate *on page 284*

Esidrix® see Hydrochlorothiazide *on page 172*

Eskalith® see Lithium *on page 205*

Esmolol Hydrochloride (ess' moe lol)
Brand Names Brevibloc®
Use Supraventricular tachycardia
Pregnancy Risk Factor C
Usual Dosage Adult: I.V.: 50-200 μg/kg/minute; average dose is 100 μg/kg/minute; loading dose: 500 μg/kg over one minute. Follow with a 50 μg/kg/minute infusion for four minutes. If an adequate therapeutic response has not been achieved, rebolus with another 500 mg/kg loading dose over one minute, and increase the maintenance infusion to 100 μg/kg/minute. Repeat this process until a therapeutic effect has been achieved.

E-Solve®2 see Erythromycin, Topical *on this page*

Estinyl® see Ethinyl Estradiol *on page 138*

Estivin® II [OTC] see Naphazoline Hydrochloride *on page 246*

Estrace® see Estradiol *on this page*

Estraderm® see Estradiol *on this page*

Estradiol (ess tra dye' ole)
Brand Names Delestrogen®; depGynogen®; Depo®-Estradiol; Depogen®; Dioval®; Dura-Estrin®; Duragen®; E-Cypionate®; Estrace®; Estraderm®; Estro-Cyp®; Estrofem®; Estroject-L.A.®; Estronol-LA®; Ru-Est-Span®; Valergen®
(Continued)

Estradiol *(Continued)*

Synonyms Estradiol Cypionate; Estradiol Valerate
Use Treatment of atrophic vaginitis, atrophic dystrophy of vulva, menopausal symptoms, female hypogonadism, ovariectomy, primary ovarian failure, inoperable breast cancer, inoperable prostatic cancer, mild to severe vasomotor symptoms associated with menopause
Pregnancy Risk Factor X
Usual Dosage Adult:

Menopausal symptoms:
Oral: 1-2 mg/day in cycles of 21 days on and seven days off or five days on and two days off
I.M.: 0.2-1 mg weekly; 1-5 mg every 3-4 weeks
Transdermal: One patch on trunk of body twice weekly; three weeks on and one week off

Atrophic vaginitis: Intravaginal: 2-4 g daily for 1-2 weeks; maintenance dosage 1 g 1-3 times a week

Female hypogonadism: I.M.: 1.5-2 mg at monthly intervals

Inoperable breast cancer: Oral: 10 mg three times a day for three months

Inoperable prostatic cancer: Oral: 1-2 mg three times a day

Estradiol and Fluoxymesterone

Brand Names Halodrin®
Synonyms Fluoxymesterone and Estradiol
Use Moderate to severe vasomotor symptoms of menopause, postpartum breast engorgement
Pregnancy Risk Factor X
Usual Dosage 1-2 tablets at bedtime given cyclically, three weeks on and one week off

Estradiol Cypionate *see* Estradiol *on previous page*

Estradiol Valerate *see* Estradiol *on previous page*

Estradurin® *see* Polyestradiol Phosphate *on page 290*

Estramustine Phosphate *(ess tra muss' teen)*

Brand Names Emcyt®
Use Palliative treatment of prostatic carcinoma
Pregnancy Risk Factor C
Usual Dosage One capsule for each 22 lb per day, in 3-4 divided doses

Estro-Cyp® *see* Estradiol *on previous page*

Estrofem® *see* Estradiol *on previous page*

Estrogen, Conjugated *(ess' troe jen)*

Brand Names Premarin®
Synonyms C.E.S.; Estrogenic Substances, Conjugated
Use Atrophic vaginitis; hypogonadism; primary ovarian failure; vasomotor symptoms of menopause; prostatic carcinoma; osteoporosis prophylactic

Pregnancy Risk Factor X
Usual Dosage Adult:

Atrophic vaginitis: Vaginally: 2-4 g/day for 21 days, off seven days and repeat

Ovarian failure: Oral: 1.25 mg/day for 21 days, off seven days and repeat

Hypogonadism: Oral: 2.5-7.5 mg/day for 20 days, off 10 days and repeat until menses occur

Menopausal symptoms: Oral: 0.3-1.25 mg/day for 21 days, off seven days and repeat

Prostatic carcinoma: Oral: 1.25-2.5 mg three times a day

Osteoporosis: Oral: 0.625 mg/day for 21 days, off seven days and repeat

Estrogenic Substance Aqueous *see* Estrone *on this page*

Estrogenic Substances, Conjugated *see* Estrogen, Conjugated *on previous page*

Estrogens With Methyltestosterone
Brand Names Premarin® With Methyltestosterone
Use Atrophic vaginitis; hypogonadism; primary ovarian failure; vasomotor symptoms of menopause; prostatic carcinoma; osteoporosis prophylactic
Pregnancy Risk Factor X
Usual Dosage Lowest dose that will control symptoms should be chosen, normally given three weeks on and one week off

Estroject-L.A.® *see* Estradiol *on page 135*

Estrone (ess' trone)
Brand Names Theelin®
Synonyms Estrogenic Substance Aqueous
Use Atrophic vaginitis; hypogonadism; primary ovarian failure; vasomotor symptoms of menopause; prostatic carcinoma; osteoporosis prophylactic
Pregnancy Risk Factor X
Usual Dosage Adult: I.M.:

Vasomotor symptoms, atrophic vaginitis: 0.1-0.5 mg 2-3 times weekly

Primary ovarian failure, hypogonadism: 0.1-1 mg weekly, up to 2 mg weekly

Prostatic carcinoma: 2-4 mg 2-3 times weekly

Estronol-LA® *see* Estradiol *on page 135*

Estropipate (ess' troe pih pate)
Brand Names Ogen®
Synonyms Piperazine Estrone Sulfate
Use Atrophic vaginitis; hypogonadism; primary ovarian failure; vasomotor symptoms of menopause; prostatic carcinoma; osteoporosis prophylactic
(Continued)

Estropipate *(Continued)*
Pregnancy Risk Factor X
Usual Dosage Oral: 0.625-5 mg/day

Estrovis® *see* Quinestrol *on page 311*

ETH *see* Terpin Hydrate *on page 344*

Ethacrynic Acid (eth a krin' ik)
Brand Names Edecrin®
Use Management of edema secondary to congestive heart failure, hepatic or renal disease
Pregnancy Risk Factor B
Usual Dosage

Adult:
  Oral: 50-200 mg/day in 1-2 divided doses
  I.V.: 50-100 mg (0.5-1 mg/kg)

Children:
  Oral: 25 mg/day to start, increase by 25 mg/day until response is obtained
  I.V.: The manufacturer does not recommend administration to children

Infants: Dosage has not been established

Ethambutol Hydrochloride (e tham' byoo tole)
Brand Names Myambutol®
Use Treatment of tuberculosis and other mycobacterial diseases in conjunction with other antituberculosis agents
Pregnancy Risk Factor B
Usual Dosage Oral:

Adult: 15-25 mg/kg/day

Children: 10-15 mg/kg/day

ETH and C *see* Terpin Hydrate and Codeine *on page 344*

Ethanoic Acid *see* Acetic Acid *on page 6*

Ethanol *see* Alcohol, Ethyl *on page 11*

Ethchlorvynol (eth klor vi' nole)
Brand Names Placidyl®
Use Short-term management of insomnia
Restrictions C-IV
Pregnancy Risk Factor C
Usual Dosage 500-1000 mg at bedtime

Ethinyl Estradiol (eth' in il ess tra dye' ole)
Brand Names Estinyl®
Use Atrophic vaginitis; hypogonadism; primary ovarian failure; vasomotor symptoms of menopause; prostatic carcinoma; osteoporosis prophylactic
Pregnancy Risk Factor X

Usual Dosage Adult:

Hypogonadism: 0.05 mg 1-3 times day for two weeks

Vasomotor symptoms: 0.02-0.05 mg for 21 days, off seven days and repeat

Prostatic carcinoma: 0.15-2 mg/day

Ethinyl Estradiol and Ethynodiol Diacetate

Brand Names Demulen® 1/35; Demulen® 1/50

Synonyms Ethynodiol Diacetate and Ethinyl Estradiol

Use Oral contraceptive

Pregnancy Risk Factor X

Usual Dosage For 21 tablet cycle packs, with 21 active tablets (28 day packs have 21 active tablets and 7 inert tablets): Take one tablet daily starting on the fifth day of menstrual cycle, with day one being the first day of menstruation; begin taking a new cycle pack on the eighth day after taking the last tablet from the previous pack

Ethinyl Estradiol and Levonorgestrel

Brand Names Nordette®

Synonyms Levonorgestrel and Ethinyl Estradiol

Use Prevention of pregnancy

Pregnancy Risk Factor X

Usual Dosage

Contraception: Oral: One tablet daily, beginning on day five of menstrual cycle (first day of menstrual flow is day one). With 20-tablet and 21-tablet packages, new dosing cycle begins seven days after last tablet taken. With 28-tablet packages, dosage is one tablet daily without interruption; extra tablets are placebos or contain iron. If next menstrual period does not begin on schedule, rule out pregnancy before starting new dosing cycle. If menstrual period begins, start new dosing cycle seven days after last tablet was taken. if all doses have been taken on schedule and one menstrual period is missed, continue dosing cycle. If two consecutive menstrual periods are missed, pregnancy test is required before new dosing cycle is started.

Biphasic oral contraceptive (Ortho-Novum™ 10/11): One color tablet daily for 10 days, then next color tablet for 11 days

Triphasic oral contraceptive (Ortho-Novum™ 7/7/7, Tri-Norinyl®, Triphasil®): One tablet daily in the sequence specified by the manufacturer

Ethinyl Estradiol and Norethindrone Acetate

Brand Names Loestrin® 1.5/30; Norlestrin® 2.5/50

Synonyms Norethindrone Acetate and Ethinyl Estradiol

Use Prevention of pregnancy

Pregnancy Risk Factor X

Usual Dosage For 21 tablet cycle packs, with 21 active tablets (28 day packs have 21 active tablets and 7 inert tablets): Take one tablet daily starting on the fifth day of menstrual cycle, with day one being the first day of menstruation; begin taking a new cycle pack on the eighth day after taking the last tablet from the previous pack

Ethinyl Estradiol and Norgestrel
Brand Names Lo/Ovral®; Ovral®
Synonyms Norgestrel and Ethinyl Estradiol
Use Prevention of pregnancy
Pregnancy Risk Factor X
Usual Dosage

Contraception: Oral: One tablet daily, beginning on day five of menstrual cycle (first day of menstrual flow is day one). With 20-tablet and 21-tablet packages, new dosing cycle begins seven days after last tablet taken; with 28-tablet packages, dosage is one tablet daily without interruption; extra tablets are placebos or contain iron. If next menstrual period does not begin on schedule, rule out pregnancy before starting new dosing cycle; if menstrual period begins, start new dosing cycle seven days after last tablet was taken; if all doses have been taken on schedule and one menstrual period is missed, continue dosing cycle; if two consecutive menstrual periods are missed, pregnancy test is required before new dosing cycle is started.

Biphasic oral contraceptive (Ortho-Novum™ 10/11): One color tablet daily for 10 days, then next color tablet for 11 days

Triphasic oral contraceptive (Ortho-Novum™ 7/7/7, Tri-Norinyl®, Triphasil®): One tablet daily in the sequence specified by the manufacturer

Ethiodized Oil (eth eye' oh dyzd)
Brand Names Ethiodol®
Use Radiographic exploration for lymphography and hysterosalpingography
Usual Dosage Dose varies with procedure

Ethiodol® see Ethiodized Oil on this page

Ethionamide (e thye on am' ide)
Brand Names Trecator®-SC
Use Used in conjunction with other antituberculosis agents in the treatment of tuberculosis and other mycobacterial diseases
Pregnancy Risk Factor C
Usual Dosage Oral:

Adult: 500-1000 mg/day in 2-4 divided doses

Children: 15-20 mg/kg/day in three divided doses, not to exceed 1 g/day

Ethopropazine Hydrochloride (eth oh proe' pa zeen)
Brand Names Parsidol®
Use Treatment of Parkinsonism, drug induced extrapyramidal reactions, and congenital athetosis
Usual Dosage Adult: Oral: 50-600 mg/day

Ethosuximide (eth oh sux' i mide)
Brand Names Zarontin®
Use Management of absence (petit mal) seizures, myoclonic seizures, and akinetic epilepsy

Pregnancy Risk Factor C
Usual Dosage Oral:

Adult: 250 mg twice daily to start, increase as needed up to 1.5 g/day in two divided doses

Children:
> 6 years: 250 mg twice daily to start, increase as needed up to 1.5 g/day in two divided doses
3-6 years: 20 mg/kg/day in divided doses

Ethotoin
Brand Names Peganone®
Synonyms Ethylphenylhydantoin
Use Generalized tonic-clonic or complex-partial seizures
Pregnancy Risk Factor D
Usual Dosage Oral:

Adult: 250 mg four times a day after meals, may be increased up to 3 g/day in divided doses four times daily

Children: 250 mg twice a day, up to 250 mg four times a day

Ethoxynaphthamido Penicillin Sodium *see* Nafcillin Sodium *on page 244*

Ethrane® *see* Enflurane *on page 130*

Ethril® *see* Erythromycin *on page 134*

Ethyl Aminobenzoate *see* Benzocaine *on page 40*

Ethyl Chloride (eth' il)
Synonyms Chloroethane
Use Local anesthetic in minor operative procedures and to relieve pain caused by insect stings and burns and irritation caused by myofascial and visceral pain syndromes
Pregnancy Risk Factor C
Usual Dosage Dosage varies with use

Ethyl Chloride and Dichlorotetrafluoroethane
Brand Names Fluro-Ethyl®
Synonyms Dichlorotetrafluoroethane and Ethyl Chloride
Use Topical refrigerant anesthetic to control pain associated with minor surgical procedures, dermabrasion, injections, contusions, and minor strains
Pregnancy Risk Factor C
Usual Dosage Press gently on side of spray valve allowing the liquid to emerge as a fine mist approximately 2-4 inches from site of application

Ethylnorepinephrine Hydrochloride (eth il nor ep i nef' rin)
Brand Names Bronkephrine®
Use Bronchial asthma and reversible bronchospasm
Pregnancy Risk Factor C
(Continued)
141

Ethylnorepinephrine Hydrochloride *(Continued)*

Usual Dosage I.M., S.C.:

Adult: 0.5-1 mL

Children: Usually 0.1-0.5 mL

Ethylphenylhydantoin *see* Ethotoin *on previous page*

Ethynodiol and Mestranol *see* Mestranol and Ethynodiol *on page 221*

Ethynodiol Diacetate and Ethinyl Estradiol *see* Ethinyl Estradiol and Ethynodiol Diacetate *on page 139*

Etidocaine Hydrochloride (e ti' doe kane)

Brand Names Duranest®
Use Infiltration anesthesia; peripheral nerve blocks; central neural blocks
Pregnancy Risk Factor B
Usual Dosage Varies with procedure

Etidronate Disodium (e ti droe' nate)

Brand Names Didronel®
Synonyms EHDP; Sodium Etidronate
Use Symptomatic treatment of Paget's disease and heterotopic ossifica-tion due to spinal cord injury or after total hip replacement
Pregnancy Risk Factor B
Usual Dosage Adult: Oral:

Paget's disease: 5 mg/kg/day for no more than six months; may give 10 mg/kg/day for up to three months

Heterotopic ossification with spinal cord injury: 20 mg/kg/day for two weeks, then 10 mg/kg/day for 10 weeks

Heterotopic ossification after total hip replacement: 20 mg/kg/day for four weeks preoperatively and for 12 weeks postoperatively

Etomidate (e tom' i date)

Brand Names Amidate®
Use Induction of general anesthesia
Pregnancy Risk Factor C
Usual Dosage Adult and Children: I.V.: > 10 years of age: 0.2-0.6 mg/kg over period of 30-60 seconds

Etoposide (e toe poe' side)

Brand Names VePesid®
Synonyms EPEG; VP-16
Use Treatment testicular and lung carcinomas
Pregnancy Risk Factor D
Usual Dosage I.V.:

Testicular cancer: 50-100 mg/m^2/day on days 1-5 to 100 mg/m^2/day on days 1, 3 and 5 every 3-4 weeks for 3-4 courses

Infant: Malignant tumor: 3 mg/kg

Children: 50-100 mg/m^2 per protocol

Investigational doses: 80-150 mg/m^2/day per protocol

Etrafon® *see* Amitriptyline and Perphenazine *on page 20*

Etretinate (e tret' i nate)
Brand Names Tegison®
Use Treatment of severe recalcitrant psoriasis in patients intolerant of or unresponsive to standard therapies
Pregnancy Risk Factor X
Usual Dosage Adult: Oral: Individualized - initial 0.75-1 mg/kg/day in divided doses up to 1.5 mg/kg/day; maintenance dose established after 8-10 weeks of therapy 0.5-0.75 mg/kg/day

ETS-2%® *see* Erythromycin, Topical *on page 135*

Eucerin® *see* Emollient Cream *on page 129*

Eulexin® *see* Flutamide *on page 153*

Eurax® *see* Crotamiton *on page 91*

Euthroid® *see* Liotrix *on page 205*

Eutonyl® *see* Pargyline Hydrochloride *on page 270*

Eutron® *see* Methyclothiazide and Pargyline *on page 230*

Evac-Q-Kit® [OTC] *see* Magnesium Citrate, Bisacodyl and Phenolphthalein *on page 210*

Evac-U-Gen® [OTC] *see* Phenolphthalein *on page 280*

Evac-U-Lax® [OTC] *see* Phenolphthalein *on page 280*

Everone® *see* Testosterone *on page 345*

E-Vista® *see* Hydroxyzine *on page 178*

E-Vital® [OTC] *see* Vitamin E *on page 378*

Exelderm® *see* Sulconazole Nitrate *on page 335*

Ex-Lax® [OTC] *see* Phenolphthalein *on page 280*

Eye-Sed® [OTC] *see* Zinc Sulfate *on page 382*

Eye-Zine® [OTC] *see* Tetrahydrozoline Hydrochloride *on page 347*

EZ-Detect® [OTC] *see* Diagnostic Test for Blood in Feces *on page 107*

F₃T *see* Trifluridine *on page 362*

Fact® [OTC] *see* Diagnostic Test for Pregnancy *on page 108*

Factor IX Complex (Human)
Brand Names Konyne®-HT; Profilnine® Heat-Treated; Proplex® SX-T; Proplex® T
Use To control bleeding in patients with Factor IX deficiency (Hemophilia B or Christmas Disease); prevention/control of bleeding in hemophilia A patients with inhibitors to factor VIII a
Pregnancy Risk Factor C
Usual Dosage I.V. only:

Factor IX deficiency: 1 unit/kg raises IX levels 1%
Highly individualized. 75 units/kg ideal body weight; repeat dose in 8-12 hours if necessary
(Continued)

143

Factor IX Complex (Human) *(Continued)*

Anticoagulant overdosage: I.V.: 15 units/kg

units required to raise blood level %: 1 unit/kg x body weight (kg) x desired increase (% of normal)

Factor VIII *see* Antihemophilic Factor, Human *on page 26*

Factrel® *see* Gonadorelin *on page 161*

Famotidine (fa moe' ti deen)

Brand Names Pepcid®

Use Therapy and treatment of duodenal ulcer, active benign ulcer, and pathological hypersecretory conditions

Pregnancy Risk Factor B

Usual Dosage Adult: Oral: 40 mg every day at bedtime for 4-8 weeks, then 20 mg at bedtime; Cl_{cr} < 10 mL/minute dose may have to be reduced to 20 mg at bedtime

Fansidar® *see* Sulfadoxine and Pyrimethamine *on page 337*

Fastin® *see* Phentermine Hydrochloride *on page 280*

Fat Emulsion

Brand Names Intralipid®; Liposyn®; Nutrilipid®; Soyacal®

Synonyms Intravenous Fat Emulsion

Use Source of calories and essential fatty acids for patients requiring parenteral nutrition of extended duration

Pregnancy Risk Factor C

Usual Dosage

Source of calories:

Adult: I.V.: 1 mL/min for 15-30 minutes (10% emulsion), if no adverse reaction occurs increase rate to 500 mL over next 4-6 hours; not to exceed 2.5 g/day

Children: I.V.: 0.1 mL/minute (10%) or 0.05 mL/min (20%) for first 10-15 minutes, if no adverse reaction occurs increase rate to deliver 1 g/kg over four hours, give up to 4 g/kg/day; this should supply 60% of daily caloric intake, protein - carbohydrate should supply the other 40% in TPN therapy. Do not exceed 50 mL/hour (20%) or 100 mL/hour (10%); do not exceed a daily dosage of 4 g/kg.

Fatty acid deficiency: Adult and Children: 8-10% of total caloric intake

Prevention of fatty acid deficiency:

Adult: 500 mL twice weekly at rate of 1 mL/minute for 30 minutes, then increase to 500 mL over 4-6 hours

Children: 5-10 mL/kg/day at 0.1 mL/minute then up to 100 mL/hour

5-FC *see* Flucytosine *on page 149*

Feen-A-Mint® [OTC] *see* Phenolphthalein *on page 280*

Feldene® *see* Piroxicam *on page 287*

Femstat® *see* Butoconazole Nitrate *on page 51*

Fenfluramine Hydrochloride (fen flure' a meen)
Brand Names Pondimin®
Use Short term adjunct in exogenous obesity
Restrictions C-IV
Pregnancy Risk Factor C
Usual Dosage Adult: Oral: 20 mg three times a day before meals or food, up to 40 mg three times daily

Fenoprofen Calcium (fen oh proe' fen)
Brand Names Nalfon®
Use Symptomatic treatment of acute and chronic rheumatoid arthritis and osteoarthritis; relief of mild to moderate pain
Pregnancy Risk Factor B/D
Usual Dosage Oral:

Adult:
Arthritis: 300-600 mg 3-4 times a day up to 3.2 g/day
Pain: 200 mg every 4-6 hours as needed

Children: Juvenile arthritis: 900 mg/m²/day, then increase over four weeks to 1.8 g/m²/day

Fentanyl and Droperidol see Droperidol and Fentanyl
on page 124

Fentanyl Citrate (fen' ta nil)
Brand Names Sublimaze®
Use As analgesic adjunct given in incremental doses in maintenance of anesthesia with barbiturate or NO_2 or a primary anesthetic agent for the induction of anesthesia in patients undergoing general surgery in which endotracheal intubation and mechanical ventilation are required
Restrictions C-II
Pregnancy Risk Factor C
Usual Dosage

Adult:
Sedation for minor procedures/analgesia: > 12 years of age: 0.5-1 μg/kg/dose;may repeat after 30-60 minutes
Preoperative, adjunct to regional anesthesia, postoperative; I.M., I.V.: 50-100 μg
Adjunct to general anesthesia: I.M., I.V.: 2-50 μg/kg
Provide general anesthesia without additional anesthetic agents: I.V. 50-100 μg/kg in conjunction with O_2 and a skeletal muscle relaxant

Children:
Sedation for minor procedures/analgesia: I.M., I.V.: 1-3 years: 2-3 μg/kg/dose; may repeat after 30-60 minutes; 3-12 years: 1-2 μg/kg/dose; may repeat after 30-60 minutes
Continuous analgesia: 1-3 μg/kg/hour

Feosol® [OTC] see Ferrous Sulfate on next page
Feosol® Spansules® [OTC] see Ferrous Sulfate on next page
Fergon® see Ferrous Gluconate on next page

Fer-In-Sol® [OTC] *see* Ferrous Sulfate *on this page*

Fermycin® Soluble *see* Chlortetracyline Hydrochloride
on page 77

Fero-Grad 500® [OTC] *see* Ferrous Sulfate and Ascorbic Acid
on this page

Ferro-Sequels® [OTC] *see* Ferrous Fumarate *on this page*

Ferrous Fumarate (fyoo' ma rate)
Brand Names Ferro-Sequels® [OTC]
Use Prevention and treatment of iron deficiency anemias
Pregnancy Risk Factor A
Usual Dosage

Adult: 200 mg 3-4 times a day

Children: 3 mg/kg three times a day

Ferrous Gluconate (gloo' koe nate)
Brand Names Fergon®
Use Prevention and treatment of iron deficiency anemias
Pregnancy Risk Factor A
Usual Dosage Oral:

Adult: 200 mg 3-4 times a day

Children: 3 mg/kg three times a day

Ferrous Sulfate
Brand Names Feosol® [OTC]; Feosol® Spansules® [OTC]; Fer-In-Sol®
[OTC]
Use Prevention and treatment of iron deficiency anemias
Pregnancy Risk Factor A
Usual Dosage Oral:

Adult: 200 mg 3-4 times a day

Children: 3 mg/kg three times a day

Ferrous Sulfate and Ascorbic Acid
Brand Names Fero-Grad 500® [OTC]
Synonyms Ascorbic Acid and Ferrous Sulfate
Use Treatment of iron deficiency in nonpregnant adults; treatment and
prevention of iron deficiency in pregnant adults
Pregnancy Risk Factor A
Usual Dosage Adult: Oral: One tablet daily

Ferrous Sulfate, Ascorbic Acid, and Vitamin B-Complex
Brand Names Iberet®-Liquid [OTC]
Use Conditions of iron deficiency with an increased needed for B-complex
vitamins and vitamin C
Pregnancy Risk Factor A

Usual Dosage Oral:

Adult and Children: > 4 years: 10 mL three times daily after meals
Children: 1-3 years: 5 mL twice daily after meals

Ferrous Sulfate, Ascorbic Acid, Vitamin B-Complex and Folic Acid

Brand Names Iberet-Folic-500®

Use Treatment of iron deficiency and prevention of concomitant folic acid deficiency where there is an associated deficient intake or increased need for B-complex vitamins

Pregnancy Risk Factor A

Usual Dosage Adult: Oral : One tablet daily

Festal®II [OTC] *see* Pancrelipase *on page 267*

Fevernol™ [OTC] *see* Acetaminophen *on page 4*

FiberCon® [OTC] *see* Calcium Polycarbophil *on page 55*

Fibrinolysin and Desoxyribonuclease (fye bri noe lye' sin)

Brand Names Elase®; Elase-Chloromycetin®

Synonyms Desoxyribonuclease and Fibrinolysin

Use Debriding agent; cervicitis; and irrigating agent in infected wounds

Pregnancy Risk Factor C

Usual Dosage

Ointment: 2-3 times daily
Wet dressing: 3-4 times daily

Fioricet® *see* Butalbital Compound *on page 51*

Fiorinal® *see* Butalbital Compound *on page 51*

Fiorinal® With Codeine *see* Butalbital and Codeine Compound *on page 51*

First Response® [OTC] *see* Diagnostic Test for Pregnancy *on page 108*

First Response® Ovulation Predictor [OTC] *see* Diagnostic Test for Ovulation *on page 107*

Fisalamine *see* Mesalamine *on page 220*

Flagyl® *see* Metronidazole *on page 234*

Flavorcee® [OTC] *see* Ascorbic Acid *on page 29*

Flavoxate (fla vox' ate)

Brand Names Urispas®

Use An antispasmodic to provide symptomatic relief of dysuria, nocturia, suprapubic pain, urgency, and incontinence

Pregnancy Risk Factor B

Usual Dosage Adult and Children: > 12 years: 100-200 mg 3-4 times daily

Flaxedil® *see* Gallamine Triethiodide *on page 155*

Flecainide Acetate (fle kay' nide)
Brand Names Tambocor®
Use Controlling supraventricular tachycardias in infants and children; prevention and suppression of documented life-threatening ventricular arrhythmias (ie, sustained ventricular tachycardia), symptomatic nonsustained ventricular tachycardia, frequent premature ventricular complexes (PVCs), uniform and multiform PVCs and or coupled PVCs
Pregnancy Risk Factor C
Usual Dosage 50-100 mg every 12 hours up to 400-600 mg until response is obtained

Fleet® Babylax® [OTC] see Glycerin on page 159

Fleet® Bisacodyl Prep [OTC] see Bisacodyl on page 45

Fleet® Enema [OTC] see Sodium Phosphate on page 329

Fleet® Mineral Oil Enema [OTC] see Mineral Oil on page 237

Fleet® Phospho®-Soda [OTC] see Sodium Phosphate on page 329

Flexeril® see Cyclobenzaprine Hydrochloride on page 93

Flint SSD® see Silver Sulfadiazine on page 324

Florinef® Acetate see Fludrocortisone Acetate on next page

Florone® see Diflorasone Diacetate on page 113

Floropryl® see Isoflurophate on page 192

Floxuridine (flox yoor' i deen)
Brand Names FUDR®
Synonyms Fluorodeoxyuridine
Use Palliative management of carcinomas of head, neck, and brain as well as liver, gallbladder, and bile ducts
Pregnancy Risk Factor C
Usual Dosage Intra-artery: 0.1-0.6 mg/kg/day

Fluconazole (floo koe' na zole)
Brand Names Diflucan®
Use Treatment of oropharyngeal and esophageal candidiasis; treatment of systemic candidal infections including urinary tract infection, peritonitis, and pneumonia; treatment of cryptococcal meningitis
Restrictions Restricted level 3
Pregnancy Risk Factor C

Indication	Day 1	Daily Therapy	Minimum Duration of Therapy
Oropharyngeal candidiasis	200 mg	100 mg	14 d
Esophageal candidiasis	200 mg	100 mg	21 d
Systemic candidiasis	400 mg	200 mg	28 d
Cryptococcal meningitis acute	400 mg	200 mg	10–12 wk after CSF culture becomes negative
relapse	200 mg	200 mg	

Usual Dosage The daily dose of fluconazole is the same for oral and intravenous administration

Efficacy of fluconazole has not been established in children; a small number of patients from age 3-13 years have been treated with fluconazole using doses of 3-6 mg/kg/day

Adult doses of fluconazole: Oral, I.V. once daily: See table.

Flucytosine (floo sye' toe seen)
Brand Names Ancobon®
Synonyms 5-FC; 5-Flurocytosine
Use Treatment of susceptible fungal infections, usually of the *Candida* or *Cryptococcus* strains

Pregnancy Risk Factor C
Usual Dosage Oral: 50-150 mg/kg/day in divided doses every 6 hours; for patients with renal impairment, the dosage interval needs to be increased to every 12 hours for > 50% decrease in renal function or every 24 hours for > 90% decrease in renal function

Fludrocortisone Acetate (floo droe kor' ti sone)
Brand Names Florinef® Acetate
Synonyms Fluohydrisone Acetate; Fluohydrocortisone Acetate; 9α-Fluorohydrocortisone Acetate
Use Addison's disease; partial replacement therapy for adrenal insufficiency and for treatment of salt losing forms of congenital adrenogenital syndrome
Pregnancy Risk Factor C
Usual Dosage Oral:

Adult: 0.1-0.2 mg daily

Children: 0.05-0.1 mg daily

Flunisolide (floo niss' oh lide)
Brand Names AeroBid®; Nasalide®
Use Steroid-dependent asthma; nasal solution is used for seasonal or perennial rhinitis
Pregnancy Risk Factor C
Usual Dosage

Adult:
Oral: Two inhalations twice a day up to eight inhalations/day
Nasal: 2 sprays each nostril twice a day to a maximum dosage of 8 sprays in each nostril per day

Children:
Oral: > 6 years of age: One inhalation twice a day up to four inhalations daily
Nasal: 6-14 years: 1 spray each nostril 2-3 times/day, not to exceed 4 sprays each nostril per day

Fluocinolone Acetonide (floo oh sin' oh lone)
Brand Names Fluonid®; Synalar®; Synemol®
Use Relief of susceptible inflammatory dermatosis
Pregnancy Risk Factor C
Usual Dosage Apply 2-4 times daily

Fluocinonide (floo oh sin' oh nide)
Brand Names Lidex®; Lidex® E
Use Anti-inflammatory, antipruritic, relief of inflammatory and pruritic manifestations
Pregnancy Risk Factor C
Usual Dosage Apply thin layer of ointment, cream or gel to affected area 3-4 times a day

Fluogen® *see* Influenza Virus Vaccine *on page 185*

Fluohydrisone Acetate *see* Fludrocortisone Acetate *on previous page*

Fluohydrocortisone Acetate *see* Fludrocortisone Acetate *on previous page*

Fluonid® *see* Fluocinolone Acetonide *on this page*

Fluoracaine® *see* Proparacaine With Fluorescein *on page 303*

Fluorescein Sodium (flure' e seen)
Brand Names Fluorescite®; Fluor-I-Strips®
Use Demonstrates defects of corneal epithelium; diagnostic aid in ophthalmic angiography
Pregnancy Risk Factor C
Usual Dosage Moisten strip with sterile water or irrigating solution, touch conjunctiva with moistened tip, blink several times after application

Fluorescite® *see* Fluorescein Sodium *on this page*

Fluoride
Brand Names Luride®; Luride®-SF F Lozi-Tabs®; Pediaflor®
Use Prevention of dental caries; treating osteoporosis and relieve bone pain in some neoplastic bone diseases
Pregnancy Risk Factor C
Usual Dosage Adult: Osteoporosis: Oral: Up to 60 mg/day; 2.2 mg of sodium fluoride is equivalent to 1 mg of fluoride. See table.

Fluoride Content of Drinking Water	Daily Dose, Oral (mg)
< 0.3 ppm Birth – 2 y	0.25–0.5
2–3 y	0.5
3–12 y	1
0.3–0.7 ppm Birth – 2 y	0.13
2–3 y	0.25
3–12 y	0.25–0.75

Fluori-Methane® *see* Dichlorodifluoromethane and Trichloromonofluoromethane *on page 110*

Fluor-I-Strips® *see* Fluorescein Sodium *on previous page*

Fluorodeoxyuridine *see* Floxuridine *on page 148*

Fluorometholone (flure oh meth' oh lone)
Brand Names FML®

Use Inflammatory conditions of the eye, including keratitis, iritis, cyclitis, and conjunctivitis

Pregnancy Risk Factor C

Usual Dosage 1-2 drops into conjunctival sac every hour during day, every two hours at night until favorable response is obtained, then use one drop every four hours; in mild or moderate inflammation: 1-2 drops into conjunctival sac 2-4 times/day. Ointment may be applied every 4 hours in severe cases or 1-3 times daily in mild to moderate cases.

Fluoroplex® *see* Fluorouracil *on this page*

Fluorouracil (flure oh yoor' a sill)
Brand Names Adrucil®; Efudex®; Fluoroplex®

Synonyms 5-Fluorouracil; 5-FU

Use Treatment of colon, breast, rectal, gastric, and pancreatic carcinomas; also used topically for management of multiple actinic keratoses

Pregnancy Risk Factor C

Usual Dosage Do not mix with I.V. additives or other chemotherapeutic agents; daily dosage must not exceed 800 mg regardless of patient's weight

Adult: I.V.: 12 mg/kg/day for 1-4 days, then 6 mg/kg every other day for four doses

Children: I.V. 50 mg/m^2 per protocol

5-Fluorouracil *see* Fluorouracil *on this page*

Fluostigmin *see* Isoflurophate *on page 192*

Fluothane® *see* Halothane *on page 166*

Fluoxetine Hydrochloride (floo ox' e teen)
Brand Names Prozac®

Use Treatment of depression in patients whose diagnosis are in the DSM lll category

Pregnancy Risk Factor C

Usual Dosage Oral: 20 mg/day in the morning up to 80 mg/day

Fluoxymesterone (floo ox i mes' te rone)
Brand Names Android-F®; Halotestin®; Ora-Testryl®
Use Replacement of endogenous testicular hormone; in female used as palliative treatment of breast cancer, postpartum breast engorgement
Pregnancy Risk Factor X
Usual Dosage Adult: Oral:

Male:
Hypogonadism: 5-20 mg/day
Delayed puberty: 2.5-20 mg/day for 4-6 months

Female:
Breast carcinoma: 10-40 mg/day in divided doses
Breast engorgement: 2.5 mg after delivery, 5-10 mg/day in divided doses for 4-5 days

Fluoxymesterone and Estradiol *see* Estradiol and Fluoxymesterone *on page 136*

Fluphenazine (floo fen' a zeen)
Brand Names Prolixin®; Prolixin Decanoate®; Prolixin Enanthate®
Synonyms Fluphenazine Decanoate; Fluphenazine Enanthate; Fluphenazine Hydrochloride
Use Management of manifestations of psychotic disorders
Pregnancy Risk Factor C
Usual Dosage Adult:
Oral: 0.5-10 mg/day
I.M.: 2.5-10 mg/day
I.M., S.C. (Decanoate®): 12.5 mg every three weeks
I.M., S.C. (Enanthate®): 12.5-25 mg every three weeks

Fluphenazine Decanoate *see* Fluphenazine *on this page*
Fluphenazine Enanthate *see* Fluphenazine *on this page*
Fluphenazine Hydrochloride *see* Fluphenazine *on this page*

Flurandrenolide (flure an dren' oh lide)
Brand Names Cordran®
Synonyms Flurandrenolone
Use Inflammation of corticosteroid-responsive dermatoses
Pregnancy Risk Factor C
Usual Dosage

Adult: Cream, lotion, ointment: Apply 2-3 times daily

Children:
Ointment or cream: Apply 1-2 times daily
Tape: Apply once daily

Flurandrenolone *see* Flurandrenolide *on this page*

Flurazepam Hydrochloride (flure az' e pam)
Brand Names Dalmane®
Use Short-term treatment of insomnia
Restrictions C-IV

Pregnancy Risk Factor D
Usual Dosage Adult: Oral: 15-30 mg at bedtime

Flurbiprofen Sodium (flure bi' proe fen)
Brand Names Ansaid®; Ocufen® Liquifilm®
Use For inhibition of intraoperative miosis; acute or long term treatment of signs of symptoms of rheumatoid arthritis and osteoarthritis
Pregnancy Risk Factor C
Usual Dosage
    Ophthalmic: One drop every 30 minutes, two hours prior to surgery
    Oral: Adult: 200-300 mg daily in divided doses 2, 3 or 4 times daily

5-Flurocytosine see Flucytosine on page 149

Fluro-Ethyl® see Ethyl Chloride and Dichlorotetrafluoroethane on page 141

Flutamide (floo' ta mide)
Brand Names Eulexin®
Use In combination therapy in treatment of metastatic prostatic carcinoma
Pregnancy Risk Factor D
Usual Dosage Oral: Two capsules every eight hours

Fluzone® see Influenza Virus Vaccine on page 185

FML® see Fluorometholone on page 151

Foille Plus® [OTC] see Benzocaine on page 40

Folacin see Folic Acid on this page

Folate see Folic Acid on this page

Folex® see Methotrexate on page 227

Folic Acid (foe' lik)
Brand Names Folvite®
Synonyms Folacin; Folate; Pteroylglutamic Acid
Use Treatment of megaloblastic and macrocytic anemias due to folate deficiency
Pregnancy Risk Factor A/C
Usual Dosage
    Adult:
        Oral, I.M., I.V., S.C.: 1 mg/day initial dosage
        Maintenance dose: 0.4 mg/day; pregnant and lactating women: 0.8 mg/day
    Children:
        Oral, I.M., I.V., S.C.: 1 mg/day initial dosage
        Maintenance dose: > 4 years of age: 0.4 mg/day
    Infant: 0.1 mg/day

Folinic Acid see Leucovorin Calcium on page 200

Follutein® see Chorionic Gonadotropin on page 78

Folvite® see Folic Acid on previous page

Footwork® [OTC] see Tolnaftate on page 357

Forane® see Isoflurane on page 192

5-Formyl Tetrahydrofolate see Leucovorin Calcium
on page 200

Fortal® see Pentazocine on page 275

Fortaz® see Ceftazidime on page 64

Fortel® Ovulation Test [OTC] see Diagnostic Test for Ovulation
on page 107

Fostex® [OTC] see Sulfur and Salicylic Acid on page 339

Fototar® [OTC] see Coal Tar on page 85

Fructose
Synonyms Fruit Sugar; Levulose
Use Source of calories and water for hydration
Pregnancy Risk Factor C
Usual Dosage Dosage depends on caloric needs; 1000 mL of 10% solution yields 375 calories

Fruit Sugar see Fructose on this page

Frusemide see Furosemide on next page

5-FU see Fluorouracil on page 151

FUDR® see Floxuridine on page 148

Fulvicin® P/G see Griseofulvin on page 161

Fulvicin-U/F® see Griseofulvin on page 161

Fungatin® [OTC] see Tolnaftate on page 357

Fungizone® see Amphotericin B on page 23

Furacin® see Nitrofurazone on page 253

Furadantin® see Nitrofurantoin on page 253

Furazolidone (fur a zoe' li done)
Brand Names Furoxone®
Use Treatment of bacterial or protozoal diarrhea and enteritis caused by susceptible organisms
Pregnancy Risk Factor C
Usual Dosage Oral:

Adult: 100 mg four times/day

Children:
5-12 years of age: 100 mg four times/day
1-4 years: 17-25 mg four times/day
1 month - 1 year: 8-17 mg four times/day

Furazosin see Prazosin Hydrochloride on page 293

Furomide® see Furosemide on next page

Furosemide (fur oh' se mide)
Brand Names Furomide®; Lasix®
Synonyms Frusemide
Use Management of edema associated with congestive heart failure and hepatic or renal disease; used alone or in combination with antihypertensives in treatment of hypertension
Pregnancy Risk Factor C
Usual Dosage Oral, I.M., I.V.:

Adult: 20-80 mg/day up to 600 mg/day

Children: 1-2 mg/kg/day up to 6 mg/kg/day

Furoxone® see Furazolidone on previous page

Gallamine Triethiodide (gal' a meen)
Brand Names Flaxedil®
Use Produce skeletal muscle relaxation during surgery after general anesthesia has been induced
Pregnancy Risk Factor C
Usual Dosage I.V.: 1 mg/kg then repeat dose of 0.5-1 mg/kg in 30-40 minutes for prolonged procedures

Gamastan® see Immune Globulin on page 183

Gamimune® N see Immune Globulin on page 183

Gamma Benzene Hexachloride see Lindane on page 204

Gammagard® see Immune Globulin on page 183

Gamma Globulin see Immune Globulin on page 183

Gammar® see Immune Globulin on page 183

Gamulin® Rh see Rho(D) Immune Globulin on page 315

Ganciclovir (gan sye' kloe vir)
Brand Names Cytovene®
Synonyms DHPG Sodium; GCV Sodium; Nordeoxyguanosine
Use CMV retinitis treatment of immunocompromised individuals, including patients with acquired immunodeficiency syndrome; investigational use in treatment of CMV pneumonia in marrow transplant recipients has not been rewarding, promising results have been achieved in AIDS patients and organ transplant recipients with CMV colitis, pneumonitis, and multiorgan involvement
Pregnancy Risk Factor C
Usual Dosage Initial dose for patients with normal renal function is 5 mg/kg (given I.V. at a constant rate of one hour) every 12 hours for 14-21 days

Gantanol® see Sulfamethoxazole on page 337

Gantrisin® see Sulfisoxazole on page 339

Garamycin® see Gentamicin Sulfate on page 157

Gastrografin® *see* Sodium Diatrizoate and Meglumine Diatrizoate
on page 328

Gastrosed™ *see* Hyoscyamine Sulfate *on page 180*

Gas-X® [OTC] *see* Simethicone *on page 324*

Gaviscon® Foamtabs [OTC] *see* Aluminum Hydroxide,
Magnesium Trisilicate, Sodium Bicarbonate and Alginic Acid
on page 15

GCV Sodium *see* Ganciclovir *on previous page*

Gelatin, Absorbable
Brand Names Gelfoam® [OTC]
Synonyms Absorbable gelatin sponge
Use As an adjunct to provide hemostasis in surgery; also used in oral and
dental surgery; in open prostatic surgery
Usual Dosage Hemostasis: Apply packs or sponges dry or saturated
with sodium chloride. When applied dry, hold in place with moderate
pressure. When applied wet, squeeze to remove air bubbles. Prostatec-
tomy cones are designed for use with the Foley bag catheter. The powder is applied as a paste prepared by adding about 4 mL of sterile saline
solution to the powder.

Gelatin, Pectin and Methylcellulose
Brand Names Orabase® Plain [OTC]
Use For temporary relief from minor oral irritations
Usual Dosage Press small dabs into place until the involved area is coat-
ed with a thin film; do not try to spread onto area; may be used as often
as needed

Gelfoam® [OTC] *see* Gelatin, Absorbable *on this page*

Gelucast® *see* Zinc Gelatin *on page 382*

Gelusil® [OTC] *see* Aluminum Hydroxide, Magnesium Hydroxide
and Simethicone *on page 15*

Gemfibrozil (jem fi' broe zil)
Brand Names Lopid®
Synonyms CI-719
Use Hypertriglyceridemia in types IV and V hyperlipidemia; increases HDL
cholesterol
Pregnancy Risk Factor B
Usual Dosage 1200 mg/day in two divided doses, 30 minutes before
breakfast and supper

Gemonil® *see* Metharbital *on page 225*

Genabid® *see* Papaverine Hydrochloride *on page 268*

Genagesic® *see* Propoxyphene and Acetaminophen
on page 304

Genapax® *see* Gentian Violet *on next page*

Genasal® Nasal Solution [OTC] *see* Oxymetazoline Hydrochloride *on page 265*

Genaspor® [OTC] *see* Tolnaftate *on page 357*

Genatuss® [OTC] *see* Guaifenesin *on page 162*

Generlac® *see* Lactulose *on page 199*

Genoptic® *see* Gentamicin Sulfate *on this page*

Genpril® [OTC] *see* Ibuprofen *on page 181*

Gentacidin® *see* Gentamicin Sulfate *on this page*

Gentafair® *see* Gentamicin Sulfate *on this page*

Gentak® *see* Gentamicin Sulfate *on this page*

Gentamicin and Prednisolone *see* Prednisolone and Gentamicin *on page 295*

Gentamicin Sulfate (jen ta mye' sin)
Brand Names Garamycin®; Genoptic®; Gentacidin®; Gentafair®; Gentak®; Gentrasul®; I-Gent®; Ocumycin®
Use Treatment of susceptible bacterial infections, normally gram-negative *Bacillus* and *Staphylococcus*; treatment of bone infections, CNS infections, respiratory tract infections, skin and soft tissue infections, as well as abdominal and urinary tract infections, endocarditis, and septicemia
Pregnancy Risk Factor C
Usual Dosage

Adult:
    I.M., I.V.: 3-5 mg/kg/day in divided doses every eight hours
    Topical: Apply 3-4 times daily
    Ophthalmic: Solution: 1-2 drops every 2-4 hours; ointment: 2-3 times daily

Children:
    I.M., I.V.: 6-7.5 mg/kg/day in divided doses every eight hours; infusion should be over a period of 30 minutes to two hours
    Topical: Apply 3-4 times daily
    Ophthalmic: Solution: 1-2 drops every 2-4 hours; ointment: 2-3 times daily; peak and trough serum concentrate should be determined periodically

Infant and Neonate: I.M., I.V.: 7.5 mg/kg/day

Premature Infant and Neonate: < 1 week: I.M., I.V.: 2.5 mg/kg every 12 hours

Gentian Violet (jen' shun)
Brand Names Genapax®
Synonyms Crystal Violet; Methylrosaniline Chloride
Use Treatment of cutaneous or mucocutaneous infections caused by *Candida albicans* and other superficial skin infections
Pregnancy Risk Factor C
Usual Dosage Apply with cotton to lesion 2-3 times daily for three days; do not swallow

Gentle Nature® [OTC] *see* Senna *on page 322*

Gentran® *see* Dextran *on page 103*

Gentrasul® *see* Gentamicin Sulfate *on previous page*

Geocillin® *see* Carbenicillin *on page 58*

Geopen® *see* Carbenicillin *on page 58*

Geridium® *see* Phenazopyridine Hydrochloride *on page 278*

Germinal® *see* Ergoloid Mesylates *on page 133*

Gesterol® *see* Progesterone *on page 299*

Gesterol® L.A. *see* Hydroxyprogesterone Caproate *on page 177*

Gevrabon® [OTC] *see* Vitamin B Complex *on page 377*

GG *see* Guaifenesin *on page 162*

GG-Cen® [OTC] *see* Guaifenesin *on page 162*

Glibenclamide *see* Glyburide *on next page*

Glipizide (glip' i zide)
Brand Names Glucotrol®
Synonyms Glydiazinamide
Use Management of noninsulin-dependent diabetes mellitus (type II)
Pregnancy Risk Factor C
Usual Dosage Adult: Oral: 2.5-40 mg/day; doses larger than 15-20 mg/day should be divided and given twice daily

Glucagon (gloo' ka gon)
Use Hypoglycemia; diagnostic aid in the radiologic examination of GI tract when a hypnotic state is needed; used with some success as a cardiac stimulant in management of severe cases of beta-adrenergic blocking agent overdosage
Pregnancy Risk Factor B
Usual Dosage

Adult:
Hypoglycemia: I.M., I.V., S.C.: 0.5-1 mg may repeat, 1-2 times
Insulin shock therapy: I.M., I.V., S.C., after coma of one hour: 0.5-1 mg, may repeat dose once
Diagnostic aid: I.M., I.V.: 0.25-2 mg 10 minutes prior to procedure

Children: I.M., I.V., S.C.: 1.10 units/vial; dose → 0.5-1 unit

Glucose *see* Dextrose in Water *on page 105*

Glucose, Instant (gloo' kose)
Brand Names Glutose® [OTC]
Use Management of hypoglycemia
Usual Dosage Oral: 10-20 g

Glucostix® [OTC] *see* Diagnostic Test for Glucose in Blood *on page 107*

Glucotrol® *see* Glipizide *on previous page*

Glukor® *see* Chorionic Gonadotropin *on page 78*

Glutamic Acid Hydrochloride (gloo tam' ik)
Brand Names Acidulin® [OTC]
Use Treatment of hypochlorhydria and achlorhydria
Pregnancy Risk Factor C
Usual Dosage Adult: Oral: 340 mg - 1.02 g three times a day before meals or food

Glutethimide (gloo teth' i mide)
Brand Names Doriden®
Use Short term treatment of insomnia
Restrictions C-III
Pregnancy Risk Factor C
Usual Dosage Oral:

Adult: 250-500 mg at bedtime, dose may be repeated but not less than four hours before intended awakening; up to 1 g daily dose

Elderly/debilitated patients: Total daily dose should not exceed 500 mg

Glutose® [OTC] *see* Glucose, Instant *on previous page*

Glyate® *see* Guaifenesin *on page 162*

Glyburide (glye' byoor ide)
Brand Names Diaβeta®; Micronase®
Synonyms Glibenclamide
Use Management of noninsulin-dependent diabetes mellitus (type II)
Pregnancy Risk Factor B
Usual Dosage Oral: 2.5-5 mg to start then 1.25-20 mg maintenance dose

Glycerin (gli' ser in)
Brand Names Fleet® Babylax® [OTC]; Ophthalgan®; Osmoglyn®
Synonyms Glycerol
Use Constipation; reduction of intraocular pressure; reduction of corneal edema
Pregnancy Risk Factor C
Usual Dosage

Constipation:
Adult and Children: > 6 years of age: 2-3 g as a suppository or 5-15 mL as an enema
Children: < 6 years of age: 1-1.5 g as a suppository or 2-5 mL as an enema
Neonate: 0.5 mL/kg/dose

Reduction of intraocular pressure: Adult: Oral: 1-1.8 g/kg 1-1.5 hours pre-operatively

Reduction of corneal edema: 1-2 drops in eye(s) every 3-4 hours; ophthalmic administration may cause pain/irritation; apply a topical anesthetic before administration of glycerin

Glycerin, Lanolin and Peanut Oil
Brand Names Massé® Breast Cream [OTC]
Use Nipple care of pregnant and nursing women
Usual Dosage Apply as often as needed

Glycerol *see* Glycerin *on previous page*

Glyceryl Guaiacolate *see* Guaifenesin *on page 162*

Glyceryl Trinitrate *see* Nitroglycerin *on page 253*

Glycopyrrolate (glye koe pye' roe late)
Brand Names Robinul®
Synonyms Glycopyrronium Bromide
Use Management of peptic ulcer disease; inhibit salivation and excessive secretions in respiratory tract preoperatively
Pregnancy Risk Factor B
Usual Dosage

Adult:
　Peptic ulcer: Oral: 1-2 mg 2-3 times daily; I.M., I.V.: 0.1-0.2 mg 3-4 times daily
　Preoperative: I.M.: 4.4 μg/kg 30-60 minutes before procedure

Children: Preoperative: I.M.:
　> 2 years: 4.4 μg/kg 30-60 minutes before procedure
　< 2 years: 4.4-8.8 μg/kg 30-60 minutes before procedure

Glycopyrronium Bromide *see* Glycopyrrolate *on this page*

Glycotuss® [OTC] *see* Guaifenesin *on page 162*

Glydiazinamide *see* Glipizide *on page 158*

Gly-Oxide® [OTC] *see* Carbamide Peroxide *on page 58*

Glytuss® [OTC] *see* Guaifenesin *on page 162*

Gold Sodium Thiomalate
Brand Names Myochrysine®
Use Treatment of progressive rheumatoid arthritis
Pregnancy Risk Factor C
Usual Dosage

Adult: I.M.: 10 mg first week; 25 mg 2nd week; then 25-50 mg weekly until 1 g cumulative dose has been given. If improvement occurs without adverse reactions, give 25-50 mg every 2-3 weeks, then every 3-4 weeks.

Children: I.M.: Initial: 0.25 mg/kg/dose first week; increment 0.25 mg/kg/dose, increasing with each weekly dose; maintenance: 0.75-1 mg/kg/dose weekly not to exceed 25 mg/dose to a total of 20 doses, then every 2-4 weeks

GoLYTELY® *see* Polyethylene Glycol-Electrolyte Solution *on page 290*

Gonadorelin (goe nad oh rell' in)
Brand Names Factrel®
Use Evaluation of the functional capacity and response of gonadotrophic hormones
Pregnancy Risk Factor B
Usual Dosage Adult and Children: > 12 years of age: I.V., S.C.: 100 µg, administered in women during early phase of menstrual cycle (day 1-7)

Gonak® [OTC] *see* Hydroxypropyl Methylcellulose *on page 178*

Gonic® *see* Chorionic Gonadotropin *on page 78*

Goniosol® [OTC] *see* Hydroxypropyl Methylcellulose *on page 178*

Gramicidin, Neomycin and Polymyxin B (gram i si' din)
Brand Names Neosporin® Ophthalmic Solution
Use Treatment of superficial ocular infection, infection prophylaxis in minor skin abrasions
Pregnancy Risk Factor C
Usual Dosage Ophthalmic: Drops: 1-2 drops 4-6 times daily

Granulex
Use Treatment of decubitus ulcers, varicose ulcers, debridement of eschar, dehiscent wounds and sunburn
Usual Dosage Apply a minimum of twice daily or as often as necessary

Grifulvin V® *see* Griseofulvin *on this page*

Grisactin® *see* Griseofulvin *on this page*

Grisactin® Ultra *see* Griseofulvin *on this page*

Griseofulvin (gri see oh ful' vin)
Brand Names Fulvicin® P/G; Fulvicin-U/F®; Grifulvin V®; Grisactin®; Grisactin® Ultra; Gris-PEG®
Synonyms Griseofulvin Microsize; Griseofulvin Ultramicrosize
Use Treatment of susceptible tinea infections of the skin, hair, and nails
Pregnancy Risk Factor C
Usual Dosage Oral:

Adult:
Microsize: 500-1000 mg/day in single or divided doses
Ultramicrosize: 330-375 mg/day in single or divided doses

Children:
Microsize: 10-11 mg/kg/day in single or divided doses
Ultramicrosize: > 2 years of age: 7.3 mg/kg/day in single or divided doses

Griseofulvin Microsize *see* Griseofulvin *on this page*

Griseofulvin Ultramicrosize *see* Griseofulvin *on this page*

Gris-PEG® *see* Griseofulvin *on this page*

Guaifenesin (gwye fen' e sin)

Brand Names Amonidrin® [OTC]; Breonesin® [OTC]; Cremacoat®2 [OTC]; Genatuss® [OTC]; GG-Cen® [OTC]; Glyate®; Glycotuss® [OTC]; Glytuss® [OTC]; Guaituss® [OTC]; Humibid® L.A.; Humibid® Sprinkle; Hytuss® [OTC]; Hytuss-2X® [OTC]; Malotuss® [OTC]; Medi-Tuss® [OTC]; Mytussin® [OTC]; Naldecon® Senior EX [OTC]; Nortussin® [OTC]; Robafen® [OTC]; Robitussin® [OTC]

Synonyms GG; Glyceryl Guaiacolate

Use Temporary control of cough due to minor throat and bronchial irritation

Pregnancy Risk Factor C

Usual Dosage

Adult and Children: > 12 years of age: Oral: 200-400 mg (10-20 mL) every 4 hours to a maximum of 2.4 g/day

Children: Oral:

6-11 years: 100-200 mg (5-10 mL) every 4 hours, not to exceed 1.2 g/day

2-5 years: 50-100 mg (2.5-5 mL) every 4 hours, not to exceed 600 mg/day

< 2 years: 12 mg/kg/day in 6 divided doses

Guaifenesin and Codeine

Brand Names Robitussin® A-C

Synonyms Codeine and Guaifenesin

Use Temporary control of cough due to minor throat and bronchial irritation

Restrictions C-V

Pregnancy Risk Factor C

Usual Dosage Oral:

Adult: 10 mL every 6-8 hours

Children:

> 12 years of age: 10 mL every four hours, up to 60 mL in a 24-hour period

6-12 years: 5 mL every four hours, not to exceed 30 mL in a 24-hour period

Guaifenesin and Dextromethorphan

Brand Names Robitussin-DM® [OTC]

Synonyms Dextromethorphan and Guaifenesin

Use Temporary control of cough due to minor throat and bronchial irritation

Pregnancy Risk Factor C

Usual Dosage Oral:

Adult: 10 mL every 6-8 hours

Children:

> 12 years: 10 mL every 6-8 hours

6-12 years: 5 mL every 6-8 hours; alternatively 6-11 years: 100-200 mg every four hours, not to exceed 1.25 daily

2-5 years: 50-100 mg every four hours, not to exceed 600 mg daily

Guaifenesin and Hydrocodone *see* Hydrocodone and Guaifenesin *on page 173*

Guaifenesin and Phenylpropanolamine
Brand Names Entex® LA; Triaminic® Expectorant [OTC]
Synonyms Phenylpropanolamine and Guaifenesin
Use Symptomatic relief of those respiratory conditions where tenacious mucous plugs and congestion complicate the problem such as sinusitis, pharyngitis, bronchitis, asthma, and as an adjunctive therapy in serous otitis media
Pregnancy Risk Factor C
Usual Dosage Oral:

Adult and Children: > 12 years of age: One tablet every 12 hours or 10 mL every four hours

Children:
6-12 years of age: 1/2 tablet every 12 hours or 5 mL every four hours
2-6 years: 2.5 mL every four hours

Guaifenesin and Pseudoephedrine
Brand Names Robitussin-PE® [OTC]
Synonyms Pseudoephedrine and Guaifenesin
Use Enhance the output of respiratory tract fluid and reduce mucosal congestion and edema in the nasal passage
Pregnancy Risk Factor C
Usual Dosage Oral:

Adult and Children. > 12 years of age: 10 mL every four hours not to exceed 60 mL in 24 hours

Children:
6-12 years: 5 mL every four hours not to exceed 30 mL in 24 hours
2-6 years: 2.5 mL every four hours not to exceed 15 mL in 24 hours

Guaifenesin, Phenylpropanolamine and Dextromethorphan
Brand Names Robitussin-CF® [OTC]
Use Temporarily relieves nasal congestion and controls cough due to minor throat and bronchial irritation; helps loosen phlegm and thin bronchial secretions to make coughs more productive
Pregnancy Risk Factor C
Usual Dosage Oral:

Adult and Children: > 12 years of age: 10 mL every four hours not to exceed 60 mL in 24 hours

Children:
6-12 years: 5 mL every four hours not to exceed 30 mL in 24 hours
2-6 years: 2.5 mL every four hours not to exceed 15 mL in 24 hours

Guaifenesin, Phenylpropanolamine and Phenylephrine
Brand Names Contuss®; Entex®
Use Symptomatic relief of sinusitis, bronchitis, pharyngitis associated with nasal congestion and thick mucous secretions in lower respiratory tract
(Continued)

Guaifenesin, Phenylpropanolamine and Phenylephrine (Continued)

Pregnancy Risk Factor C
Usual Dosage Adult and Children: > 12 years of age: One capsule four times daily (every six hours) with food or fluid

Guaifenesin, Pseudoephedrine and Codeine

Brand Names Robitussin®-DAC
Use Temporarily relieves nasal congestion and controls cough due to minor throat and bronchial irritation; helps loosen phlegm and thin bronchial secretions to make coughs more productive
Restrictions C-V
Pregnancy Risk Factor C
Usual Dosage Oral:

Adult and Children: > 12 years of age: 10 mL every four hours, not to exceed 40 mL in 24 hours

Children: 6-12 years: 5 mL every four hours, not to exceed 20 mL in 24 hours

Guaituss® [OTC] *see* Guaifenesin *on page 162*

Guanabenz Acetate (gwahn' a benz)

Brand Names Wytensin®
Use Management of hypertension
Pregnancy Risk Factor C
Usual Dosage 4 mg twice daily up to 32 mg twice daily

Guanadrel Acetate (gwahn' a drel)

Brand Names Hylorel®
Use Step 2 agent in stepped-care treatment of hypertension, usually with a diuretic
Pregnancy Risk Factor B
Usual Dosage Initially 10 mg/day (5 mg twice a day); adjust dosage until blood pressure is controlled, usually dosage is 20-75 mg/day, given twice a day

Guanethidine Sulfate (gwahn eth' i deen)

Brand Names Ismelin®
Use Treatment of moderate to severe hypertension
Pregnancy Risk Factor C
Usual Dosage

Adult: 25-50 mg/day in three divided doses

Children: Up to 3 mg/kg/24 hours

Guanfacine Hydrochloride (gwahn' fa seen)

Brand Names Tenex®
Use Management of hypertension
Pregnancy Risk Factor B
Usual Dosage 1 mg usually at bedtime, may increase if needed; 1 mg every day is most common dose

Gyne-Lotrimin® *see* Clotrimazole *on page 84*

Gyne-Sulf® *see* Sulfabenzamide, Sulfacetamide, and Sulfathiazole *on page 336*

Gynol II® *see* Nonoxynol 9 *on page 254*

Haemophilus b Conjugate Vaccine (hee mof' il us)
Brand Names ProHIBiT®
Use Routine immunization of children 18 months to 5 years of age against invasive diseases caused by *H. influenzae* type B
Usual Dosage I.M.: 0.5 mL in outer aspect area of the vastus lateralis (midthigh) or deltoid

Haemophilus b Conjugate Vaccine *see Haemophilus* b Vaccine *on this page*

Haemophilus b Oligosaccharide Conjugate Vaccine *see Haemophilus* b Vaccine *on this page*

Haemophilus b Polysaccharide Vaccine *see Haemophilus* b Vaccine *on this page*

Haemophilus b Vaccine
Brand Names β-Capsa I®; Hib-Imune®; HibTITER®; PedavaxHIB®; Pro-HIBiT®
Synonyms Diphtheria CRM₁₉₇ Protein Conjugate; Diphtheria Toxoid Conjugate; *Haemophilus* b Conjugate Vaccine; *Haemophilus* b Oligosaccharide Conjugate Vaccine; *Haemophilus* b Polysaccharide Vaccine; HbCV; Hib Polysaccharide Conjugate; PRP-D
Use For immunization of children 24 months to six years of age against diseases caused by *H. influenzae* type b
Usual Dosage Children: 24 months - 6 years of age: S.C.: 0.5 mL (25 µg) single administration only

Halcinonide (hal sin' oh nide)
Brand Names Halog®
Use Inflammation of corticosteroid-responsive dermatoses
Pregnancy Risk Factor C
Usual Dosage Adult and Children: Apply sparingly 1-3 times a day, occlusive dressing may be used for severe or resistant dermatoses

Halcion® *see* Triazolam *on page 361*

Haldol® *see* Haloperidol *on this page*

Haldol® Decanoate *see* Haloperidol *on this page*

Haldrone® *see* Paramethasone Acetate *on page 270*

Halodrin® *see* Estradiol and Fluoxymesterone *on page 136*

Halog® *see* Halcinonide *on this page*

Haloperidol (ha loe per' i dole)
Brand Names Haldol®; Haldol® Decanoate
Use Treatment of psychoses, Tourette's disorder; severe behavioral problems in children
(Continued)

165

Haloperidol *(Continued)*

Pregnancy Risk Factor C
Usual Dosage

Adult:
Oral: 0.5-5 mg 2-3 times daily
I.M.: 2-5 mg every 4-8 hours as needed

Children: Oral: 3-12 years:
Agitation or hyperkinesia: 0.01-0.03 mg/kg/day
Tourette's disorder: 0.05-0.075 mg/kg/day in 2-3 divided doses
Psychotic disorders: 0.05-0.15 mg/kg/day in 2-3 divided doses

Children: I.M.: 1-3 mg/dose every 4-8 hours to a maximum of 0.1 mg/kg/day

Haloprogin (ha loe proe' jin)
Brand Names Halotex®
Use Treatment of topical fungus infection
Pregnancy Risk Factor C
Usual Dosage Adult: Twice daily for 2-3 weeks

Halotestin® *see* Fluoxymesterone *on page 152*

Halotex® *see* Haloprogin *on this page*

Halothane (ha' loe thane)
Brand Names Fluothane®
Use General induction and maintenance of anesthesia (inhalation)
Usual Dosage Maintenance concentration varies from 0.5-1.5%

Haltran® [OTC] *see* Ibuprofen *on page 181*

Hamamelis Water *see* Witch Hazel *on page 380*

Hartmann's Solution *see* Ringer's Injection, Lactated *on page 316*

HbCV *see* Haemophilus b Vaccine *on previous page*

HBIG *see* Hepatitis B Immune Globulin *on next page*

H-BIG® *see* Hepatitis B Immune Globulin *on next page*

25-HCC *see* Calcifediol *on page 52*

hCG *see* Chorionic Gonadotropin *on page 78*

HCTZ *see* Hydrochlorothiazide *on page 172*

HDCV *see* Rabies Virus Vaccine, Human Diploid *on page 313*

Healon® *see* Sodium Hyaluronate *on page 328*

Hemabate™ *see* Carboprost *on page 60*

Hema-Chek® [OTC] *see* Diagnostic Test for Blood in Feces *on page 107*

Hema-Combistix [OTC] *see* Diagnostic Test for Blood, Glucose, pH, and Protein in Urine *on page 107*

Hemastix® [OTC] *see* Diagnostic Test for Blood in Urine
on page 107

Hematest® [OTC] *see* Diagnostic Test for Blood in Feces
on page 107

Hemiacidrin *see* Citric Acid Bladder Mixture *on page 80*

Hemin (hee' min)
Brand Names Panhematin®
Use Treatment of recurrent attacks of acute intermittent porphyria (AIP) only after an appropriate period of alternate therapy has been tried
Usual Dosage I.V.: 1-4 mg/kg/day administered over 10-15 minutes for 3-14 days; may be repeated no earlier than every 12 hours; not to exceed 6 mg/kg in any 24 hour period

Hemocult® II [OTC] *see* Diagnostic Test for Blood in Feces
on page 107

Hemocult® Slides *see* Diagnostic Test for Blood in Feces
on page 107

Hemofil® M *see* Antihemophilic Factor, Human *on page 26*

Heparin (hep' a rin)
Brand Names Calciparine®; HepFlush®; Hep-Lock®; Liquaemin®
Synonyms Heparin Lock Flush; Heparin Sodium, Heparin Calcium
Use Prophylaxis and treatment of thromboembolic disorders
Pregnancy Risk Factor C
Usual Dosage

Adult:
I.V. bolus: 10,000 units to start, 5000-10,000 units every 4-6 hours; I.V. intermittently or as constant infusion
I.V. infusion: 5000 units in bolus, then 20,000-40,000 units in one liter of I.V. solution over 24 hours
S.C.: 8000-10,000 units every eight hours; prophylaxis: S.C.: 5000 units every 8-12 hours

Children:
Intermittent I.V.: 50 units/kg to start, 50-100 units/kg/dose every four hours
I.V. infusion: 50 units/kg to start, then 10-25 units/kg/hour as continuous infusion

Heparin Lock Flush *see* Heparin *on this page*

Heparin Sodium, Heparin Calcium *see* Heparin *on this page*

HepatAmine® *see* Amino Acid Injection *on page 17*

Hepatitis B Immune Globulin
Brand Names H-BIG®; Hep-B-Gammagee®; HyperHep®
Synonyms HBIG
Use Provide passive immunity to hepatitis B infection to those individuals exposed
(Continued)

167

Hepatitis B Immune Globulin *(Continued)*
Pregnancy Risk Factor C
Usual Dosage I.M.:

Adult: 0.06 mL/kg, usual dose is 3-5 mL

Children: 0.06 mL/kg

Hepatitis B Vaccine
Brand Names Energix®; Heptavax-B®; Recombivax HB®
Use Immunization against infection caused by all known subtypes of hepatitis B virus
Pregnancy Risk Factor C
Usual Dosage I.M.:

Adult and Children: > 10 years of age: 10 µg/dose

Neonates and Children: < 10 years: 5 µg/dose; repeat in one month and in six months

Hep-B-Gammagee® *see* Hepatitis B Immune Globulin *on previous page*

HepFlush® *see* Heparin *on previous page*

Hep-Lock® *see* Heparin *on previous page*

Heptavax-B® *see* Hepatitis B Vaccine *on this page*

Herplex® *see* Idoxuridine *on page 181*

HES *see* Hetastarch *on this page*

Hespan® *see* Hetastarch *on this page*

Hetastarch (het' a starch)
Brand Names Hespan®
Synonyms HES; Hydroxyethyl Starch
Use Blood volume expander used in treatment of shock or impending shock when blood or blood products are not available
Pregnancy Risk Factor C
Usual Dosage Up to 1500 mL/day

Hexa-Betalin® *see* Pyridoxine Hydrochloride *on page 309*

Hexachlorophene (hex a klor' oh feen)
Brand Names pHisoHex®; pHiso® Scrub; Septisol®
Use As surgical scrub and as a bacteriostatic skin cleanser; to control an outbreak of gram-positive infection when other procedures have been unsuccessful

Hexafluorenium (hex a flure en' ee um)
Brand Names Mylaxen®
Use Adjunct for use with succinylcholine to prolong neuromuscular blockade
Pregnancy Risk Factor C
Usual Dosage I.V.: Administer in a ratio of 2 mg to each 1 mg of succinylcholine

Hexamethylmelamine
Synonyms HMM; HXM
Use Ovarian carcinoma; lung cancer
Restrictions NCI investigational drug
Pregnancy Risk Factor D
Usual Dosage Adult: Oral: 4-12 mg/kg/day in divided doses for 21-90 days on 240-320 mg/m^2/day in divided doses for 21 days, repeated every six weeks

Hexocyclium Methylsulfate
Brand Names Tral®
Use Adjunctive therapy in peptic ulcer and other GI disorders
Pregnancy Risk Factor C
Usual Dosage Adult: Oral: 25 mg four times a day before meals or food and at bedtime

Hexylresorcinol (hex il re zor' si nole)
Brand Names Sucrets® [OTC]
Use Minor antiseptic and local anesthetic for sore throat
Usual Dosage May be used as needed, allow to dissolve slowly in mouth

Hibiclens® [OTC] see Chlorhexidine Gluconate on page 70

Hib-Imune® see Haemophilus b Vaccine on page 165

Hib Polysaccharide Conjugate see Haemophilus b Vaccine on page 165

HibTITER® see Haemophilus b Vaccine on page 165

Hiprex® see Methenamine on page 226

Hismanal® see Astemizole on page 31

Histadyl® E.C. see Chlorpheniramine, Pseudoephedrine and Codeine on page 75

Histaject® see Brompheniramine Maleate on page 48

Histalog™ see Betazole Hydrochloride on page 43

Histamine Phosphate (hiss' ta meen)
Use Diagnostic test for achlorhydria and pheochromocytoma test
Usual Dosage Adult:

Gastric: S.C.: 0.0275 mg/kg

Pheochromocytoma: I.V.: 10 µg, then 50 µg five minutes later if no response after first dose

Histerone® see Testosterone on page 345

Histolyn-CYL® see Histoplasmin on this page

Histoplasmin (hiss toe plaz' min)
Brand Names Histolyn-CYL®
Use Diagnosing histoplasmosis; to assess cell-mediated immunity
Pregnancy Risk Factor C
(Continued)

169

Histoplasmin *(Continued)*

Usual Dosage Adult: Intradermally: 0.1 mL of 1:100 dilution 5-10 cm apart into volar surface of forearm

HMM *see* Hexamethylmelamine *on previous page*

HMS Liquifilm® *see* Medrysone *on page 216*

HN₂ *see* Mechlorethamine Hydrochloride *on page 214*

Homatropine and Hydrocodone *see* Hydrocodone and Homatropine *on page 173*

Homatropine Hydrobromide *(hoe ma' troe peen)*

Brand Names Isopto® Homatropine
Use Producing cycloplegia and mydriasis for refraction; treatment of acute inflammatory conditions of the uveal tract
Pregnancy Risk Factor C
Usual Dosage

Adult:
Refraction: 1-2 drops of a 2% solution or one drop of a 5% solution; repeat in 5-10 minutes if needed
Uveitis: 1-2 drops of a 2 or 5% solution 2-3 times a day or as often as every 3-4 hours

Children:
Refraction: One drop of a 2% solution; may repeat at 10 minute intervals as necessary
Uveitis: One drop of a 2% solution 2-3 times daily

Horse Anti-human Thymocyte Gamma Globulin *see* Lymphocyte Immune Globulin *on page 208*

H.P. Acthar® Gel *see* Corticotropin *on page 89*

Humate-P® *see* Antihemophilic Factor, Human *on page 26*

Humatin® *see* Paromomycin Sulfate *on page 270*

Humibid® L.A. *see* Guaifenesin *on page 162*

Humibid® Sprinkle *see* Guaifenesin *on page 162*

Humorsol® *see* Demecarium Bromide *on page 99*

Humulin® L *see* Insulin, Zinc Suspension *on page 186*

Humulin® N *see* Insulin, Isophane Suspension *on page 185*

Humulin® R *see* Insulin, Regular *on page 186*

Humulin® U *see* Insulin, Zinc Suspension, Extended *on page 186*

Hurricaine® *see* Benzocaine *on page 40*

HXM *see* Hexamethylmelamine *on previous page*

Hyaluronidase *(hye al yoor on' i dase)*

Brand Names Wydase®
Use Increase the dispersion and absorption of other drugs; increase rate of absorption of parenteral fluids given by hypodermoclysis

Pregnancy Risk Factor C
Usual Dosage

Absorption and dispersion of drugs: Add 150 units to the injection solution

Hypodermoclysis: 150 units will facilitate absorption of 1000 mL or more of solution

Hybolin® Decanoate *see* Nandrolone *on page 246*

Hybolin® Improved *see* Nandrolone *on page 246*

Hycodan® *see* Hydrocodone and Homatropine *on page 173*

Hycomine® *see* Hydrocodone and Phenylpropanolamine *on page 174*

Hycotuss® Expectorant Liquid *see* Hydrocodone and Guaifenesin *on page 173*

Hydeltrasol® *see* Prednisolone *on page 294*

Hydeltra-T.B.A.® *see* Prednisolone *on page 294*

Hydergine® *see* Ergoloid Mesylates *on page 133*

Hydergine® LC *see* Ergoloid Mesylates *on page 133*

Hydralazine and Hydrochlorothiazide
Brand Names Apresazide®
Synonyms Hydrochlorothiazide and Hydralazine
Use Management of moderate to severe hypertension and treatment of congestive heart failure
Pregnancy Risk Factor C
Usual Dosage Adult: One capsule twice daily

Hydralazine and Reserpine
Brand Names Serpasil®-Apresoline®
Use Hypertensive disorders
Pregnancy Risk Factor C
Usual Dosage
Dosage is individualized
Normal adult dose: Oral: One or two tablets three times daily

Hydralazine Hydrochloride (hye dral' a zeen)
Brand Names Apresoline®
Use Management of moderate to severe hypertension
Pregnancy Risk Factor C
Usual Dosage

Adult:
Oral: 10-100 mg four times a day
I.M., I.V.: 20-40 mg every 4-6 hours as needed

Children:
Oral: 0.1875 mg/kg four times a day; may increase to 1.875 mg/kg four times a day
I.M., I.V.: 1.7-3.5 mg/kg/day in 4-6 divided doses

Hydralazine, Hydrochlorothiazide, and Reserpine
Brand Names Ser-Ap-Es®
Use Hypertensive disorders
Pregnancy Risk Factor C
Usual Dosage Adult: Oral: One or two tablets three times daily

Hydrated Chloral *see* Chloral Hydrate *on page 68*

Hydrea® *see* Hydroxyurea *on page 178*

Hydroactive Dressing, Flexible
Brand Names DuoDerm®
Use Local management of dermal ulcers, pressure sores, leg ulcers, minor wounds, and occlusive dressing
Usual Dosage Apply as directed

Hydrochlorothiazide (hye droe klor oh thye' a zide)
Brand Names Aquazide-H®; Diaqua®; Esidrix®; HydroDIURIL®; Hydro-T®; Micrin®; Oretic®; Thiuretic®
Synonyms HCTZ
Use Management of mild to moderate hypertension; treatment of edema in congestive heart failure and nephrotic syndrome
Pregnancy Risk Factor B
Usual Dosage Oral:

Adult: 25-100 mg/day in 1-2 doses

Children:
> 6 months: 2.2 mg/kg/day in two divided doses
< 6 months: Up to 3.3 mg/kg in two divided doses

Hydrochlorothiazide and Amiloride *see* Amiloride and Hydrochlorothiazide *on page 17*

Hydrochlorothiazide and Hydralazine *see* Hydralazine and Hydrochlorothiazide *on previous page*

Hydrochlorothiazide and Methyldopa *see* Methyldopa and Hydrochlorothiazide *on page 230*

Hydrochlorothiazide and Reserpine
Brand Names Hydropres®
Synonyms Reserpine and Hydrochlorothiazide
Use Management of mild to moderate hypertension; treatment of edema in congestive heart failure and nephrotic syndrome
Pregnancy Risk Factor C
Usual Dosage Adult: Oral: 1-2 tablets once or twice daily

Hydrochlorothiazide and Spironolactone
Brand Names Aldactazide®
Synonyms Spironolactone and Hydrochlorothiazide
Use Management of mild to moderate hypertension; treatment of edema in congestive heart failure and nephrotic syndrome
Pregnancy Risk Factor C

Usual Dosage Oral:

Adult: 1-8 tablets in 1-2 divided doses

Children: 1.66-3.3 mg/kg/day (of spironolactone) in 2-4 divided doses

Hydrochlorothiazide and Triamterene

Brand Names Dyazide®; Maxzide®

Synonyms Triamterene and Hydrochlorothiazide

Use Management of mild to moderate hypertension; treatment of edema in congestive heart failure and nephrotic syndrome

Pregnancy Risk Factor C

Usual Dosage Adult: 1-2 capsules twice daily after meals

Hydrocil® [OTC] see Psyllium on page 308

Hydrocodone and Acetaminophen (hye droe koe' done)

Brand Names Vicodin®

Synonyms Acetaminophen and Hydrocodone

Use Relief of moderate to severe pain

Restrictions C-III

Pregnancy Risk Factor C

Usual Dosage 1-2 tablets every 4-6 hours

Hydrocodone and Chlorpheniramine Polistirex

Brand Names Tussionex®

Use Symptomatic relief of cough

Restrictions C-III

Pregnancy Risk Factor C

Usual Dosage Oral:

Adult: 5 mL every 12 hours; do not exceed 10 mL in 24 hours

Children: 6-12 years: 2.5 mL every 12 hours; do not exceed 5 mL in 24 hours

Hydrocodone and Guaifenesin

Brand Names Hycotuss® Expectorant Liquid

Synonyms Guaifenesin and Hydrocodone

Use Symptomatic relief of nonproductive coughs associated with upper and lower respiratory tract congestion

Restrictions C-III

Pregnancy Risk Factor C

Usual Dosage Oral:

Adult: 5 mL every four hours, after meals and at bedtime, up to 30 mL in 24 hours

Children:
> 12 years: 5 mL every four hours, after meals and at bedtime
2-12 years: 2.5 mL every four hours, after meals and at bedtime
< 2 years: 0.3 mg/kg/day (hydrocodone) in four divided doses

Hydrocodone and Homatropine

Brand Names Hycodan®

Synonyms Homatropine and Hydrocodone

Use Symptomatic relief of cough

(Continued)

Hydrocodone and Homatropine *(Continued)*

Restrictions C-III
Pregnancy Risk Factor C
Usual Dosage (Based on hydrocodone component) Oral:

Adult: 5-10 mg every 4-6 hours, a single dose should not exceed 15 mg; do not administer more frequently than every four hours

Children: 0.6 mg/kg/day in 3-4 divided doses; do not administer more frequently than every four hours

A single dose should not exceed 10 mg in children older than 12, 5 mg in children 2-12 years, and 1.25 mg in children < 2 years of age

Hydrocodone and Phenylpropanolamine

Brand Names Hycomine®
Synonyms Phenylpropanolamine and Hydrocodone
Use Symptomatic relief of cough and nasal congestion
Restrictions C-III
Pregnancy Risk Factor C
Usual Dosage Oral:

Adult: 5 mL every four hours, up to 6 doses/24 hours

Children: 6-12 years: 2.5 mL every four hours, up to 6 doses/24 hours

Hydrocortisone (hye droe kor' ti sone)

Brand Names A-hydroCort®; Cortef®; Hydrocortone®; Solu-Cortef®
Synonyms Compound F; Cortisol; Hydrocortisone Acetate; Hydrocortisone Cypionate; Hydrocortisone Sodium Phosphate; Hydrocortisone Sodium Succinate
Use Management of adrenocortical insufficiency; relief of inflammation of corticosteroid-responsive dermatoses; adjunctive treatment of ulcerative colitis
Pregnancy Risk Factor C
Usual Dosage

Adult: Apply to affected area twice a day or four times a day (also for children ≥ 2 years of age)
Oral: 10-320 mg/day in 2-4 divided doses
I.M., I.V.: 100-500 mg every 2-10 hours (succinate); 15-240 mg every 12 hours (phosphate)
Rectal: 10-100 mg 1-2 times daily
Topical: Apply 3-4 times daily
Ophthalmic: Apply 1/2" ribbon 2-4 times daily

Children:
Shock: I.M., I.V.: 50 mg/kg, then 50-75 mg/kg/day every six hours
Topical: Apply 3-4 times daily
Ophthalmic: Apply 1/2" ribbon 2-4 times daily
Physiological replacement: 12.5 mg/m²/day I.M.; 25 mg/m²/day orally every eight hours
Status asthmaticus: Loading 4-8 mg/kg/dose, then 10 mg/kg/day every six hours

Hydrocortisone Acetate *see* Hydrocortisone *on previous page*

Hydrocortisone Alcohol and Benzoyl Peroxide
Brand Names Vanoxide-HC®
Use Treatment of acne vulgaris and oily skin
Pregnancy Risk Factor C
Usual Dosage Shake well; apply thin film 1-3 times daily, gently massage into skin

Hydrocortisone and Dibucaine *see* Dibucaine and Hydrocortisone *on page 110*

Hydrocortisone and Iodochlorhydroxyquin *see* Iodochlorhydroxyquin and Hydrocortisone *on page 189*

Hydrocortisone and Lidocaine
Brand Names Lida-Mantle HC®
Use Topical anti-inflammatory and anesthetic for skin disorders
Usual Dosage Apply 2-4 times daily

Hydrocortisone and Polymyxin B
Brand Names Otobiotic® Otic
Use Treatment of superficial bacterial infections of external ear canal
Pregnancy Risk Factor C
Usual Dosage Four drops 3-4 times daily

Hydrocortisone and Pramoxine
Brand Names Pramosone®; Proctofoam®-HC
Synonyms Pramoxine and Hydrocortisone
Use Treatment of severe anorectal inflammation
Pregnancy Risk Factor C
Usual Dosage Apply to affected areas 3-4 times daily

Hydrocortisone and Urea
Brand Names Carmol-HC®
Synonyms Urea and Hydrocortisone
Use Inflammation of corticosteroid-responsive dermatoses
Pregnancy Risk Factor C
Usual Dosage Apply thin film and rub in well 1-4 times daily

Hydrocortisone Cypionate *see* Hydrocortisone *on previous page*

Hydrocortisone, Neomycin and Colistin
Brand Names Coly-Mycin® S Otic Drops
Use Treatment of superficial and susceptible bacterial infections of the external auditory canal; for treatment of susceptible bacterial infections of mastoidectomy and fenestration cavities
Pregnancy Risk Factor C
Usual Dosage

Adult: Four drops in affected ear 3-4 times a day

Children: Three drops in affected ear 3-4 times a day

Hydrocortisone Sodium Phosphate *see* Hydrocortisone
on page 174

Hydrocortisone Sodium Succinate *see* Hydrocortisone
on page 174

Hydrocortone® *see* Hydrocortisone *on page 174*

HydroDIURIL® *see* Hydrochlorothiazide *on page 172*

Hydro-Ergoloid® *see* Ergoloid Mesylates *on page 133*

Hydroflumethiazide (hye droe floo meth eye' a zide)
Brand Names Saluron®
Use Management of mild to moderate hypertension; treatment of edema
in congestive heart failure and nephrotic syndrome
Pregnancy Risk Factor B
Usual Dosage One tablet 1-2 times daily

Hydroflumethiazide and Reserpine
Brand Names Salutensin®
Use Management of hypertension
Pregnancy Risk Factor C
Usual Dosage As determined by individual titration, usually one tablet
once or twice daily

Hydrogenated Ergot Alkaloids *see* Ergoloid Mesylates
on page 133

Hydromagnesium aluminate *see* Magaldrate *on page 209*

Hydromorphone Hydrochloride (hye droe mor' fone)
Brand Names Dilaudid®
Synonyms Dihydromorphinone
Use Management of moderate to severe pain, antitussive at lower doses
Restrictions C-II
Pregnancy Risk Factor C
Usual Dosage Adult:
Oral, I.M., S.C.: 2-4 mg every 4-6 hours as needed
Rectal: 3 mg every 6-8 hours as needed

Hydropres® *see* Hydrochlorothiazide and Reserpine
on page 172

Hydroquinone (hye' droe kwin one)
Brand Names Solaquin Forte®
Use Gradual bleaching of hyperpigmented skin conditions
Usual Dosage Apply thin layer and rub in twice a day

Hydro-T® *see* Hydrochlorothiazide *on page 172*

Hydrous Wool Fat *see* Lanolin *on page 199*

Hydroxacen® *see* Hydroxyzine *on page 178*

Hydroxyamphetamine Hydrobromide
(hye drox ee am fe' ta meen)
Brand Names Paredrine®
Use Produce mydriasis in diagnostic eye examination
Usual Dosage 1-2 drops into conjunctival sac

Hydroxychloroquine Sulfate (hye drox ee klor' oh kwin)
Brand Names Plaquenil®
Use Suppress and treat acute attacks of malaria, as well as treatment of systemic lupus erythematosus and rheumatoid arthritis
Pregnancy Risk Factor C
Usual Dosage Oral:

Adult:

Suppression: Two tablets weekly on same day each week; begin two weeks before exposure; continue for 6-8 weeks after leaving epidemic area

Acute attack: Four tablets first dose day one; two tablets in six hours day one; two tablets in one dose day two; and two tablets in one dose on day three

Rheumatoid arthritis: 2-3 tablets daily to start; increase dose until optimum response level is reached; usually after 4-12 weeks dose should be reduced by 1/2 and continue on that dose

Lupus erythematosus: Two tablets every day or twice daily for several weeks depending on response; for prolonged dose usually 200-400 mg daily is sufficient

Children:

Suppression: 5 mg/kg weekly; should not exceed the recommended adult dose

Acute attack: 10 mg/kg initial dose; followed by 5 mg/kg in six hours on day one; 5 mg/kg in one dose on day two and on day three

Hydroxydaunomycin Hydrochloride *see* Doxorubicin
Hydrochloride *on page 123*

Hydroxyethyl Starch *see* Hetastarch *on page 168*

Hydroxyprogesterone Caproate
(hye drox ee proe jess' te rone)
Brand Names Duralutin®; Gesterol® L.A.; Hy-Gestrone®; Hylutin®; Hypro-gest®
Use For treatment of amenorrhea, abnormal uterine bleeding, submucous fibroids, endometriosis, uterine carcinoma, and testing of estrogen production
Pregnancy Risk Factor X
Usual Dosage Adult: I.M.:

Amenorrhea: 375 mg; if no bleeding begin cyclic treatment with estradiol valerate

Endometriosis: Start cyclic therapy with estradiol valerate

Uterine carcinoma: 1 g once or more times daily (1-7 g/week) for up to 12 weeks

(Continued)

177

Hydroxyprogesterone Caproate *(Continued)*

Test for endogenous estrogen production: 250 mg anytime; bleeding 7-14 days after injection indicate positive test

Hydroxypropyl Methylcellulose (hye drox ee proe' pill)

Brand Names Gonak® [OTC]; Goniosol® [OTC]; Occucoat™

Use Ophthalmic surgical aid in cataract extraction and intraocular implantation; gonioscopic examinations

Usual Dosage Introduced into anterior chamber of eye with 20 gauge or larger cannula

Hydroxyurea (hye drox' ee yoo ree ah)

Brand Names Hydrea®

Use Treatment of malignant neoplasms including melanoma, granulocytic leukemia, and ovarian carcinomas; also used with radiation in treatment of squamous cell carcinoma of the head and neck

Pregnancy Risk Factor C

Usual Dosage

Adult: Oral:

Solid tumors: Intermittent therapy: 80 mg/kg every third day; continuous therapy: 20-30 mg/kg every day

Concomitant therapy with irradiation: 80 mg every third day

Resistant chronic myelocytic leukemia: 20-30 mg/kg every day

Children: No dosage regimens have been established; consult the Hematology Service for doses

25-Hydroxyvitamin D₃ *see* Calcifediol *on page 52*

Hydroxyzine (hye drox' i zeen)

Brand Names Anxanil®; Atarax®; E-Vista®; Hydroxacen®; Hy-Pam®; Quiess®; Vistaril®; Vistazine®

Synonyms Hydroxyzine Hydrochloride; Hydroxyzine Pamoate

Use Treatment of anxiety, as a preoperative sedative, an antipruritic, an antiemetic, and in alcohol withdrawal symptoms

Pregnancy Risk Factor C

Usual Dosage

Adult:

Alcohol withdrawal: I.M.: 50-100 mg every 4-6 hours

Antiemetic: I.M.: 25-100 mg

Anxiety: Oral: 50-100 four times a day

Preoperative sedation: Oral: 50-100 mg; I.M.: 25-100 mg

Management of pruritus: Oral: 25 mg 3-4 times daily

Children:

Antiemetic: I.M.: 1.1 mg/kg

Anxiety: > 6 years: 50-100 mg in 3-4 divided doses; < 6 years: 50 mg in divided doses

Preoperative sedation: Oral: 0.6 mg/kg; I.M.: 1.1 mg/kg

Management of pruritus: > 6 years: 50-100 mg in divided doses; < 6 years: 50 mg/day in divided doses

Hydroxyzine Hydrochloride *see* Hydroxyzine *on previous page*

Hydroxyzine Pamoate *see* Hydroxyzine *on previous page*

Hy-Gestrone® *see* Hydroxyprogesterone Caproate *on page 177*

Hygroton® *see* Chlorthalidone *on page 77*

Hylorel® *see* Guanadrel Acetate *on page 164*

Hylutin® *see* Hydroxyprogesterone Caproate *on page 177*

Hyoscine Hydrobromide *see* Scopolamine *on page 321*

Hyoscyamine, Atropine, Scopolamine and Phenobarbital

Brand Names Donnatal®; Kinesed®

Use As an adjunct in treatment of peptic ulcer disease, irritable bowel, spastic colitis, spastic bladder, and renal colic

Pregnancy Risk Factor C

Usual Dosage Oral:

Adult: 0.125-0.25 mg (1-2 capsules or tablets) 3-4 times daily; or 0.375-0.75 mg (1 Donnatal® Extentab®) in sustained release form every 12 hours; or 5-10 mL elixir 3-4 times/day or every eight hours

Children: Kinesed® dose: 1/2-1 tablet 3-4 times/day
10 lbs: 0.5 mL every four hours or 0.75 mL every six hours to start
20 lbs: 1 mL every four hours or 1.5 mL every six hours to start
30 lbs: 1.5 mL every four hours or 2 mL every six hours to start
50 lbs: 2.5 mL every four hours or 3.75 mL every six hours to start
75 lbs: 3.75 mL every four hours or 5 mL every six hours to start
100 lbs: 5 mL every four hours or 7.5 mL every six hours to start

Hyoscyamine, Atropine, Scopolamine, Kaolin and Pectin

Brand Names Donnagel®

Use Antidiarrheal; also used in gastritis, enteritis, colitis, and acute gastrointestinal upsets, and nausea which may accompany any of these conditions

Pregnancy Risk Factor C

Usual Dosage Oral:

Adult:
Diarrhea: 30 mL at once and 15-30 mL with each loose stool
Other conditions: 15 mL every three hours as needed

Children:
> 30 pounds: 5-10 mL
20-30 pounds: 5 mL
10-20 pounds: 2.5 mL

Hyoscyamine, Atropine, Scopolamine, Kaolin, Pectin and Opium

Brand Names Donnagel®-PG

Use Treatment of diarrhea

Restrictions C-V

(Continued)

179

Hyoscyamine, Atropine, Scopolamine, Kaolin, Pectin and Opium *(Continued)*

Pregnancy Risk Factor C
Usual Dosage

Adult and Children: > 12 years of age: 30 mL (1 fluid ounce) initially, followed by 15 mL every three hours

Children: 6-12 years of age: 10 mL initially and 5-10 mL every three hours thereafter

Dosage recommendations (body weight/dosage): 10 lb/2.5 mL; 20 lb/5 mL; 30 lb and over/5-10 mL. Do not administer more than four doses in any 24-hour period

Hyoscyamine Sulfate *(hye oh sye' a meen)*

Brand Names Anaspaz®; Cystospaz®; Gastrosed™; Levsin®; Levsinex®; Neoquess®

Synonyms *l*-Hyoscyamine Sulfate

Use GI tract disorders caused by spasm, adjunctive therapy for peptic ulcers

Pregnancy Risk Factor C
Usual Dosage

Adult:
Oral or S.L.: 0.125-0.25 mg 3-4 times daily before meals or food and at bedtime; 0.375-0.75 mg (timed release) every 12 hours
I.M., I.V., S.C.: 0.25-0.5 mg every six hours

Children:
2-10 years of age: 1/2 adult dosage
< 2 years: 1/4 adult dosage

Hy-Pam® *see* Hydroxyzine *on page 178*

Hypaque®-M *see* Sodium Diatrizoate and Meglumine Diatrizoate *on page 328*

Hyperab® *see* Rabies Immune Globulin, Human *on page 313*

HyperHep® *see* Hepatitis B Immune Globulin *on page 167*

Hyperstat® I.V. *see* Diazoxide *on page 110*

Hyper-Tet® *see* Tetanus Immune Globulin, Human *on page 345*

HypRho®-D *see* Rh$_o$(D) Immune Globulin *on page 315*

Hyprogest® *see* Hydroxyprogesterone Caproate *on page 177*

Hyskon® *see* Dextran *on page 103*

Hytakerol® *see* Dihydrotachysterol *on page 115*

Hytrin® *see* Terazosin *on page 342*

Hytuss® [OTC] *see* Guaifenesin *on page 162*

Hytuss-2X® [OTC] *see* Guaifenesin *on page 162*

Ibenzmethyzin *see* Procarbazine Hydrochloride *on page 298*

Iberet-Folic-500® *see* Ferrous Sulfate, Ascorbic Acid, Vitamin B-Complex and Folic Acid *on page 147*

Iberet®-Liquid [OTC] *see* Ferrous Sulfate, Ascorbic Acid, and Vitamin B-Complex *on page 146*

Ibidomide Hydrochloride *see* Labetalol Hydrochloride *on page 198*

Ibuprin® [OTC] *see* Ibuprofen *on this page*

Ibuprofen (eye byoo proe' fen)
Brand Names Advil® [OTC]; Genpril® [OTC]; Haltran® [OTC]; Ibuprin® [OTC]; Ibu-Tab®; Medipren® [OTC]; Menadol® [OTC]; Midol® 200 [OTC]; Motrin®; Motrin® IB [OTC]; Nuprin® [OTC]; Pamprin IB® [OTC]; Pedia-Profen™; Rufen®; Saleto-200® [OTC]; Saleto-400®; Trendar® [OTC]; Uni-Pro® [OTC]
Synonyms *p*-Isobutylhydratropic Acid
Use Management of inflammatory disorders, as an analgesic in the treatment of mild to moderate pain and as an antipyretic
Pregnancy Risk Factor B/D
Usual Dosage Oral:

Adult:
 Analgesia: 200-400 mg every 4-6 hours
 Inflammatory diseases: 300-800 mg 3-4 times daily

Children:
 > 40 kg: Adult dosage
 30-40 kg: Maximum 800 mg/day
 20-30 kg: Maximum 600 mg/day
 < 20 kg: Maximum 400 mg/day

Ibu-Tab® *see* Ibuprofen *on this page*

I-Chlor® *see* Chloramphenicol *on page 69*

Ictotest® [OTC] *see* Diagnostic Test for Bilirubin in the Urine *on page 106*

Idoxuridine (eye dox yoor' i deen)
Brand Names Herplex®; Stoxil®
Synonyms IDU; IUdR
Use Treatment of herpes simplex keratitis
Pregnancy Risk Factor C
Usual Dosage
 Solution: One drop in eye(s) every hour during day and two hours at night, continue until definite improvement is noted, then reduce daytime dose to one drop every two hours and every four hours at night; continue for 3-5 days after healing appears complete
 Ointment: Use five times daily (every four hours) with last dose at bedtime; continue therapy for 3-5 days after healing appears complete

IDU *see* Idoxuridine *on this page*

Ifex® *see* Ifosfamide *on next page*

IFLrA *see* Interferon Alfa-2a *on page 187*

IFN *see* Interferon Alfa-2a *on page 187*

IFN-alpha 2 *see* Interferon Alfa-2b *on page 187*

Ifosfamide (eye foss' fa mide)
Brand Names Ifex®

Use In combination with certain other antineoplastics in treatment of lung cancer, Hodgkin's and non-Hodgkin's lymphoma, breast cancer, acute and chronic lymphocytic leukemia, ovarian cancer, testicular cancer, and sarcomas

Pregnancy Risk Factor C

Usual Dosage Dosages may vary with protocols normally given 700-1000 mg/m^2/day for five days; 2400 mg/m^2/day for three days; or up to 5000 mg/m^2 as a single dose

IG *see* Immune Globulin *on next page*

I-Gent® *see* Gentamicin Sulfate *on page 157*

IGIM *see* Immune Globulin *on next page*

IGIV *see* Immune Globulin *on next page*

Ilopan® *see* Dexpanthenol *on page 103*

Ilopan-Choline® *see* Dexpanthenol *on page 103*

Ilosone® *see* Erythromycin *on page 134*

Ilotycin® *see* Erythromycin *on page 134*

Ilotycin® Gluceptate *see* Erythromycin *on page 134*

Ilozyme® *see* Pancrelipase *on page 267*

Imferon® *see* Iron Dextran Complex *on page 191*

Imipenem/Cilastatin (i mi pen' em)
Brand Names Primaxin®

Use Treatment of susceptible bacterial infections; most active against gram-positive aerobic cocci and many gram-negative *Bacillus* and numerous other bacteria including anaerobes

Pregnancy Risk Factor C

Usual Dosage

Adult: I.V.: 250-1000 mg every six hours; infuse each 250-500 mg dose over 20-30 minutes; infuse each one gram dose over 40-60 minutes

Children: 15-25 mg/kg/dose every six hours (3 months - 13 years of age)

Imipramine (im ip' ra meen)
Brand Names Janimine®; Tofranil®; Tofranil-PM®

Synonyms Imipramine Hydrochloride; Imipramine Pamoate

Use Treatment of various forms of depression, often in conjunction with psychotherapy

Pregnancy Risk Factor D

Usual Dosage

Adult: Oral, I.M.: 25-50 mg 3-4 times daily, total dose may be given at bedtime

Children: Oral: > 6 years: 25 mg one hour before bedtime; increase by 25 mg at weekly intervals up to 50 mg for children < 12 years and to 75 mg for children > 12 years; gradually taper dose to prevent relapse

Imipramine Hydrochloride *see* Imipramine *on previous page*

Imipramine Pamoate *see* Imipramine *on previous page*

Immune Globulin
Brand Names Gamastan®; Gamimune® N; Gammagard®; Gammar®; Sandoglobulin®; Venoglobulin®-I
Synonyms Gamma Globulin; IG; IGIM; IGIV; Immune Globulin Intramuscular; Immune Globulin Intravenous; Immune Serum Globulin; ISG
Use Prophylaxis against hepatitis A, measles, varicella, and possibly rubella and immunoglobulin deficiency
Pregnancy Risk Factor C
Usual Dosage I.M.:

Hepatitis A: 0.02 mL/kg

IgG: 1.3 mL/kg then 0.66 mL/kg in 3-4 weeks

Measles: 0.25 mL/kg

Rubella: 0.55 mL/kg

Varicella: 0.6-1.2 mL/kg

Immune Globulin Intramuscular *see* Immune Globulin *on this page*

Immune Globulin Intravenous *see* Immune Globulin *on this page*

Immune Serum Globulin *see* Immune Globulin *on this page*

Imodium® *see* Loperamide Hydrochloride *on page 206*

Imodium® A-D [OTC] *see* Loperamide Hydrochloride *on page 206*

Imovax® *see* Rabies Virus Vaccine, Human Diploid *on page 313*

Imuran® *see* Azathioprine *on page 34*

I-Naphline® *see* Naphazoline Hydrochloride *on page 246*

Inapsine® *see* Droperidol *on page 124*

Indameth® *see* Indomethacin *on next page*

Indapamide (in dap' a mide)
Brand Names Lozol®
Use Management of mild to moderate hypertension; treatment of edema in congestive heart failure and nephrotic syndrome
Pregnancy Risk Factor B
Usual Dosage Adult: Oral: 2.5-5 mg every day

Inderal® *see* Propranolol Hydrochloride *on page 304*

Inderal® LA *see* Propranolol Hydrochloride *on page 304*

Inderide® *see* Propranolol and Hydrochlorothiazide
on page 304

Indian Gum
Synonyms Karaya Powder; Sterculia Gum
Use Sterilized powder for ostomy use

Indigo Carmine *see* Indigotindisulfonate Sodium *on this page*

Indigotindisulfonate Sodium (in di goe tin dye sul' foe nate)
Synonyms Indigo Carmine
Use For localizing ureteral orifices during cystoscopy and ureteral cathe-
terization, marker dye to identify severed ureters and fistulous communi-
cations
Usual Dosage I.V. (preferred), I.M.: Usually 5 mL; smaller doses in infants
and children

Indocin® *see* Indomethacin *on this page*

Indocin® I.V. *see* Indomethacin *on this page*

Indocin® SR *see* Indomethacin *on this page*

Indocyanine Green (in doe sye' a neen)
Brand Names Cardio-Green®
Use For determining hepatic function, cardiac output and liver blood flow
and for ophthalmic angiography
Usual Dosage Varies with procedure

Indo-Lemmon® *see* Indomethacin *on this page*

Indometacin *see* Indomethacin *on this page*

Indomethacin (in doe meth' a sin)
Brand Names Indameth®; Indocin®; Indocin® I.V.; Indocin® SR; Indo-
Lemmon®
Synonyms Indometacin
Use Management of inflammatory disorders, as an analgesic in the treat-
ment of mild to moderate pain and as an antipyretic; I.V. form used as an
alternate to surgery in management of patent ductus arteriosus in pre-
mature neonates
Pregnancy Risk Factor B/D
Usual Dosage

Adult: Oral, rectal: 25-50 mg 2-3 times daily or 75 mg sustained-release
once or twice daily

Children: Oral: 2-14 years: 2-4 mg/kg/day in 2-4 divided doses

Neonate: I.V.: 0.2 mg/kg to start, 2 doses of 0.1 mg/kg at 12-24 hour intervals; age < 48 hours at time of first dose, 0.2 mg/kg; 2-7 days old at
time of first dose, or 0.25 mg/kg if over 7 days at time of initial dose

I-N-Ethyl Sisomicin *see* Netilmicin Sulfate *on page 250*

Infant Nutritional Formulas
Brand Names Isomil®; Pedialyte®

Inflamase® _see_ Prednisolone _on page 294_

Inflamase® Mild _see_ Prednisolone _on page 294_

Influenza Virus Vaccine (in floo en' za)
Brand Names Fluogen®; Fluzone®
Use Provide active immunity to influenza virus strains contained in the vaccine
Pregnancy Risk Factor C
Usual Dosage The following table summarizes vaccine and dosage recommendations by age group.

Influenza Vaccine

Age	Product Type	Dosage (mL)	Number of Doses
Over 12 y	Whole virus or split virus	0.5	1
3–12 y	Split virus only	0.5	2†
6–35 mo	Split virus only	0.25	2†

†Four weeks or more between doses

INH _see_ Isoniazid _on page 192_

Innovar® _see_ Droperidol and Fentanyl _on page 124_

Inocor® _see_ Amrinone Lactate _on page 24_

Insect Sting Kit
Brand Names Ana-Kit®
Use Anaphylaxis emergency treatment of insect bites or stings by the sensitive patient that may occur within minutes of insect sting or exposure to to an allergic substance

Insta-Char® [OTC] _see_ Charcoal _on page 68_

Insta® Kit _see_ Diagnostic Test for Streptococci _on page 108_

Insulatard® NPH _see_ Insulin, Isophane Suspension _on this page_

Insulatard® NPH Human _see_ Insulin, Isophane Suspension _on this page_

Insulin Injection _see_ Insulin, Regular _on next page_

Insulin, Isophane Suspension
Brand Names Beef NPH Iletin® II; Humulin® N; Insulatard® NPH; Insulatard® NPH Human; Novolin® N; NPH Iletin®I; NPH Purified Pork; Pork NPH Iletin® II
Synonyms NPH
Use Treatment of insulin-dependent diabetes mellitus, also noninsulin-dependent diabetes mellitus unresponsive to treatment with diet and/or oral hypoglycemics
(Continued)
185

Insulin, Isophane Suspension *(Continued)*

Pregnancy Risk Factor B

Usual Dosage Dose requires continuous medical supervision.

Insulin, Isophane Suspension and Insulin Injection

Brand Names Mixtard®; Mixtard® Human 70/30; Novolin® 70/30

Use Treatment of insulin-dependent diabetes mellitus, also noninsulin-dependent diabetes mellitus unresponsive to treatment with diet and/or oral hypoglycemics

Pregnancy Risk Factor B

Usual Dosage Dose requires continuous medical supervision

Insulin, Protamine Zinc Suspension

Brand Names Protamine, Zinc and Iletin®I; Protamine, Zinc and Iletin® II (Beef); Protamine, Zinc and Iletin® II (Pork)

Synonyms PZI

Use Treatment of insulin-dependent diabetes mellitus, also noninsulin-dependent diabetes mellitus unresponsive to treatment with diet and/or oral hypoglycemics

Pregnancy Risk Factor B

Usual Dosage Dose requires continuous medical supervision

Insulin, Regular (in' su lin)

Brand Names Beef Regular Iletin® II; Humulin® R; Novolin® R; Novolin® R Penfill; Pork Regular Iletin® II; Regular Iletin® I; Regular Purified Pork; Velosulin®; Velosulin® Human

Synonyms Insulin Injection

Use Treatment of insulin-dependent diabetes mellitus, also noninsulin-dependent diabetes mellitus unresponsive to treatment with diet and/or oral hypoglycemics

Pregnancy Risk Factor B

Usual Dosage Dose requires continuous medical supervision

Insulin, Zinc Suspension

Brand Names Humulin® L; Lente® Iletin®I; Lente® Iletin® II (Beef); Lente® Iletin® II (Pork); Lente® Purified Pork Insulin; Novolin® L

Synonyms Lente®

Use Treatment of insulin-dependent diabetes mellitus, also noninsulin-dependent diabetes mellitus unresponsive to treatment with diet and/or oral hypoglycemics

Pregnancy Risk Factor B

Usual Dosage Dose requires continuous medical supervision

Insulin, Zinc Suspension, Extended

Brand Names Humulin® U; Ultralente® Iletin®I; Ultralente® Purified Beef

Synonyms Ultralente®

Use Treatment of insulin-dependent diabetes mellitus, also noninsulin-dependent diabetes mellitus unresponsive to treatment with diet and/or oral hypoglycemics

Pregnancy Risk Factor B

Usual Dosage Dose requires continuous medical supervision

Insulin, Zinc Suspension, Prompt
Brand Names Semilente® Iletin®I; Semilente® Purified Pork
Synonyms Semilente®
Use Treatment of insulin-dependent diabetes mellitus, also noninsulin-dependent diabetes mellitus unresponsive to treatment with diet and/or oral hypoglycemics
Pregnancy Risk Factor B
Usual Dosage Dose requires continuous medical supervision

Intal® see Cromolyn Sodium on page 91

α-2-interferon see Interferon Alfa-2b on this page

Interferon Alfa-2a (in ter feer' on)
Brand Names Roferon-A®
Synonyms IFLrA; IFN; rIFN-A
Use To induce hairy-cell leukemia remission; treatment of AIDS-related Kaposi's sarcoma
Pregnancy Risk Factor C
Usual Dosage Adult: I.M., S.C. induction:

Hairy-cell leukemia: Three million units daily for 16-24 weeks; maintenance dose three million units three times per week

AIDS-related Kaposi's sarcoma: 36 million units daily for 10-12 weeks; maintenance 36 million units three times a week if tolerated

Interferon Alfa-2b
Brand Names Intron® A
Synonyms IFN-alpha 2; α-2-interferon; rLFN-α2
Use To induce hairy-cell leukemia remission; treatment of AIDS-related Kaposi's sarcoma; condylomata acuminata
Pregnancy Risk Factor C
Usual Dosage Adult:

Hairy-cell leukemia: I.M., S.C.: Two million units/m^2

AIDS-related Kaposi's sarcoma: I.M., S.C.: 30 million units/m^2 three times per week

Condylomata acuminata: Intralesionally: One million units/lesion three times per week for three weeks

Intestinex® [OTC] see Lactobacillus acidophilus and Lactobacillus bulgaricus on page 199

Intralipid® see Fat Emulsion on page 144

Intravenous Fat Emulsion see Fat Emulsion on page 144

Intron® A see Interferon Alfa-2b on this page

Intropin® see Dopamine Hydrochloride on page 122

Inulin (in' yoo lin)
Use For measurement of glomerular filtration rate (GFR)
Usual Dosage Dose varies

Inversine® *see* Mecamylamine Hydrochloride *on page 214*

Invert Sugar and Water
Use Nonelectrolyte fluid replacement and caloric supplementation solution, has same caloric value as dextrose but is more rapidly utilized
Pregnancy Risk Factor C
Usual Dosage I.V.: Infusion rate should not exceed 1 g/kg/hour

Iodinated Glycerol (eye' oh di nay ted gli' ser ole)
Brand Names Iophen®; Organidin®; R-Gen®
Use As a mucolytic expectorant in an adjunctive treatment of bronchitis, bronchial asthma, pulmonary emphysema, cystic fibrosis, or chronic sinusitis
Pregnancy Risk Factor X
Usual Dosage 20 drops in fruit juice or other liquid four times daily

Iodinated Glycerol With Dextromethorphan
Brand Names Tussi-Organidin® DM
Use Symptomatic relief of irritating, nonproductive cough associated with respiratory tract conditions
Pregnancy Risk Factor X
Usual Dosage

Adult: 5-10 mL every four hours

Children: 2.5-5 mL every four hours

Iodine (eye' oh din)
Synonyms Lugol's Solution; Strong Iodine Solution
Use Used preoperatively to reduce vascularity of the thyroid gland prior to thyroidectomy; management of thyrotoxic crisis or recurrent hyperthyroidism
Usual Dosage Oral:

Reduce vascularity of the thyroid gland preoperatively: 0.1-0.3 mL three times/day; dilute with water or juice

Thyrotoxic crisis: 1 mL three times/day; dilute with water or juice

Graves' disease in neonates: 1 drop every 8 hours

Iodine *see* Trace Metals *on page 358*

Iodipamide Meglumine (eye oh di' pa mide)
Brand Names Cholografin® Meglumine
Use Used in cholangiography and cholecystography
Usual Dosage I.V.: 10.3% - 100 mL by slow infusion over 30-45 minutes; 52% - 20 mL by slow injection over 10 minutes

Iodipamide Meglumine and Diatrizoate Meglumine *see*
Diatrizoate Meglumine and Iodipamide Meglumine
on page 109

Iodochlorhydroxyquin (eye oh doe klor' hye drox ee kwin)
Brand Names Vioform® [OTC]
Synonyms Clioquinol
Use Used topically in the treatment of tinea pedis, tinea cruris, and skin infections caused by dermatophytic fungi (ring worm)
Usual Dosage Apply 2-3 times daily; do not use over seven days

Iodochlorhydroxyquin and Hydrocortisone
Brand Names Vioform-HC®
Synonyms Hydrocortisone and Iodochlorhydroxyquin
Use Contact or atopic dermatitis; eczema; neurodermatitis; anogenital pruritus; mycotic dermatoses; moniliasis
Usual Dosage Apply in a thin film 3-4 times daily

Iodo-Pak® see Trace Metals on page 358

Iodopen® see Trace Metals on page 358

Iodoquinol (eye oh. doe kwin' ole)
Brand Names Yodoxin®
Synonyms Diiodohydroxyquin
Use Treatment of acute and chronic intestinal amebiasis; asymptomatic cyst passers; *Blastocystis hominis* infections
Pregnancy Risk Factor C
Usual Dosage
  Adult: 650 mg 2-3 times daily after meals for 20 days; not to exceed 2 g daily
  Children: 30-40 mg/kg/day in 2-3 divided doses for 20 days; not to exceed 1.95 g daily

Iodoquinol and Hydrocortisone
Brand Names Vytone®
Use Treatment of eczema; infectious dermatitis; chronic eczematoid otitis externa; mycotic dermatoses
Usual Dosage Apply 3-4 times daily

Iohexol (eye oh hex' ole)
Brand Names Omnipaque®
Use For various intrathecal and intravascular radiographic procedures
Usual Dosage Dose varies with procedure

Ionamin® see Phentermine Hydrochloride on page 280

Ionil® [OTC] see Salicylic Acid on page 319

Iopanoic Acid (eye oh pa noe' ik)
Brand Names Telepaque®
Use For oral cholecystography and cholangiography
Usual Dosage 3 g

Iophen® see Iodinated Glycerol on previous page

Iopidine® *see* Apraclonidine Hydrochloride *on page 28*

Iosat® *see* Potassium Iodide *on page 291*

Iothalamate Meglumine (eye oh thal a' mate)
Brand Names Conray®
Use For use in cystography and cystourethrography, retrograde pyelography (43%) as well as many other procedures where a parenteral agent is needed
Usual Dosage Dose varies with procedure

Iothalamate Sodium
Brand Names Angio-Conray®
Synonyms Sodium Iothalamate
Use Parenteral radiopaque agent used in urography, angiocardiography, and aortography
Usual Dosage Dose varies with procedure

Ipecac Syrup (ip' e kak)
Use Treatment of acute oral drug overdosage and in certain poisonings
Pregnancy Risk Factor C
Usual Dosage Oral:

Adult: 30 mL followed by 200-300 mL of water; repeat dose one time if vomiting does not occur within 20 minutes

Children:
1-12 years of age: 15 mL followed by 10-20 mL/kg of water; repeat dose one time if vomiting does not occur within 20 minutes
6-12 months: 5-10 mL followed by 10-20 mL/kg of water; repeat dose one time if vomiting does not occur within 20 minutes

I-Phrine® Ophthalmic Solution *see* Phenylephrine Hydrochloride *on page 282*

I-Pilocarpine® *see* Pilocarpine Hydrochloride *on page 285*

Ipodate Sodium (eye' poe date)
Brand Names Oragrafin®
Use Diagnostic aid (radiopaque medium) in oral cholecystography
Usual Dosage Adult: Oral: 3 g

Ipratropium Bromide (i pra troe' pee um)
Brand Names Atrovent®
Use A bronchodilator used in bronchospasm associated with COPD, bronchitis, and emphysema
Pregnancy Risk Factor B
Usual Dosage Two inhalations four times a day up to 12 inhalations in 24 hours

I-Pred® *see* Prednisolone *on page 294*

Iproveratril Hydrochloride *see* Verapamil Hydrochloride *on page 374*

IPV *see* Poliovirus Vaccine, Inactivated *on page 289*

Iron Dextran Complex
Brand Names Imferon®
Use Treatment of iron deficiency anemia
Pregnancy Risk Factor C
Usual Dosage I.M., I.V.:

Iron deficient anemia:

$$0.3 \times \text{weight (lb)} \times (100 - \frac{\text{hemoglobin in g\% } \times 100}{14.8}) = \frac{\text{mg iron}}{50} = \text{total dose mL}$$

ISD *see* Isosorbide Dinitrate *on page 194*

ISDN *see* Isosorbide Dinitrate *on page 194*

ISG *see* Immune Globulin *on page 183*

Ismelin® *see* Guanethidine Sulfate *on page 164*

Ismotic® *see* Isosorbide *on page 193*

Isobamate *see* Carisoprodol *on page 61*

Iso-Bid® *see* Isosorbide Dinitrate *on page 194*

Isocal® [OTC] *see* Nutritional Formula, Enteral/Oral
on page 258

Isocarboxazid (eye soe kar box' a zid)
Brand Names Marplan®
Use Symptomatic treatment of depressed patients refractory to or intoler-ant to tricyclic antidepressants or electroconvulsive therapy
Pregnancy Risk Factor C
Usual Dosage 10 mg three times a day; reduce to 10-20 mg daily in divid-ed doses when condition improves

Isodine® [OTC] *see* Povidone-Iodine *on page 292*

Isoethadione *see* Paramethadione *on page 269*

Isoetharine (eye soe eth' a reen)
Brand Names Arm-a-Med® Isoetharine; Beta-2®; Bronkometer®; Bronko-sol®; Dey-Lute® Isoetharine
Synonyms Isoetharine Hydrochloride; Isoetharine Mesylate
Use Bronchodilator in bronchial asthma and for reversible bronchospasm occurring with bronchitis and emphysema
Pregnancy Risk Factor C
Usual Dosage Treatments are usually not repeated more often than every four hours, except in severe cases.

Hydrochloride: Hand nebulizer: 3-7 inhalations undiluted; oxygen aerol-ization

IPPB: 0.25-0.5 mL diluted 1:3 with sterile normal saline or other diluent

Mesylate: Metered dose inhalator (MDI): 1-2 inhalations every four hours if necessary
(Continued)

Isoetharine *(Continued)*

1% solution:
Adult: 0.5 mL in 2-4 mL of normal saline every 2-4 hours
Children: 0.01-0.02 mL/kg in 1.5-2 mL normal saline with a maximum
dose of 0.5 mL/dose given every 2-6 hours

Isoetharine Hydrochloride *see* Isoetharine *on previous page*

Isoetharine Mesylate *see* Isoetharine *on previous page*

Isoflurane (eye soe flure' ane)
Brand Names Forane®
Use General induction and maintenance of anesthesia (inhalation)
Usual Dosage 1.5-3%

Isoflurophate (eye soe flure' oh fate)
Brand Names Floropryl®
Synonyms DFP; Diisopropyl Fluorophosphate; Dyflos; Fluostigmin
Use Treat primary open-angle glaucoma and conditions that obstruct
aqueous outflow and to treat accommodative convergent strabismus
Usual Dosage

Glaucoma: 1/4" strip in eye every 8-72 hours

Strabismus: 1/4" strip to each eye every night for two weeks

Isomil® *see* Infant Nutritional Formulas *on page 184*

Isonate® *see* Isosorbide Dinitrate *on page 194*

Isoniazid (eye soe nye' a zid)
Brand Names Laniazid®; Nydrazid®
Synonyms INH; Isonicotinic Acid Hydrazide
Use In treatment of susceptible tuberculosis infections and prophylactical-
ly to those individuals exposed to tuberculosis
Pregnancy Risk Factor C
Usual Dosage Oral, I.M.:

Adult: 5-10 mg/kg/day, maximum 300 mg/day; or 15 mg/kg 2-3 times
weekly, maximum 900 mg twice weekly

Children: 10-20 mg/kg/day, maximum 300-500 mg/day; or 20-40 mg/kg
two times weekly, maximum 900 mg twice weekly. When used in conjunction with rifampin (15 mg/kg/day) limit isoniazid to 10 mg/kg/day to
minimize risk of hepatotoxicity

Isonicotinic Acid Hydrazide *see* Isoniazid *on this page*

Isonipecaine Hydrochloride *see* Meperidine Hydrochloride
on page 218

Isoprenaline Hydrochloride *see* Isoproterenol *on next page*

Isopro® *see* Isoproterenol *on next page*

Isopropamide Iodide (eye soe proe' pa mide)
Brand Names Darbid®
Use Adjunctive therapy for peptic ulcer, irritable bowel syndrome
Pregnancy Risk Factor C
Usual Dosage Adult and Children: > 12 years: Oral: 5-10 mg every 12 hours

Isoproterenol (eye soe proe ter' e nole)
Brand Names Aerolone®; Dey-Dose® Isoproterenol; Dispos-a-Med® Isoproterenol; Isopro®; Isuprel®; Medihaler-Iso®; Norisodrine®; Vapo-Iso®
Synonyms Isoprenaline Hydrochloride; Isoproterenol Hydrochloride; Isoproterenol Sulfate
Use Treatment of reversible airway obstruction as in asthma or COPD; used parenterally in A-V nodal block or shock
Pregnancy Risk Factor C
Usual Dosage

Adult:
Bronchodilation: (using 1:200 inhalation solution) 0.25-0.5 mL diluted with normal saline to 2 mL; give every four hours as needed
Cardiac arrhythmias: 5 μg/minute initially, titrate to patient response (2-20 μg/minute)
Shock: I.V.: 0.5-5 μg/minute; adjust according to response

Children:
Bronchodilation: (using 1:200 inhalation solution) 0.01 mL/kg/dose every four hours as needed (maximum 0.05 mL/dose) diluted with NS to 2 mL
Cardiac arrhythmias: Start 0.1 μg/kg/minute (usual effective dose 0.2-2 μg/kg/minute)

Isoproterenol Hydrochloride *see* Isoproterenol *on this page*

Isoproterenol Sulfate *see* Isoproterenol *on this page*

Isoptin® *see* Verapamil Hydrochloride *on page 374*

Isopto® Atropine *see* Atropine Sulfate *on page 32*

Isopto® Carbachol *see* Carbachol *on page 57*

Isopto® Carpine® *see* Pilocarpine Hydrochloride *on page 285*

Isopto® Eserine *see* Physostigmine Salicylate *on page 284*

Isopto® Frin Ophthalmic Solution *see* Phenylephrine Hydrochloride *on page 282*

Isopto® Homatropine *see* Homatropine Hydrobromide *on page 170*

Isopto® Hyoscine *see* Scopolamine *on page 321*

Isordil® *see* Isosorbide Dinitrate *on next page*

Isosorbide (eye soe sor' bide)
Brand Names Ismotic®
Use Short-term emergency treatment of acute angle-closure glaucoma
Pregnancy Risk Factor C
Usual Dosage Adult: Oral: Initially 1.5 g/kg with a usual range of 1-3 g/kg 2-4 times daily

Isosorbide Dinitrate
Brand Names Dilitrate®-SR; Iso-Bid®; Isonate®; Isordil®; Isotrate®; Sorbitrate®

Synonyms ISD; ISDN

Use Prevention and treatment of angina pectoris

Pregnancy Risk Factor C

Usual Dosage Adult:
   Oral: 5-30 mg four times a day or 40 mg every 6-12 hours in sustained-released dosage form
   Sublingual: 2.5-10 mg every 4-6 hours
   Chew: 5-10 mg every 2-3 hours

Isotrate® see Isosorbide Dinitrate on this page

Isotretinoin (eye soe tret' i noyn)
Brand Names Accutane®

Synonyms 13-cis-Retinoic Acid

Use Treatment of severe recalcitrant cystic and/or conglobate acne unresponsive to conventional therapy

Pregnancy Risk Factor X

Usual Dosage 0.5-2 mg/kg/day in two divided doses for 15-20 weeks; investigational use: 100 mg/m^2/day has been used

Isoxsuprine Hydrochloride (eye sox' syoo preen)
Brand Names Vasodilan®

Use Treatment of peripheral vascular diseases, such as arteriosclerosis obliterans and Raynaud's disease

Pregnancy Risk Factor C

Usual Dosage 10-20 mg 3-4 times daily

Isuprel® see Isoproterenol on previous page

I-Tropine® see Atropine Sulfate on page 32

IUdR see Idoxuridine on page 181

Ivadantin® see Nitrofurantoin on page 253

I-White® Ophthalmic Solution see Phenylephrine Hydrochloride on page 282

Janimine® see Imipramine on page 182

Kabikinase® see Streptokinase on page 333

Kanamycin Sulfate (kan a mye' sin)
Brand Names Kantrex®

Use Treatment of susceptible bacterial infection including gram-negative aerobes, gram-positive *Bacillus* as well as some mycobacteria

Pregnancy Risk Factor D

Usual Dosage

Adult:
   Infections: I.M., I.V.: 15 mg/kg/day in divided doses every 8-12 hours
   Preoperative intestinal antisepsis: Oral: 1 g every 4-6 hours for 36-72 hours

Children: I.M., I.V.: Infections: 15 mg/kg/day in divided doses every 8-12 hours

Kantrex® *see* Kanamycin Sulfate *on previous page*

Kanular® *see* Pancrelipase *on page 267*

Kaochlor® S-F *see* Potassium Chloride *on page 291*

Kaolin and Pectin (kay' oh lin)
Brand Names Kao-tin® [OTC]; K-Pek® [OTC]
Synonyms Pectin and Kaolin
Use Treatment of uncomplicated diarrhea
Pregnancy Risk Factor C
Usual Dosage Oral:

Adult: 60-120 mL after each loose stool

Children:
6-12 years: 30-60 mL after each loose stool
3-6 years: 15-30 mL after each loose stool

Kaolin and Pectin With Opium
Brand Names Parepectolin®
Use Symptomatic relief of diarrhea
Restrictions C-V
Pregnancy Risk Factor C
Usual Dosage Oral:

Adult and Children: > 12 years of age: 15-30 mL with each loose bowel movement, not to exceed 120 mL in 12 hours

Children:
6-12 years: 5-10 mL with each loose bowel movement, not to exceed 40 mL in 12 hours
3-6 years: 7.5 mL with each loose bowel movement, not to exceed 30 mL in 12 hours

Kaon® *see* Potassium Gluconate *on page 291*

Kaopectate® [OTC] *see* Attapulgite *on page 32*

Kao-tin® [OTC] *see* Kaolin and Pectin *on this page*

Karaya Powder *see* Indian Gum *on page 184*

Kato® *see* Potassium Chloride *on page 291*

Kayexalate® *see* Sodium Polystyrene Sulfonate *on page 329*

K-Dur® 20 *see* Potassium Chloride *on page 291*

Keflet® *see* Cephalexin Monohydrate *on page 66*

Keflex® *see* Cephalexin Monohydrate *on page 66*

Keflin® *see* Cephalothin Sodium *on page 66*

Keftab® *see* Cephalexin Monohydrate *on page 66*

Kefurox® *see* Cefuroxime *on page 65*

Kefzol® *see* Cefazolin Sodium *on page 63*

Kemadrin® *see* Procyclidine Hydrochloride *on page 299*

Kenacort® Syrup *see* Triamcinolone *on page 359*

Kenacort® Tablet *see* Triamcinolone *on page 359*

Kenalog® Injection *see* Triamcinolone *on page 359*

Keralyt® *see* Salicylic Acid and Propylene Glycol *on page 320*

Keri® *see* Emollient Cream *on page 129*

Keri® Lotion [OTC] *see* Emollient Lotion *on page 129*

Ketalar® *see* Ketamine Hydrochloride *on this page*

Ketamine Hydrochloride (keet' a meen)
Brand Names Ketalar®
Use Induction of anesthesia; short procedures; supplement nitrous oxide
Pregnancy Risk Factor D
Usual Dosage
    I.V.: Initial: 1-4.5 mg/kg (0.5-2 mg/lb)
    I.M.: Initial: 6.5-13 mg/kg (3-6 mg/lb)/10 mg/kg (5 mg/lb) will usually produce 12-25 minutes of anesthesia
    Maintenance: Increments of one-half to the full induction dose may be repeated as needed

    Adult: I.V.: 1-2 mg/kg at a rate of 0.5 mg/minute for induction of anesthesia

    Children:
        I.V. bolus: Dilute 100 mg/mL solution 1:1 with sterile water, normal saline, or D_5W or use the 10 or 50 mg/mL solution without further dilution
        I.M.: 5-7 mg/kg/dose
        I.V. 2-3 mg/kg/dose

Ketoconazole (kee toe koe' na zole)
Brand Names Nizoral®
Use Treatment of susceptible fungal infections, including candidiasis, oral thrush, blastomycosis, histoplasmosis as well as dermatophytoses and superficial mycoses
Pregnancy Risk Factor C
Usual Dosage Oral:

    Adult: 200-400 mg every day

    Children: 3.3-6.6 mg/kg/day in single dose

Keto-Diastix® [OTC] *see* Diagnostic Test for Glucose and Ketones in Urine *on page 107*

Ketoprofen (kee toe proe' fen)
Brand Names Orudis®
Use Acute or long term treatment of rheumatoid arthritis and osteoarthritis; primary dysmenorrhea; mild to moderate pain
Pregnancy Risk Factor B/D in third trimester
Usual Dosage Adult and Children: > 12 years: Oral: 50-75 mg 3-4 times a day up to 300 mg/daily

Ketorolac Tromethamine (kee' toe role ak)
Brand Names Toradol®
Use Short-term management of pain
Pregnancy Risk Factor B
Usual Dosage Adult: I.M.: 30 mg initially then 15 mg every 6 hours thereafter, or 60 mg initially, then 30 mg every 6 hours thereafter; a maximum dose in the first 24 hours is 150 mg with 120 mg per 24 hours thereafter

Ketostix® [OTC] see Diagnostic Test for Acetone in Urine on page 106

Key-Pred® see Prednisolone on page 294

Key-Pred-SP® see Prednisolone on page 294

KI see Potassium Iodide on page 291

Kidrolase® see Asparaginase on page 30

Kinesed® see Hyoscyamine, Atropine, Scopolamine and Phenobarbital on page 179

Kinevac® see Sincalide on page 325

Klonopin™ see Clonazepam on page 83

K-Lor™ see Potassium Chloride on page 291

Kloromin® [OTC] see Chlorpheniramine Maleate on page 74

K-Lyte/CL® see Potassium Chloride on page 291

KMnO₄ see Potassium Permanganate on page 292

Koate®-HS see Antihemophilic Factor, Human on page 26

Koate®-HT see Antihemophilic Factor, Human on page 26

Konakion® see Phytonadione on page 285

Kondremul® [OTC] see Mineral Oil on page 237

Konsyl® [OTC] see Psyllium on page 308

Konsyl-D® [OTC] see Psyllium on page 308

Konyne®-HT see Factor IX Complex (Human) on page 143

Kool Foot® [OTC] see Zinc Undecylenate on page 382

K-Pek® [OTC] see Kaolin and Pectin on page 195

K-Phos® Modified Formula see Potassium Acid Phosphate on page 291

K-PHOS® Neutral [OTC] see Phosphorus Replacement Products on page 284

K-Phos® Neutral see Potassium Phosphate and Sodium Phosphate on page 292

Kutrase® see Pancrelipase on page 267

Ku-Zyme® see Pancrelipase on page 267

Kwell® see Lindane on page 204

K-Y® Jelly [OTC] see Lubricating Jelly on page 208

L-3-Hydroxytyrosine *see* Levodopa *on page 201*

Labetalol Hydrochloride (la bet' a lole)
Brand Names Normodyne®; Trandate®
Synonyms Ibidomide Hydrochloride
Use Treatment of mild to severe hypertension
Pregnancy Risk Factor C
Usual Dosage

Adult:
 Oral: 100 mg twice daily, may increase as needed every 2-3 days by
   100 mg until desired response is obtained; usual dose is 200-400 mg
   twice daily; not to exceed 2.4 g/day
 I.V.: 20 mg or 1-2 mg/kg whichever is lower, IVP over 2 minutes, may
   give 40-80 mg at 10-minute intervals, up to 300 mg
 I.V. infusion: May start at 2 mg/minute

Children: Oral: Initial: 4 mg/kg/day in 2 divided doses

LaBID® *see* Theophylline *on page 348*

Labstix® [OTC] *see* Diagnostic Test for Acetone, Blood, Glucose,
 pH, and Protein in Urine *on page 106*

Lac-Hydrin® *see* Lactic Acid With Ammonium Hydroxide
 on this page

Lacri-Lube® [OTC] *see* Ocular Lubricant *on page 259*

Lactaid® [OTC] *see* Lactase *on this page*

Lactase
Brand Names Lactaid® [OTC]; Lactrase® [OTC]
Use To help digest lactose in milk for patients with lactose intolerance
Usual Dosage Capsules: 1-2 capsules

Lactated Ringer's *see* Ringer's Injection, Lactated
 on page 316

Lactic Acid and Salicylic Acid *see* Salicylic Acid and Lactic
 Acid *on page 319*

Lactic Acid and Sodium-PCA (lak' tik)
Brand Names LactiCare® [OTC]
Synonyms Sodium-PCA and Lactic Acid
Use Lubricate and moisturize the skin counteracting dryness and itching
Usual Dosage Apply as needed

Lactic Acid With Ammonium Hydroxide
Brand Names Lac-Hydrin®
Use Treatment of moderate to severe xerosis and ichthyosis vulgaris
Usual Dosage Shake well; apply to affected areas, use twice daily, rub in
 well

LactiCare® [OTC] *see* Lactic Acid and Sodium-PCA
 on this page

Lactinex® [OTC] *see Lactobacillus acidophilus* and *Lactobacillus bulgaricus on this page*

Lactobacillus acidophilus and *Lactobacillus bulgaricus*

Brand Names Bacid® [OTC]; Enterodophilus® [OTC]; Intestinex® [OTC]; Lactinex® [OTC]; More-Dophilus® [OTC]

Use Uncomplicated diarrhea particularly that caused by antibiotic therapy; re-establish normal physiologic and bacterial flora of the intestinal tract

Usual Dosage

Granules: One packet added to or taken with cereal, food, milk, fruit juice, or water, 3-4 times daily

Tablet, chewable: Four tablets 3-4 times daily; may follow each dose with a small amount of milk, fruit juice, or water

Lactoflavin *see Riboflavin on page 316*

Lactrase® [OTC] *see Lactase on previous page*

Lactulose (lak' tyoo lose)

Brand Names Cephulac®; Cholac®; Chronulac®; Constilac®; Constulose®; Duphalac®; Enulose®; Generlac®; Lactulose PSE®

Use Adjunct in the prevention and treatment of portal-systemic encephalopathy; treatment of chronic constipation

Pregnancy Risk Factor C

Usual Dosage Oral:

Adult: 30-40 mL, 3-4 times daily; adjust dosage daily to produce 2-3 soft stools; doses of 30-45 mL may be given hourly to cause rapid laxation, then reduce to recommended dose

Children (little information on use with children): Older children: Daily dose of 40-50 mL; if initial dose causes diarrhea, then reduce it immediately

Infants: 2.5-10 mL in divided doses

Lactulose PSE® *see Lactulose on this page*

Ladakamycin *see Azacitidine on page 33*

Lamprene® *see Clofazimine on page 83*

Laniazid® *see Isoniazid on page 192*

Lanolin (lan' oh lin)

Synonyms Hydrous Wool Fat; Refined Wool Fat; Wool Fat

Lanoxicaps® *see Digoxin on page 113*

Lanoxin® *see Digoxin on page 113*

Lantrisul® *see Sulfadiazine, Sulfamethazine and Sulfamerazine on page 336*

Lariam® *see Mefloquine Hydrochloride on page 216*

Larodopa® *see* Levodopa *on next page*

Larotid® *see* Amoxicillin *on page 21*

Lasan® *see* Anthralin *on page 26*

Lasix® *see* Furosemide *on page 155*

Lassar's Zinc Paste *see* Zinc Oxide *on page 382*

Latamoxef Disodium *see* Moxalactam Disodium *on page 241*

LAtest ASO® *see* Diagnostic Test for Streptococci *on page 108*

LAtest-CRP® *see* Diagnostic Test for C-Reactive Protein *on page 107*

LAtest-RF® *see* Diagnostic Test for Rheumatoid Factor *on page 108*

Lavacol® **[OTC]** *see* Alcohol, Ethyl *on page 11*

Lax-Pills® **[OTC]** *see* Phenolphthalein *on page 280*

***l*-Bunolol Hydrochloride** *see* Levobunolol Hydrochloride *on next page*

L-Carnitine *see* Levocarnitine *on next page*

L.C.D. *see* Coal Tar *on page 85*

LCR *see* Vincristine Sulfate *on page 376*

L-Deprenyl *see* Selegiline Hydrochloride *on page 322*

***L*-Dopa** *see* Levodopa *on next page*

Ledercillin® **VK** *see* Penicillin V Potassium *on page 274*

Lederplex® **[OTC]** *see* Vitamin B Complex *on page 377*

Legatrin® **[OTC]** *see* Quinine Sulfate *on page 312*

Lente® *see* Insulin, Zinc Suspension *on page 186*

Lente® **Iletin**®**I** *see* Insulin, Zinc Suspension *on page 186*

Lente® **Iletin**® **II (Beef)** *see* Insulin, Zinc Suspension *on page 186*

Lente® **Iletin**® **II (Pork)** *see* Insulin, Zinc Suspension *on page 186*

Lente® **Purified Pork Insulin** *see* Insulin, Zinc Suspension *on page 186*

Leucovorin Calcium (loo koe vor' in)
  Brand Names Wellcovorin®
  Synonyms Calcium Leucovorin; Citrovorum Factor; Folinic Acid; 5-Formyl Tetrahydrofolate
  Use Antidote for folic acid antagonists, treatment of megaloblastic anemias when folate is deficient as in infancy, sprue, pregnancy, and nutritional deficiency when oral folate therapy is not possible
Pregnancy Risk Factor C
Usual Dosage Adult:
    Rescue dose: Oral, I.V.: 10 mg/m² to start, then 10 mg/m² every six hours orally for 72 hours

Megaloblastic anemia: I.M.: 1 mg every day

Leukeran® *see* Chlorambucil *on page 69*

Leuprolide Acetate (loo proe' lide)
Brand Names Lupron®
Synonyms Leuprorelin Acetate
Use Palliative treatment of advanced prostate carcinoma, precocious puberty
Pregnancy Risk Factor B
Usual Dosage S.C.:

Adult: Advanced prostatic carcinoma: 1 mg/day

Children: Precocious puberty: 35-40 µg/kg/day

Leuprorelin Acetate *see* Leuprolide Acetate *on this page*

Leurocristine *see* Vincristine Sulfate *on page 376*

Levamisole (lee vam' i sole)
Brand Names Tramisol
Use Adjuvant treatment with fluorouracil in Dukes stage C colon cancer
Usual Dosage Oral: 50 mg every 8 hours for 3 days initially, then 50 mg every 8 hours for 3 days every 2 weeks (Fluorouracil is always given concomitantly)

Levarterenol Bitartrate *see* Norepinephrine Bitartrate
on page 255

Levobunolol Hydrochloride (lee voe byoo' noe lole)
Brand Names Betagan® Liquifilm®
Synonyms *l*-Bunolol Hydrochloride
Use To lower intraocular pressure in chronic open-angle glaucoma or ocular hypertension
Pregnancy Risk Factor C
Usual Dosage Adult: One (1) drop in eye(s) 1-2 times a day

Levocarnitine (lee voe kar' ni teen)
Brand Names Carnitor®; Vitacarn®
Synonyms L-Carnitine
Use Therapy in patients with primary systemic carnitine deficiency
Pregnancy Risk Factor B
Usual Dosage Oral:

Adult: 940 mg 2-3 times daily

Children: 50-100 mg/kg/day

Levodopa (lee voe doe' pa)
Brand Names Dopar®; Larodopa®
Synonyms *L*-3-Hydroxytyrosine; *L*-Dopa
Use Treatment of Parkinson's disease; used as a diagnostic agent for growth hormone deficiency
(Continued)

Levodopa *(Continued)*
Pregnancy Risk Factor C
Usual Dosage Oral:

Adult: 500-1000 mg/day in divided doses every 6-12 hours; increase by 100-750 mg/day every 3-7 days until response or total dose of 8000 is reached

Children:
> 70 lbs: 500 mg
30-70 lbs: 250 mg
< 30 lbs: 125 mg

Levodopa and Carbidopa
Brand Names Sinemet®
Synonyms Carbidopa and Levodopa
Use Treatment of Parkinsonian syndrome
Pregnancy Risk Factor C
Usual Dosage Adult: Oral: 75/300 to 150/1500 mg/day in 3-4 divided doses; can increase up to 200/2000 mg/day

Levo-Dromoran® *see* Levorphanol Tartrate *on this page*

Levomepromazine *see* Methotrimeprazine Hydrochloride *on page 228*

Levonorgestrel and Ethinyl Estradiol *see* Ethinyl Estradiol and Levonorgestrel *on page 139*

Levophed® *see* Norepinephrine Bitartrate *on page 255*

Levoprome® *see* Methotrimeprazine Hydrochloride *on page 228*

Levorphanol Tartrate *(lee vor' fa nole)*
Brand Names Levo-Dromoran®
Synonyms Levorphan Tartrate
Use Relief of moderate to severe pain; also used parenterally for preoperative sedation and an adjunct to nitrous oxide/oxygen anesthesia
Restrictions C-II
Pregnancy Risk Factor B/D
Usual Dosage Adult: Oral, S.C.: 2 mg, up to 3 mg if necessary

Levorphan Tartrate *see* Levorphanol Tartrate *on this page*

Levothroid® *see* Levothyroxine Sodium *on this page*

Levothyroxine Sodium *(lee voe thye rox' een)*
Brand Names Levothroid®; Levoxine®; Synthroid®; Synthrox®; Syroxine®
Synonyms *L*-Thyroxine Sodium; T_4 Thyroxine Sodium
Use Replacement or supplemental therapy in hypothyroidism
Pregnancy Risk Factor A
Usual Dosage

Adult:
Oral: 12.5-50 µg/day to start, then increase by 25-50 µg/day at intervals of 2-4 weeks; most adults dose is 100-200 µg/day

I.V.: 75% of oral dose

Children: Oral:
   Over 12 years: Over 150 μg/day; 2-3 μg/kg/day
   6-12 years: 100-150 μg/day; 4-5 μg/kg/day
   1-5 years: 75-100 μg/day; 5-6 μg/kg/day
   6-12 months: 50-75 μg/day; 6-8 μg/kg/day
   0-6 months of age: 25-50 μg/day; 8-10 μg/kg/day

Children: I.V.: 75% of oral dose

Neonates: I.V.: 20-40 mg/day; 4 weeks - 1 year of age: 40 mg/day

Levoxine® *see* Levothyroxine Sodium *on previous page*

Levsin® *see* Hyoscyamine Sulfate *on page 180*

Levsinex® *see* Hyoscyamine Sulfate *on page 180*

Levulose *see* Fructose *on page 154*

Levulose, Dextrose and Phosphoric Acid
Brand Names Emetrol® [OTC]
Synonyms Dextrose, Levulose and Phosphoric Acid; Phosphoric Acid, Levulose and Dextrose
Use Relieve nausea associated with upset stomach that occurs with intestinal flu, pregnancy, food indiscretions, and emotional upsets
Usual Dosage

Morning sickness: 15-30 mL on arising; repeat every three hours or when nausea threatens

Motion sickness and vomiting due to drug therapy: 5 mL doses for young children; 15 mL doses for older children and adults

Regurgitation in infants: 5 or 10 mL, 10-15 minutes before each feeding; in refractory cases: 10-15 mL, 30 minutes before each feeding

Vomiting due to psychogenic factors:
   Adult: 15-30 mL; repeat dose every 15 minutes until distress subsides; do not take for more than one hour
   Children: 5-10 mL; repeat dose every 15 minutes until distress subsides; do not take for more than one hour

l-Hyoscyamine Sulfate *see* Hyoscyamine Sulfate *on page 180*

Librax® *see* Clidinium and Chlordiazepoxide *on page 81*

Libritabs® *see* Chlordiazepoxide *on page 69*

Librium® *see* Chlordiazepoxide *on page 69*

Lida-Mantle HC® *see* Hydrocortisone and Lidocaine *on page 175*

Lidex® *see* Fluocinonide *on page 150*

Lidex® E *see* Fluocinonide *on page 150*

Lidocaine and Epinephrine
Brand Names Xylocaine® With Epinephrine
Use Local infiltration anesthesia
(Continued)

Lidocaine and Epinephrine *(Continued)*
Pregnancy Risk Factor B
Usual Dosage Dosage varies with the anesthetic procedure
Children: Lidocaine dose should not exceed 7 mg/kg

Lidocaine Hydrochloride (lye' doe kane)
Brand Names Anestacon®; Baylocaine®; LidoPen®; Xylocaine®
Synonyms Lignocaine Hydrochloride
Use Local anesthetic and acute treatment of ventricular arrhythmias from myocardial infarction, cardiac manipulation, digitalis intoxication
Pregnancy Risk Factor B
Usual Dosage

Topical: Apply to affected area as needed
Injectable local anesthetic: Varies with procedure, degree of anesthesia needed, vascularity of tissue, duration of anesthesia required, and physical condition of patient

Adult: Antiarrhythmic: I.V.: 50-100 mg bolus, may repeat in five minutes; no more than 200-300 g should be administered in a one hour period; then 1-3 mg/minute infusion

Children: I.V.: 0.5-1 mg/kg bolus, not to exceed 3-5 mg/kg/dose; then 10-50 μg/kg/minute infusion

LidoPen® *see* Lidocaine Hydrochloride *on this page*

Lignocaine Hydrochloride *see* Lidocaine Hydrochloride *on this page*

Limbitrol® *see* Amitriptyline and Chlordiazepoxide *on page 20*

Lincocin® *see* Lincomycin *on this page*

Lincomycin (lin koe mye' sin)
Brand Names Lincocin®
Use Treatment of susceptible bacterial infections, mainly those caused by streptococci and staphylococci
Pregnancy Risk Factor C
Usual Dosage

Adult:
Oral: 500 mg every 6-8 hours
I.M.: 600 mg every 12-24 hours
I.V.: 600-1 g every 8-12 hours up to 8 g/day

Children: > 1 month:
Oral: 30-60 mg/kg/day in 3-4 divided doses
I.M.: 10 mg/kg every 12-24 hours
I.V.: 10-20 mg/kg/day in divided doses 2-3 times daily

Lindane (lin' dane)
Brand Names Kwell®
Synonyms Benzene Hexachloride; Gamma Benzene Hexachloride
Use Treatment of scabies and pediculosis

Pregnancy Risk Factor B
Usual Dosage

Scabies: Apply a thin layer of lotion and massage it on skin from the neck to the toes. For adults, bathe and remove the drug after 8-12 hours; for children, wash off 6 hours after application.

Pediculosis: 15-30 mL of shampoo is applied and lathered for 4-5 minutes; rinse hair thoroughly and comb with a fine tooth comb to remove nits; repeat treatment in 7 days if lice or nits are still present

Lioresal® see Baclofen on page 36

Liothyronine Sodium (lye oh thye' roe neen)
Brand Names Cytomel®
Synonyms Sodium L-Tri-iodothyronine; T₃ Thyronine Sodium
Use Replacement or supplemental therapy in hypothyroidism
Pregnancy Risk Factor A
Usual Dosage 25-75 µg/day

Liotrix (lye' oh trix)
Brand Names Euthroid®; Thyrolar®
Synonyms T₃/T₄ Liotrix
Use Replacement or supplemental therapy in hypothyroidism
Pregnancy Risk Factor A
Usual Dosage 0.5-3 grains/day

Lipancreatin see Pancrelipase on page 267

Lipomul Oral [OTC] see Corn Oil on page 89

Liposyn® see Fat Emulsion on page 144

Lipovite® [OTC] see Vitamin B Complex on page 377

Liquaemin® see Heparin on page 167

Liquapen® see Penicillin G, Parenteral on page 273

Liqui-Char® [OTC] see Charcoal on page 68

Liquid Antidote see Charcoal on page 68

Lisinopril (lyse in' oh pril)
Brand Names Prinivil®; Zestril®
Use Treatment of hypertension, either alone or in combination with other antihypertensive agents
Pregnancy Risk Factor C
Usual Dosage 20-40 mg/day in a single dose

Lithane® see Lithium on this page

Lithium (lith' ee um)
Brand Names Cibalith-S®; Eskalith®; Lithane®; Lithobid®; Lithonate®; Lithotabs®
Synonyms Lithium Carbonate; Lithium Citrate
Use Treat acute manic episodes and as a prophylaxis against their recurrence

(Continued)

205

Lithium *(Continued)*
Pregnancy Risk Factor D
Usual Dosage Oral:

Adult: 300 mg 3-4 times daily; blood level monitoring is necessary to determine proper dose

Children: Usual dosage in children has not been established; 15-60 mg/kg/day in divided doses have been administered; do not exceed usual adult dose; monitor serum levels closely

Lithium Carbonate *see* Lithium *on previous page*

Lithium Citrate *see* Lithium *on previous page*

Lithobid® *see* Lithium *on previous page*

Lithonate® *see* Lithium *on previous page*

Lithotabs® *see* Lithium *on previous page*

Lixolin® *see* Theophylline *on page 348*

8-L-Lysine Vasopressin *see* Lypressin *on page 209*

LMD® *see* Dextran *on page 103*

Lodosyn® *see* Carbidopa *on page 58*

Lodrane® *see* Theophylline *on page 348*

Loestrin® 1.5/30 *see* Ethinyl Estradiol and Norethindrone Acetate *on page 139*

Lomotil® *see* Diphenoxylate and Atropine *on page 118*

Lomustine *(loe mus' teen)*
Brand Names CeeNU®
Synonyms CCNU
Use Treatment of brain tumors and Hodgkin's disease
Pregnancy Risk Factor C
Usual Dosage Adult and Children: Oral: 130 mg/m^2 as a single dose every six weeks; readjust after initial treatment according to platelet and leukocytes

Loniten® *see* Minoxidil *on page 238*

Lo/Ovral® *see* Ethinyl Estradiol and Norgestrel *on page 140*

Loperamide Hydrochloride *(loe per' a mide)*
Brand Names Imodium®; Imodium® A-D [OTC]
Use Treatment of acute diarrhea and chronic diarrhea associated with inflammatory bowel disease; also used to decrease the volume of ileostomy discharge
Pregnancy Risk Factor B
Usual Dosage Oral:

Adult: 4 mg (two capsules) initially, followed by 2 mg after each loose stool, up to 16 mg (eight capsules) per day

Children:
Acute diarrhea: 0.4-0.8 mg/kg/day divided every 6-12 hours; 13-20 kg: 1 mg three times/day; 20-30 kg: 2 mg twice/day; > 30 kg: 2 mg three times/day
Chronic diarrhea: 0.08-0.24 mg/kg/day divided 2-3 times/day

Lopid® *see* Gemfibrozil *on page 156*

Lopremone *see* Protirelin *on page 306*

Lopressor® *see* Metoprolol Tartrate *on page 234*

Loprox® *see* Ciclopirox Olamine *on page 79*

Lopurin™ *see* Allopurinol *on page 13*

Lorazepam (lor a' ze pam)
Brand Names Ativan®
Use Management of anxiety and insomnia, preoperative sedation, and to provide amnesia
Restrictions C-IV
Pregnancy Risk Factor D
Usual Dosage

Adult:
Anxiety: Oral: 2-3 mg/day in 2-3 divided doses
Insomnia: Oral: 2 mg at bedtime
Preoperative: I.M.: 0.05 mg/kg two hours before surgery; I.V.: 0.044 mg/kg 15-20 minutes before surgery
Operative amnesia: I.V.: up to 0.05 mg/kg

Children: Anticonvulsant therapy: Dosage recommendations are not well established, but are in the 0.05-0.1 mg/kg/dose range. A May 1986 Journal of Pediatrics study suggested an initial 0.05 mg/kg/dose. This dose may be repeated at 15 minute intervals **if no response is seen**, for a total of three doses

Lorelco® *see* Probucol *on page 297*

Loroxide® [OTC] *see* Benzoyl Peroxide *on page 41*

Losec® *see* Omeprazole *on page 259*

Lotrimin® *see* Clotrimazole *on page 84*

Lotrisone® *see* Betamethasone Dipropionate and Clotrimazole *on page 43*

Lovastatin (loe' va sta tin)
Brand Names Mevacor®
Synonyms Mevinolin; Monacolin K
Use Adjunct to dietary therapy to decrease elevated serum total and LDL cholesterol concentrations in primary hypercholesterolemia
Pregnancy Risk Factor X
Usual Dosage 20 mg with evening meal initially, then adjust at four week intervals; maximum dose is 80 mg/day

Loxapine (lox' a peen)
Brand Names Loxitane®

Synonyms Loxapine Hydrochloride; Loxapine Succinate; Oxilapine Succinate

Use Management of psychotic disorders

Pregnancy Risk Factor C

Usual Dosage 10 mg twice daily, increase dose until psychotic symptoms are controlled; usual dose range is 60-100 mg/day in divided doses 2-4 times daily

Loxapine Hydrochloride see Loxapine on this page

Loxapine Succinate see Loxapine on this page

Loxitane® see Loxapine on this page

Lozol® see Indapamide on page 183

L-PAM see Melphalan on page 217

L-Sarcolysin see Melphalan on page 217

L-Thyroxine Sodium see Levothyroxine Sodium on page 202

L-Tryptophan see Tryptophan on page 367

Lubricating Jelly
Brand Names K-Y® Jelly [OTC]; Surgilube® [OTC]

Use Aid for easy insertion of rectal thermometers or tampons; a sexual lubricant

Usual Dosage Apply to area and repeat as necessary

Ludiomil® see Maprotiline Hydrochloride on page 213

Lufyllin® see Dyphylline on page 126

Lugol's Solution see Iodine on page 188

Lugol's Solution see Potassium Iodide on page 291

Luminal® see Phenobarbital on page 279

Lupron® see Leuprolide Acetate on page 201

Luride® see Fluoride on page 150

Luride®-SF F Lozi-Tabs® see Fluoride on page 150

Lymphocyte Immune Globulin
Brand Names Atgam®

Synonyms Antithymocyte Immunoglobulin; ATG; Horse Anti-human Thymocyte Gamma Globulin

Use Prevention and treatment of acute renal allograft rejection; treatment of moderate to severe aplastic anemia in patients not considered suitable candidates for bone marrow transplantation

Pregnancy Risk Factor C

Usual Dosage An intradermal skin test is recommended prior to administration of the initial dose of ATG. Use 0.1 mL of a 1:1000 dilution if ATG in normal saline

Aplastic anemia protocol: 20 mg/kg/day for 8 days

Prevention: Adult and Children: I.V.: 15 mg/kg/day every 14 days, then give every other day for seven more doses

Treatment: Adult and Children: I.V. 10-15 mg/kg/day for 14 days, then give every other day for seven more doses

Lyphocin® *see* Vancomycin Hydrochloride *on page 371*

Lypressin (lye press' in)
Brand Names Diapid®
Synonyms 8-L-Lysine Vasopressin
Use To control or prevent signs and complications of neurogenic diabetes insipidus
Pregnancy Risk Factor B
Usual Dosage Adult and Children: 1-2 sprays into one or both nostrils four tirnes a day; approximately 2 USP posterior pituitary pressor units per spray

Lysodren® *see* Mitotane *on page 239*

Maalox® [OTC] *see* Aluminum Hydroxide and Magnesium Hydroxide *on page 15*

Maalox® Plus [OTC] *see* Aluminum Hydroxide, Magnesium Hydroxide and Simethicone *on page 15*

Maalox® Therapeutic Concentrate [OTC] *see* Aluminum Hydroxide and Magnesium Hydroxide *on page 15*

Macrodantin® *see* Nitrofurantoin *on page 253*

Macrodex® *see* Dextran *on page 103*

Mafenide Acetate (ma' fe nide)
Brand Names Sulfamylon®
Use Adjunct in the treatment of 2nd and 3rd degree burns to prevent septicemia caused by susceptible organisms
Pregnancy Risk Factor C
Usual Dosage Apply once or twice daily with a sterile gloved hand; apply to a thickness of approximately 15 mm; the burned area should be covered with cream at all times

Magaldrate (mag' al drate)
Brand Names Riopan® [OTC]
Synonyms Hydromagnesium aluminate
Use Symptomatic relief of hyperacidity associated with peptic ulcer, gastritis, peptic esophagitis and hiatal hernia
Pregnancy Risk Factor C
Usual Dosage Adult: Oral: 540-1080 mg between meals and at bedtime

Magaldrate and Simethicone
Brand Names Riopan Plus® [OTC]
Synonyms Simethicone and Magaldrate
Use Relief of hyperacidity associated with peptic ulcer, gastritis, peptic esophagitis and hiatal hernia which are accompanied by symptoms of gas
(Continued)

Magaldrate and Simethicone *(Continued)*

Pregnancy Risk Factor C
Usual Dosage Adult: Oral: 5-10 mL between meals and at bedtime

Magnacal® [OTC] *see* Nutritional Formula, Enteral/Oral *on page 258*

Magnesia Magma *see* Magnesium Hydroxide *on this page*

Magnesium Chloride (mag nee' zhum)

Use To correct or prevent hypomagnesemia
Usual Dosage I.V. in TPN:

Adult: 8-24 mEq/day

Children: 2-10 mEq/day

Magnesium Citrate

Brand Names Citroma® [OTC]
Synonyms Citrate of Magnesia
Use To evaluate bowel prior to certain surgical and diagnostic procedures
Usual Dosage Oral:

Adult: ≥ 12 years of age: 1/2-1 full bottle

Children:
    < 6 years of age: 2-4 mL/kg given as a single daily dose or in divided
    doses
    6-12 years: 1/3-1/2 bottle

Magnesium Citrate, Bisacodyl and Phenolphthalein

Brand Names Evac-Q-Kit® [OTC]
Use To evaluate bowel prior to certain surgical and diagnostic procedures

Magnesium Gluconate

Brand Names Magonate® [OTC]
Use Dietary supplement for treatment of magnesium deficiencies
Usual Dosage 27-54 mg 2-3 times daily

Magnesium Hydroxide

Synonyms Magnesia Magma; Milk of Magnesia; MOM
Use Short-term treatment of occasional constipation and symptoms of hy-
    peracidity
Pregnancy Risk Factor B
Usual Dosage Oral:

Adult:
    Laxative: 30-60 mL at bedtime
    Antacid: 5-15 mL as needed

Children:
    Laxative: 6-12 years of age: 15-30 mL at bedtime; 2-6 years: 5-15 mL at
    bedtime
    Antacid: 2.5-5 mL as needed

Magnesium Hydroxide and Aluminum Hydroxide *see*
Aluminum Hydroxide and Magnesium Hydroxide
on page 15

Magnesium Oxide

Use Short-term treatment of occasional constipation and symptoms of hyperacidity

Usual Dosage Oral:

Antacid: 250-1.5 g with water or milk four times a day after meals and at bedtime

Laxative: 2-4 g at bedtime with full glass of water

Magnesium Sulfate

Synonyms Epsom Salts

Use Treatment and prevention of hypomagnesemia and in seizure prevention in severe pre-eclampsia or eclampsia, pediatric acute nephritis; also used as short-term treatment of constipation

Pregnancy Risk Factor B

Usual Dosage

Adult:
Eclampsia, pre-eclampsia: I.V.: 4 g initially then switch to I.M.; I.M.: 1-4 g every four hours
Hypomagnesemia: I.M.: 1 g every six hours for four doses; in severe hypomagnesemia as much as 250 mg/kg may be given I.M. over a four hour period, or 5 g infused slowly over a three hour period; total dosage should not exceed 30-40 grams daily
Laxative: Oral: 10-30 g

Children: Laxative: Oral:
6-12 years: 5-10 g
2-5 years: 2.5-5 g

Magonate® [OTC] *see* Magnesium Gluconate *on previous page*

Maigret-50® *see* Phenylpropanolamine Hydrochloride
on page 283

Maize Oil *see* Corn Oil *on page 89*

Malathion (mal a thye' on)

Brand Names Ovide™

Use Treatment of head lice and their ova

Pregnancy Risk Factor B

Usual Dosage Sprinkle Ovide™ lotion on dry hair and rub gently until the scalp is thoroughly moistened; pay special attention to the back of the head and neck. Allow to dry naturally - use no heat and leave uncovered. After 8-12 hours, the hair should be washed with a nonmedicated shampoo; rinse and use a fine-toothed comb to remove dead lice and eggs. If required, repeat with second application in 7-9 days. Further treatment is generally not necessary. Other family members should be evaluated to determine if infested and if so, receive treatment.

Malotuss® [OTC] *see* Guaifenesin *on page 162*

Malt Soup Extract
Brand Names Maltsupex® [OTC]
Use Short-term treatment of constipation
Usual Dosage Oral:

Adult: ≥ 12 years: 30 mL twice a day for 3-4 days, then 15-30 mL 1-2 times/day

Children: 2-11 years: 15-30 mL 1-2 times/day

Infant:
Breast fed: > 1 month: 5-10 mL in 2-4 ounces of water or fruit juice 1-2 times/day
Bottle fed: > 1 month: 7.5 mL-30 mL per day in formula for 3-4 days, then 5-10 mL daily

Maltsupex® [OTC] *see* Malt Soup Extract *on this page*

Mandelamine® *see* Methenamine *on page 226*

Mandol® *see* Cefamandole Nafate *on page 62*

Manganese (man' ga nees)
Use Supplement to I.V. solutions given for TPN
Usual Dosage

Adult: 0.15-0.8 mg/day

Children: 2-10 µg/kg/day

Manganese *see* Trace Metals *on page 358*

Manga-Pak® *see* Trace Metals *on page 358*

Mannitol (man' i tole)
Brand Names Osmitrol®
Synonyms D-Mannitol
Use Reduction of increased intracranial pressure associated with cerebral edema; promotion of diuresis in the prevention and/or treatment of oliguria or anuria due to acute renal failure; reduction of increased intraocular pressure; promoting urinary excretion of toxic substances
Pregnancy Risk Factor C
Usual Dosage

Adult:
Diuresis: I.V.: Give up to 200 g
Oliguria: I.V.: 12.5 g test dose (0.2 g/kg) over 3-5 minutes, then 50-100 g if response to test dose is adequate
Intracranial or intraocular pressure: I.V.: 1.5-2 g/kg over 30-60 minutes
Urologic irrigation: 2.5% (100 mL mannitol to 900 mL sterile water for injection)

Children: Some literature suggests an initial test dose of 0.2 g/kg over 3-5 minutes; for therapeutic purposes, 2 g/kg may be given
Edema: Use 20% solution over 2-6 hours
Cerebral or ocular edema: Use 20% solution over 30-60 minutes

Mantoux *see* Tuberculin *on page 367*

Maolate® *see* Chlorphenesin Carbamate *on page 73*

Maprotiline Hydrochloride (ma proe' ti leen)
Brand Names Ludiomil®
Use Treatment of depression and anxiety associated with depression
Pregnancy Risk Factor B
Usual Dosage 75 mg/day to start, increase by 25 mg every two weeks up to 150-225 mg/day; given in three divided doses or in a single daily dose

Marax® *see* Theophylline, Ephedrine and Hydroxyzine *on page 350*

Marbaxin® *see* Methocarbamol *on page 227*

Marcaine® *see* Bupivacaine Hydrochloride *on page 49*

Marezine® [OTC] *see* Cyclizine *on page 93*

Marinol® *see* Dronabinol *on page 124*

Marplan® *see* Isocarboxazid *on page 191*

Mar-Pred® *see* Methylprednisolone *on page 231*

Massé® Breast Cream [OTC] *see* Glycerin, Lanolin and Peanut Oil *on page 160*

Matulane® *see* Procarbazine Hydrochloride *on page 298*

Maxitrol® *see* Dexamethasone, Neomycin and Polymyxin B *on page 103*

Maxivate® *see* Betamethasone *on page 43*

Maxolon® *see* Metoclopramide *on page 233*

Maxzide® *see* Hydrochlorothiazide and Triamterene *on page 173*

MCH *see* Microfibrillar Collagen Hemostat *on page 236*

MCT Oil® [OTC] *see* Medium Chain Triglycerides *on page 215*

MD-50® *see* Diatrizoate Sodium *on page 109*

Measles and Rubella Vaccines, Combined
Brand Names M П VAX® II
Synonyms Rubella and Measles Vaccines, Combined
Use Simultaneous immunization against measles and rubella
Pregnancy Risk Factor X
Usual Dosage Inject S.C. into outer aspect of upper arm

Measles, Mumps and Rubella Vaccines, Combined
Brand Names M-M-R® II
Synonyms Mumps, Measles and Rubella Vaccines, Combines; Rubella, Measles and Mumps Vaccines, Combined
Use Measles, mumps, and rubella prophylaxis
Pregnancy Risk Factor X
Usual Dosage Give S.C. in outer aspect of the upper arm to children 15
(Continued)

213

Measles, Mumps and Rubella Vaccines, Combined
(Continued)

months or older; each dose contains 1000 TCID$_{50}$ (tissue culture infectious doses) of five attenuated measle virus vaccine, 5000 TCID$_{50}$ of live mumps virus vaccine and 1000 TCID$_{50}$ of live rubella virus vaccine

Measles Virus Vaccine, Live, Attenuated
Brand Names Attenuvax®
Synonyms More Attenuated Enders Strain; Rubeola vaccine
Use Immunization against measles (rubeola) in persons 15 months of age or older
Pregnancy Risk Factor X
Usual Dosage Adult and Children: S.C.: > 15 months of age: 0.5 mL in outer aspect of the upper arm

Measurin® [OTC] *see* Aspirin *on page 30*

Mebaral® *see* Mephobarbital *on page 219*

Mebendazole (me ben' da zole)
Brand Names Vermox®
Use Treatment of pinworms, whipworms, roundworms, and hookworms
Pregnancy Risk Factor C
Usual Dosage Adult and Children:

Pinworms: Single chewable tablet; may need to repeat after two weeks

Whipworms, roundworms, hookworms: One tablet twice daily, morning and evening on three consecutive days; if patient is not cured within 3-4 weeks, a second course of treatment may be administered

Mecamylamine Hydrochloride (mek a mill' a meen)
Brand Names Inversine®
Use Treatment of moderately severe to severe hypertension and in uncomplicated malignant hypertension
Pregnancy Risk Factor C
Usual Dosage Adult: Oral: 2.5 mg twice a day after meals for two days; increased by increments of 2.5 mg at intervals of ≥ 2 days until desired blood pressure response is achieved

Mechlorethamine Hydrochloride (me klor eth' a meen)
Brand Names Mustargen®
Synonyms HN$_2$; Mustine; Nitrogen Mustard
Use Combination therapy of Hodgkin's disease and malignant lymphomas; palliative treatment of bronchogenic, breast and ovarian carcinoma; may be used by intracavitary injection for treatment of metastatic tumors
Pregnancy Risk Factor D
Usual Dosage Adult:
　　I.V.: 0.4 mg/kg repeated every 3-6 hours
　　Intracavitary: 10-20 mg

Meclan® *see Meclocycline Sulfosalicylate on this page*

Meclizine Hydrochloride (mek' li zeen)
Brand Names Antivert®; Antirzine®; Bonine® [OTC]; Dizmiss® [OTC]; Meni-D®; Ru-Vert-M®
Synonyms Meclozine Hydrochloride
Use Prevention and treatment of motion sickness, as well as management of vertigo in the vestibular system
Pregnancy Risk Factor B
Usual Dosage Adult: Oral:

Motion sickness: 25-50 mg one hour before travel, repeat dose every 24 hours if needed

Vertigo: 25-100 mg in divided doses

Meclocycline Sulfosalicylate (me kloe sye' kleen)
Brand Names Meclan®
Use Topical treatment of inflammatory acne vulgaris
Pregnancy Risk Factor B
Usual Dosage Apply to affected areas twice daily

Meclofenamate Sodium (me kloe fen am' ate)
Brand Names Meclomen®
Use Treatment of inflammatory disorders
Pregnancy Risk Factor B/D
Usual Dosage Adult: Oral: 200-300 mg 3-4 times daily

Meclomen® *see Meclofenamate Sodium on this page*

Meclozine Hydrochloride *see Meclizine Hydrochloride on this page*

Medicinal Charcoal *see Charcoal on page 68*

Medihaler-Epi® *see Epinephrine on page 131*

Medihaler-Iso® *see Isoproterenol on page 193*

Medilax® [OTC] *see Phenolphthalein on page 280*

Medipren® [OTC] *see Ibuprofen on page 181*

Medi-Tuss® [OTC] *see Guaifenesin on page 162*

Medium Chain Triglycerides
Brand Names MCT Oil® [OTC]
Synonyms Triglycerides, Medium Chain
Use Dietary supplement for those who cannot digest long chain fats
Pregnancy Risk Factor C
Usual Dosage Oral: 15 mL 3-4 times daily

Medralone® *see Methylprednisolone on page 231*

Medrol® *see Methylprednisolone on page 231*

Medroxyprogesterone Acetate (me drox' ee proe jess' te rone)

Brand Names Depo-Provera®; Provera®

Synonyms Acetoxymethylprogesterone; Methylacetoxyprogesterone

Use Endometrial carcinoma or renal carcinoma as well as secondary amenorrhea or abnormal uterine bleeding due to hormonal imbalance

Pregnancy Risk Factor X

Usual Dosage Adult:

Carcinoma: I.M.: 400-1000 mg/week

Amenorrhea: Oral: 5-10 mg/day for 5-10 days

Abnormal uterine bleeding: Oral: 5-10 mg for 5-10 days starting on day 16 or 21 of cycle

Medrysone (me' dri sone)

Brand Names HMS Liquifilm®

Use Treatment of allergic conjunctivitis, vernal conjunctivitis, episcleritis, ophthalmic epinephrine sensitivity reaction

Pregnancy Risk Factor C

Usual Dosage Adult and Children: One (1) drop in conjunctival sac 2-4 times daily; may use every hour during first 1-2 days

Mefenamic Acid (me fe nam' ik)

Brand Names Ponstel®

Use Short term relief of mild to moderate pain including primary dysmenorrhea

Pregnancy Risk Factor C/D in third trimester

Usual Dosage Adult and Children: > 14 years of age: Oral: 500 mg to start then 250 mg every four hours as needed, maximum therapy one week

Mefloquine Hydrochloride (me' floe kwin)

Brand Names Lariam®

Use Treatment of acute malarial infections and prevention of malaria

Pregnancy Risk Factor C

Usual Dosage

Adult: Oral:

Mild to moderate malaria infection: Five tablets (1250 mg) as a single dose with at least 8 oz of water

Malaria prophylaxis: One tablet (250 mg) once weekly for 4 weeks, then one tablet every other week; start treatment 1 week prior to departure to an endemic area; to avoid development of malaria after return from an endemic area, continue prophylaxis for 4 additional weeks; for prolonged stays in an endemic area this prophylaxis be achieved by continuing the recommended dosage schedule, once weekly for 4 weeks, then once every other week, until traveler has taken 3 doses following return to a malaria-free area

Mefoxin® *see* Cefoxitin Sodium *on page 64*

Mega-B® [OTC] *see* Vitamin B Complex *on page 377*

Megace® *see* Megestrol Acetate *on next page*

Megacillin® *see* Penicillin G Benzathine, Parenteral
on page 272

Megatron® [OTC] *see* Vitamin B Complex *on page 377*

Megestrol Acetate (me jess' trole)
Brand Names Megace®
Use Palliative treatment of breast and endometrial carcinomas
Pregnancy Risk Factor X
Usual Dosage Adult: Oral:

Breast carcinoma: 40 mg four times a day

Endometrial: 40-320 mg/day in divided doses

Mellaril® *see* Thioridazine *on page 352*
Mellaril-S® *see* Thioridazine *on page 352*

Melphalan (mel' fa lan)
Brand Names Alkeran®
Synonyms L-PAM; L-Sarcolysin; Phenylalanine Mustard
Use Palliative treatment of multiple myeloma and nonresectable; epithelial ovarian carcinoma
Pregnancy Risk Factor D
Usual Dosage

Adult: Oral:
Multiple myeloma: 6 mg/day or 10 mg/day for 7-10 days or 0.15 mg/kg/day for seven days
Ovarian carcinoma: 0.2 mg/kg/day for five days, repeat in 4-5 weeks

Children: Oral: Neuroblastoma conditioning regimen (BMT): 140 mg/m^2 x 1 followed by 70 mg/m^2 x 1 24 hours later

Menadiol Sodium Diphosphate (men a dye' ole)
Brand Names Synkayvite®
Synonyms Vitamin K$_4$
Use Prevention and treatment of hypoprothrombinemia caused by vitamin K deficiency secondary to oral anti-infective therapy and salicylates and inadequate absorption and synthesis of vitamin K
Pregnancy Risk Factor C/X
Usual Dosage

Hypoprothrombinemia (vitamin K deficiency, liver disease or malabsorption): Oral, I.M., I.V., S.C.:
Adult: 5-15 mg/dose 1-2 times/day
Children: 5-10 mg/dose; repeat every 12-24 hours as needed
Infants: 2.5-5 mg/dose; repeat every 12-24 hours as needed

Minimum daily requirement not established
Adult: 0.03 µg/kg/day
Infant: 1-5 µg/kg/day

Menadol® [OTC] *see* Ibuprofen *on page 181*
Meni-D® *see* Meclizine Hydrochloride *on page 215*

Menotropins (men oh troe' pins)
Brand Names Pergonal®
Use Used sequentially with hCG to induce ovulation and pregnancy in the infertile woman with functional anovulation; used with hCG in men to stimulate spermatogenesis in those with primary hypogonadotropic hypogonadism
Pregnancy Risk Factor X
Usual Dosage

Female: I.M.: 1 ampule (75 IU of FSH and LH) daily for 9-12 days followed by 10,000 units hCG one day after the last dose; repeated at least twice at same level before increasing dosage to 2 ampules

Male: I.M.: Following pretreatment with hCG, one ampule three times weekly and hCG 2000 IU twice a week until sperm is detected in the ejaculate (4-6 months) then may be increased to 2 ampules of menotropins three times a week

Mentholatum® [OTC] see Rubs and Liniments on page 319

Mentholatum® Deep Heating Rub [OTC] see Rubs and Liniments on page 319

Mepacrine Hydrochloride see Quinacrine Hydrochloride on page 311

Mepenzolate Bromide (me pen' zoe late)
Brand Names Cantil®
Use Management of peptic ulcer disease; inhibit salivation and excessive secretions in respiratory tract preoperatively
Pregnancy Risk Factor C
Usual Dosage Adult: Oral: 25-50 mg four times a day with meal and at bedtime

Meperidine Hydrochloride (me per' i deen)
Brand Names Demerol®
Synonyms Isonipecaine Hydrochloride; Pethidine Hydrochloride
Use Management of moderate to severe pain; used as an adjunct to anesthesia and preoperative sedation
Restrictions C-II
Pregnancy Risk Factor B
Usual Dosage

Adult:
Analgesia: I.V.: 10 mg/mL by slow I.V. injection or by continuous I.V. infusion 1 mg/mL
Preop sedation: I.M., S.C.: 50-100 mg 1/2-1 1/2 hours before anesthesia
Relief of pain: Oral, I.M., S.C.: 50-150 mg every 3-4 hours, as necessary

Children:
Analgesia: I.V.: 10 mg/mL by slow I.V. injection or by continuous I.V. infusion 1 mg/mL
Preop sedation: I.M., S.C.: 1-2 mg/kg 1/2-1 1/2 hours before anesthesia (up to adult dose)
Relief of pain: Oral, I.M., S.C.: 0.5-0.8 mg/lb (0-1.8 mg/kg) up to adult dose every 3-4 hours when necessary

Mephentermine Sulfate (me fen' ter meen)
Brand Names Wyamine® Sulfate
Use Treatment of hypotension secondary to ganglionic blockade or spinal anesthesia; may be used as an emergency measure to maintain blood pressure until whole blood replacement becomes available
Pregnancy Risk Factor C
Usual Dosage

Hypotension:
Adult: I.M., I.V.: 0.5 mg/kg
Children: 0.4 mg/kg

Hypotensive emergency: I.V. infusion: 20-60 mg

Mephenytoin (me fen' i toyn)
Brand Names Mesantoin®
Synonyms Methoin; Methylphenylethylhydantoin; Phenantoin
Use Prophylactic management of tonic-clonic seizures, partial seizures
Pregnancy Risk Factor C
Usual Dosage Oral:

Adult: Usual maintenance dose: 200-800 mg/day in 3 divided doses; Initial dose: 50-100 mg/day given daily; increase by 50-100 mg at no less than weekly intervals

Children: 3-15 mg/kg/day in 3 divided doses; usual maintenance dose is 100-400 mg daily in 3 divided doses

Mephobarbital (me foe bar' bi tal)
Brand Names Mebaral®
Use Sedative; treatment of grand mal and petit mal epilepsy
Restrictions C-IV
Pregnancy Risk Factor D
Usual Dosage Oral:

Adult:
Sedation: 32-100 mg 3-4 times daily
Epilepsy: 400-600 mg daily

Children:
Sedation: 16-32 mg 3-4 times daily
Epilepsy: > 5 years: 32-64 mg 3-4 times daily; < 5 years: 16-32 mg 3-4 times daily

Mephyton® *see* Phytonadione *on page 285*

Mepivacaine Hydrochloride (me piv' a kane)
Brand Names Carbocaine®; Polocaine®
Use Local anesthesia by nerve block; infiltration in dental procedures
Usual Dosage
Topical: Apply to affected area as needed
Injectable local anesthetic: Varies with procedure, degree of anesthesia needed, vascularity of tissue, duration of anesthesia required, and physical condition of patient

Meprobamate (me proe ba' mate)
Brand Names Equanil®; Meprospan®; Miltown®; Neuramate®
Use Management of anxiety disorders
Restrictions C-IV
Pregnancy Risk Factor D
Usual Dosage Oral:

Adult: 400 mg 3-4 times daily, up to 2400 mg/day

Children: 100-200 mg 2-3 times daily

Meprobamate and Aspirin see Aspirin and Meprobamate on page 31

Meprospan® see Meprobamate on this page

Merbromin
Brand Names Mercurochrome®
Use Topical antiseptic
Usual Dosage Apply freely, until injury has healed

Mercaptopurine (mer kap toe pyoor' een)
Brand Names Purinethol®
Synonyms 6-Mercaptopurine; 6-MP
Use Treatment of leukemias
Pregnancy Risk Factor D
Usual Dosage Oral:

Adult: 1.5-2.5 mg/kg/day

Children: 60-75 mg/m^2/day given daily (give 33% of calculated dose when used concurrently with allopurinol)

6-Mercaptopurine see Mercaptopurine on this page

Mercuric Oxide
Synonyms Yellow Mercuric Oxide
Use Treatment of irritation and minor infections of the eyelids
Usual Dosage Apply small amount to inner surface of lower eyelid once or twice daily

Mercurochrome® see Merbromin on this page

Merlenate® [OTC] see Zinc Undecylenate on page 382

Meruvax® II see Rubella Virus Vaccine, Live on page 318

Mesalamine (me sal' a meen)
Brand Names Rowasa®
Synonyms 5-Aminosalicylic Acid; 5-ASA; Fisalamine; Mesalazine
Use Treatment of ulcerative colitis, proctosigmoiditis, and proctitis
Pregnancy Risk Factor B
Usual Dosage Retention enema: 60 mL (4 g) at bedtime, retained over night, approximately eight hours

Mesalazine see Mesalamine on this page

Mesantoin® *see* Mephenytoin *on page 219*

Mesna

Brand Names Mesnex™

Use Reduce the incidence of ifosfamide-induced hemorrhagic cystitis

Pregnancy Risk Factor B

Usual Dosage Adult: I.V.: As bolus equal to 20% of ifosfamide dosage (w/w) at the time of ifosfamide administration and 4 and 8 hours after each dose of mesna is 60 % of the ifosfamide

Mesnex™ *see* Mesna *on this page*

Mesoridazine Besylate (mez oh rid' a zeen)

Brand Names Serentil®

Use Symptomatic management of psychotic disorders, including schizophrenia, behavioral problems, alcoholism as well as reducing anxiety and tension occurring in neurosis

Pregnancy Risk Factor C

Usual Dosage For most patients, 25 mg initially; may repeat dose in 30-60 minutes, if necessary. The usual optimum dosage range is 25-200 mg/day. Concentrate may be diluted just prior to administration with distilled water, acidified tap water, orange or grape juice; do not prepare and store bulk dilutions. See table.

Mesoridazine

Disease State	Initial Oral Dose	Optimum Total Dosage Range (mg/d)
Schizophrenia	50 mg tid	100–400
Behavior problems in mental deficiency and chronic brain syndrome	25 mg tid	75–300
Alcoholism	25 mg bid	50–200
Psychoneurotic manifestations	10 mg tid	30–150

Mestinon® *see* Pyridostigmine Bromide *on page 309*

Mestranol and Ethynodiol (mes' tra nole)

Brand Names Ovulen®

Synonyms Ethynodiol and Mestranol

Use Prevention of pregnancy

Usual Dosage

Contraception: Oral: One (1) tablet daily, beginning on day five of menstrual cycle (first day of menstrual flow is day one). With 20-tablet and 21-tablet packages, new dosing cycle begins seven days after last tablet taken; with 28-tablet packages, dosage is one tablet daily without interruption; extra tablets are placebos or contain iron. If next men-

(Continued)

Mestranol and Ethynodiol *(Continued)*

strual period does not begin on schedule, rule out pregnancy before starting new dosing cycle; if menstrual period begins, start new dosing cycle seven days after last tablet was taken. If all doses have been taken on schedule and one menstrual period is missed, continue dosing cycle; if two consecutive menstrual periods are missed, pregnancy test is required before new dosing cycle is started.

Biphasic oral contraceptive (Ortho-Novum™ 10/11): One (1) color tablet daily for 10 days, then next color tablet for 11 days

Triphasic oral contraceptive (Ortho-Novum™ 7/7/7, Tri-Norinyl®, Triphasil®): One (1) tablet daily in the sequence specified by the manufacturer

Mestranol and Norethindrone

Brand Names Norinyl®; Ortho-Novum™ 1/50; Ortho-Novum™ 1/80
Synonyms Norethindrone and Mestranol
Use Prevention of pregnancy
Pregnancy Risk Factor X
Usual Dosage

Contraception: Oral: One (1) tablet daily, beginning on day five of menstrual cycle (first day of menstrual flow is day one). With 20-tablet and 21-tablet packages, new dosing cycle begins seven days after last tablet taken; with 28-tablet packages, dosage is one (1) tablet daily without interruption; extra tablets are placebos or contain iron. If next menstrual period does not begin on schedule, rule out pregnancy before starting new dosing cycle; if menstrual period begins, start new dosing cycle seven days after last tablet was taken. If all doses have been taken on schedule and one menstrual period is missed, continue dosing cycle; if two consecutive menstrual periods are missed, pregnancy test is required before new dosing cycle is started.

Biphasic oral contraceptive (Ortho-Novum™ 10/11): One (1) color tablet daily for 10 days, then next color tablet for 11 days

Triphasic oral contraceptive (Ortho-Novum™ 7/7/7, Tri-Norinyl®, Triphasil®): One (1) tablet daily in the sequence specified by the manufacturer

Mestranol and Norethynodrel

Brand Names Enovid®
Synonyms Norethynodrel and Mestranol
Use Prevention of pregnancy
Usual Dosage

Contraception: Oral: One (1) tablet daily, beginning on day five of menstrual cycle (first day of menstrual flow is day one). With 20-tablet and 21-tablet packages, new dosing cycle begins seven days after last tablet taken; with 28-tablet packages, dosage is one tablet daily without interruption; extra tablets are placebos or contain iron. If next menstrual period does not begin on schedule, rule out pregnancy before starting new dosing cycle; if menstrual period begins, start new dosing cycle seven days after last tablet was taken. If all doses have been taken on schedule and one menstrual period is missed, continue dosing cycle; if two consecutive menstrual periods are missed, pregnancy test is required before new dosing cycle is started.

Biphasic oral contraceptive (Ortho-Novum™ 10/11): One (1) color tablet daily for 10 days, then next color tablet for 11 days

Triphasic oral contraceptive (Ortho-Novum™ 7/7/7, Tri-Norinyl®, Triphasil®): One (1) tablet daily in the sequence specified by the manufacturer

Metacortandralone *see* Prednisolone *on page 294*

Metahydrin® *see* Trichlormethiazide *on page 361*

Metamucil® [OTC] *see* Psyllium *on page 308*

Metamucil® Instant Mix [OTC] *see* Psyllium *on page 308*

Metandren® *see* Methyltestosterone *on page 232*

Metaprel® *see* Metaproterenol Sulfate *on this page*

Metaproterenol Sulfate (met a proe ter' e nol)
Brand Names Alupent®; Dey-Dose® Metaproterenol; Metaprel®
Synonyms Orciprenaline Sulfate
Use Bronchodilator in reversible airway obstruction due to asthma or COPD
Pregnancy Risk Factor C
Usual Dosage

Adult:
Oral: 20 mg 3-4 times daily
Inhalation: 2-3 inhalations every 3-4 hours, up to 12 inhalations in 24 hours
Nebulizer: 5-15 inhalations 3-4 times daily
IPPB: 0.2-0.3 mL of 5% solution 3-4 times daily

Children:
Oral: > 9 years: 20 mg 3-4 times daily
Inhalation: > 12 years: 2-3 inhalations every 3-4 hours, up to 12 inhalations in 24 hours
Nebulizer: > 12 years: 5-15 inhalations 3-4 times daily
IPPB: > 12 years: 0.2-0.3 mL of 5% solution 3-4 times daily

Metaraminol Bitartrate (met a ram' i nole)
Brand Names Aramine®
Use Acute hypotensive crisis in the treatment of shock
Pregnancy Risk Factor C
Usual Dosage Adult:

Prevention of hypotension: I.M., S.C.: 2-10 mg

Adjunctive treatment of hypotension: I.V.: 15-100 mg in 250-500 mL NS or 5% dextrose in water

Severe shock: I.V.: 0.5-5 mg direct I.V. injection then use I.M. dose

Metasep® [OTC] *see* Parachlorometaxylenol *on page 269*

Metaxalone (me tax' a lone)
Brand Names Skelaxin®

Use Relief of discomfort associated with acute, painful musculoskeletal conditions

Pregnancy Risk Factor C

Usual Dosage Adult and Children: < 12 years of age: Oral: 800 mg 3-4 times daily

Methacholine Chloride
Brand Names Provocholine®

Use Diagnosis of bronchial airway hyperactivity in subjects who do not have clinically apparent asthma

Pregnancy Risk Factor C

Usual Dosage The following is a suggested schedule for administration of methacholine challenge. Calculate cumulative units by multiplying number of breaths by concentration given. Total cumulative units is the sum of cumulative units for each concentration given. See table.

Vial	Serial Concentration (mg/mL)	No. of Breaths	Cumulative Units per Concentration	Total Cumulative Units
E	0.025	5	0.125	0.125
D	0.25	5	1.25	1.375
C	2.5	5	12.5	13.88
B	10	5	50	63.88
A	25	5	125	188.88

Methacycline Hydrochloride (meth a sye' kleen)
Brand Names Rondomycin®

Use Treatment of susceptible bacterial infections of both gram-negative and gram-positive organisms

Usual Dosage Oral:

Adult: 150 mg four times a day or 30 mg twice daily

Children: > 8 years: 6-12 mg/kg/day into 2-4 divided doses

Methadone Hydrochloride (meth' a done)
Brand Names Dolophine®; Methadose®

Use Management of severe pain, used in narcotic detoxification mainte- nance programs

Restrictions C-II

Pregnancy Risk Factor C

Usual Dosage Adult:

Analgesia: Oral, I.M., S.C.: 2-5-10 mg every 3-4 hours, up to 5-20 mg every 6-8 hours

Detoxification: Oral: 15-40 mg/day

Maintenance: Oral: 20-120 mg/day

Methadose® see Methadone Hydrochloride *on previous page*

Methamphetamine Hydrochloride (meth am fet' a meen)
Brand Names Desoxyn®
Synonyms Desoxyephedrine Hydrochloride
Use Narcolepsy; exogenous obesity; abnormal behavioral syndrome in children (minimal brain dysfunction)
Restrictions C-II
Pregnancy Risk Factor C
Usual Dosage

Attention deficit disorder: Children: > 6 years of age: 2.5-5 mg 1-2 times daily, may increase by 5 mg increments weekly until optimum response is achieved, usually 20-25 mg/day

Exogenous obesity: Adult and Children: > 12 years of age: 5 mg, 30 minutes before each.meal, 10-15 mg in morning; treatment duration should not exceed a few weeks

Methantheline Bromide (meth an' tha leen)
Brand Names Banthine®
Synonyms Methanthelinium Bromide
Use Adjunctive treatment of peptic ulcer, irritable bowel syndrome, pancreatitis, ureteral and urinary bladder spasm; to reduce duodenal motility during diagnostic radiologic procedures and treatment of an uninhibited neurogenic bladder
Pregnancy Risk Factor C
Usual Dosage Oral:

Adult: 50-100 mg every six hours

Children:
> 1 year of age: 12.5-50 mg four times a day
< 1 year of age: 12.5-25 mg four times a day

Neonate: 12.5 mg twice a day then three times a day

Methanthelinium Bromide see Methantheline Bromide
on this page

Metharbital (meth ar' bi tal)
Brand Names Gemonil®
Use Control of grand mal, petit mal, myoclonic and mixed types of seizures
Restrictions C-III
Pregnancy Risk Factor D
Usual Dosage Oral:

Adult: 100 mg 1-3 times a day, adjust dosage to obtain optimal effect

Children: 5-15 mg/kg/day or 50 mg 1-3 times daily

Methazolamide (meth a zoe' la mide)

Brand Names Neptazane®

Use Adjunctive treatment of open-angle or secondary glaucoma; short-term therapy of narrow-angle glaucoma when delay of surgery is desired

Pregnancy Risk Factor C

Usual Dosage Oral: 50-100 mg 2-3 times daily

Methdilazine Hydrochloride (meth dill' a zeen)

Brand Names Tacaryl®

Use Symptomatic relief of pruritus associated with urticaria; neuroallergic, atopic, contact, poison ivy or eczematous dermatitis; pruritus ani or drug rash

Pregnancy Risk Factor C

Usual Dosage Oral:

Adult: 8 mg 2-4 times daily

Children: 4 mg 2-4 times daily

Methenamine (meth en' a meen)

Brand Names Hiprex®; Mandelamine®

Use Prophylaxis or suppression of recurrent urinary tract infections

Pregnancy Risk Factor C

Usual Dosage Oral:

Adult: 1 g four times a day after meals and at bedtime

Children:
6-12 years: 0.5 g four times a day
< 6 years: 0.25 g/14 kg four times a day

Methergine® *see* Methylergonovine Maleate *on page 231*

Methicillin Sodium (meth i sill' in)

Brand Names Staphcillin®

Synonyms Dimethoxyphenyl Penicillin Sodium; Sodium Methicillin

Use Systemic infections caused by penicillinase-producing staphylococci

Pregnancy Risk Factor B

Usual Dosage I.M., I.V.:

Adult: 4-12 g in divided doses every 4-6 hours

Children: 100-300 mg/kg/day in divided doses every 4-6 hours

Methimazole (meth im' a zole)

Brand Names Tapazole®

Synonyms Thiamazole

Use Palliative treatment of hyperthyroidism, return the hyperthyroid patient to a normal metabolic state prior to thyroidectomy, and to control thyrotoxic crisis that may accompany thyroidectomy

Pregnancy Risk Factor D

Usual Dosage Oral:

Adult: 1.6-10 mg every eight hours

Children: 0.067-0.133 mg/kg every eight hours

Methionine (me thye' oh neen)
Brand Names Pedameth®
Use Treatment of diaper rash and control of odor, dermatitis and ulceration caused by ammoniacal urine
Usual Dosage Oral:

Adult: 200-400 mg 3-4 times daily

Children: 75 mg in formula or other liquid 3-4 times daily for 3-5 days

Methocarbamol (meth oh kar' ba mole)
Brand Names Delaxin®; Marbaxin®; Robaxin®; Robomol®
Use Treatment of muscle spasm associated with acute painful musculoskeletal conditions; supportive therapy in tetanus
Pregnancy Risk Factor C
Usual Dosage

Adult:
  Muscle spasm: Oral: 1.5 g four times a day for 2-3 times, then decrease to 4-4.5 g/day in 3-6 divided doses; I.M., I.V.: 1 g every eight hours if oral not possible
  Tetanus: Oral: Up to 25 g/day in divided doses; I.V.: 1-2 g every six hours until NG tube can be inserted, then give oral

Children: Tetanus: I.V.: 15 mg/kg every six hours

Methohexital Sodium (meth oh hex' i tal)
Brand Names Brevital® Sodium
Use Ultra short-acting intravenous anesthetic; induction and maintenance of general anesthesia for short procedures
Restrictions C-IV
Pregnancy Risk Factor C
Usual Dosage 50-120 mg to start; 20-40 mg every 4-7 minutes

Methoin see Mephenytoin on page 219

Methosarb® see Calusterone on page 55

Methotrexate (meth oh trex' ate)
Brand Names Folex®; Mexate®; Rheumatrex®
Synonyms Amethopterin; MTX
Use Treatment of trophoblastic neoplasms, leukemias, psoriasis, rheumatoid arthritis, and breast, head, and lung carcinomas
Pregnancy Risk Factor D
Usual Dosage Adult:

Trophoblastic neoplasms: Oral, I.M.: 15-30 mg/day for five days, repeat in seven days

Leukemia: Oral, I.M., I.V.: 3.3 mg/m^2/day for 4-6 weeks, 20-30 mg/m^2 oral or I.M. two times weekly

Rheumatoid arthritis: Oral: 7.5 mg once weekly or 2.5 mg every 12 hours for 3 doses/week

Osteosarcoma:
  I.V.: < 12 years:12 g/m^2 (12-18 g); > 12 years: 8 g/m^2 (18 g maximum dose)

(Continued)

227

Methotrexate (Continued)

I.T.: 10-15 mg/m^2 (maximum dose: 15 mg) by protocol

Non-Hodgkin's lymphoma: I.V.: 200-300 mg/m^2

Methotrimeprazine Hydrochloride

(meth oh trye mep' ra zeen)

Brand Names Levoprome®

Synonyms Levomepromazine

Use Relief of moderate to severe pain in nonambulatory patients; for analgesia and sedation when respiratory depression is to be avoided, as in obstetrics; preanesthetic for producing sedation, somnolence and relief of apprehension and anxiety

Pregnancy Risk Factor C

Usual Dosage Adult: I.M.:

Sedation analgesia: 10-20 mg every 4-6 hours as needed

Preoperative medication: 2-20 mg, 45 mg 3 hours before surgery

Postoperative analgesia: 2.5-7.5 mg every 4-6 hours is suggested as necessary since residual effects of anesthetic may be present

Methoxamine Hydrochloride (meth ox' a meen)

Brand Names Vasoxyl®

Use Treatment of hypotension occurring during general anesthesia; to terminate episodes of supraventricular tachycardia; treatment of shock

Pregnancy Risk Factor C

Usual Dosage Adult:

Emergencies: I.V.: 3-5 mg

Supraventricular tachycardia: I.V.: 10 mg

During spinal anesthesia: I.M.: 10-20 mg

Methoxsalen (meth ox' a len)

Brand Names Oxsoralen®; Oxsoralen-Ultra®

Synonyms Methoxypsoralen; 8-MOP

Use For symptomatic control of severe, recalcitrant, disabling psoriasis in conjunction with long wave ultraviolet radiation; induce repigmentation in vitiligo topical repigmenting agent in conjunction with controlled doses of ultraviolet A (UVA) or sunlight

Restrictions Lotion should not be dispensed to a patient, it should be applied only under physician controlled conditions for light exposure and subsequent light shielding

Pregnancy Risk Factor C

Usual Dosage Oral:

Psoriasis: Adult: 10-70 mg 1 1/2-2 hours before exposure to ultraviolet light, 2-3 times at least 48 hours apart; dosage is based upon patient's body weight and skin type

Vitiligo: Adult and Children: > 12 years of age:
20 mg 2-4 hours before exposure to UVA light or sunlight
Topical: Apply lotion 1-2 hours before exposure to UVA light, no more than once weekly

Methoxyflurane (meth ox ee floo' rane)
Brand Names Penthrane®
Use Adjunct to provide anesthesia procedures under four hours in duration
Usual Dosage 0.3-0.8% for analgesia and anesthesia, with 0.1-2% for maintenance when used with nitrous oxide

Methoxypsoralen *see* Methoxsalen *on previous page*

Methscopolamine Bromide (meth skoe pol' a meen)
Brand Names Pamine®
Use Adjunctive therapy in the treatment of peptic ulcer
Pregnancy Risk Factor C
Usual Dosage 2.5 mg 30 minutes before meals or food and 2.5-5 mg at bedtime

Methsuximide (meth sux' i mide)
Brand Names Celontin®
Use Control of absence (petit mal) seizures; useful adjunct in refractory, partial complex seizures
Pregnancy Risk Factor C
Usual Dosage Oral:

Adult: 300 mg/day for the first week; may increase by 300 mg weekly up to 1.2 g in 2-4 divided doses per day

Children: 10-20 mg/kg/day in 2-4 divided doses

Methyclothiazide (meth i kloe thye' a zide)
Brand Names Aquatensen®; Enduron®
Use Management of mild to moderate hypertension; treatment of edema in congestive heart failure and nephrotic syndrome
Pregnancy Risk Factor B
Usual Dosage Adult: Oral:

Edema: 2.5-10 mg every day

Hypertension: 2.5-5 mg every day

Methyclothiazide and Cryptenamine Tannates
Brand Names Diutensin®
Synonyms Cryptenamine Tannates and Methyclothiazide
Use Management of hypertension
Pregnancy Risk Factor B
Usual Dosage 1-4 tablets per day

Methyclothiazide and Deserpidine
Brand Names Enduronyl®; Enduronyl® Forte
Use Management of mild to moderately severe hypertension
Pregnancy Risk Factor C
Usual Dosage Individualized, normally 1-4 tablets daily

Methyclothiazide and Pargyline
Brand Names Eutron®
Synonyms Pargyline and Methyclothiazide
Use Management of hypertension
Pregnancy Risk Factor C
Usual Dosage Individualized, normally 1-4 tablets daily

Methylacetoxyprogesterone *see* Medroxyprogesterone Acetate
on page 216

Methylcellulose (meth ill sell' yoo lose)
Brand Names Citrucel® [OTC]; Cologel® [OTC]
Use Used orally as an adjunct in treatment of constipation; used in oph-
thalmic preparations for relief of dry eyes and ocular lubricant for artificial
eyes and contact lenses
Pregnancy Risk Factor C
Usual Dosage

Adult: Oral: 5-20 mL three times a day

Children:
Oral: 5-10 mL 1-2 times daily
Ophthalmic: 0.25%-1% 1-2 drops in eye(s) 3-4 times daily

Methyldopa (meth ill doe' pa)
Brand Names Aldomet®
Use Management of moderate to severe hypertension
Pregnancy Risk Factor C
Usual Dosage

Adult:
Oral: 250-500 mg 2-3 times daily, up to 3000 mg/24 hours
I.V.: 250-1000 mg every six hours

Children:
Oral: 10-65 mg/kg/day in 2-4 divided doses
I.V.: 5-10 mg/kg every six hours

Methyldopa and Chlorothiazide *see* Chlorothiazide and
Methyldopa *on page 72*

Methyldopa and Hydrochlorothiazide
Brand Names Aldoril®
Synonyms Hydrochlorothiazide and Methyldopa
Use Management of moderate to severe hypertension
Pregnancy Risk Factor C
Usual Dosage One tablet 2-3 times daily for first 48 hours, then decrease
or increase at intervals of not less than two days until an adequate re-
sponse is achieved

Methylene Blue (meth' i leen)
Brand Names Urolene Blue®
Use Mild genitourinary antiseptic; antidote for cyanide poisoning
Pregnancy Risk Factor C

Usual Dosage
Oral: 55-130 mg three times daily with full glass of water
I.V.: 1-2 mg/kg over several minutes

Methylergometrine Maleate *see* Methylergonovine Maleate *on this page*

Methylergonovine Maleate (meth ill er goe noe' veen)
Brand Names Methergine®
Synonyms Methylergometrine Maleate
Use Prevention and treatment of postpartum and postabortion hemorrhage caused by uterine atony or subinvolution
Pregnancy Risk Factor C
Usual Dosage Adult:
Oral: 0.2-0.4 mg every 6-12 hours for 2-7 days
I.M., I.V.: 0.2 mg every 2-4 hours for five doses then change to oral dosage

Methylone® *see* Methylprednisolone *on this page*

Methylphenidate Hydrochloride (meth ill fen' i date)
Brand Names Ritalin®
Use Treatment of attention deficit disorder and symptomatic management of narcolepsy
Restrictions C-II
Pregnancy Risk Factor C
Usual Dosage Children: > 6 years:

Attention deficit disorder: Initial dose: 0.25 mg/kg/dose given before breakfast and lunch or three times/day; daily dose may be doubled each week until 2 mg/kg/day dosage is reached or 60 mg/day

Narcolepsy: 10 mg 2-3 times daily, up to 60 mg/day

Methylphenylethylhydantoin *see* Mephenytoin *on page 219*

Methylphytyl Napthoquinone *see* Phytonadione *on page 285*

Methylpolysiloxane *see* Simethicone *on page 324*

Methylprednisolone (meth ill pred niss' oh lone)
Brand Names A-methaPred®; depMedalone®; Depoject®; Depo-Medrol®; Depopred®; Duralone®; Mar-Pred®; Medralone®; Medrol®; Methylone®; Solu-Medrol®
Synonyms 6-α-Methylprednisolone; Methylprednisolone Acetate; Methylprednisolone Sodium Succinate
Use Treatment of a variety of diseases including those of hematologic, allergic, inflammatory, neoplastic, and autoimmune in origin
Pregnancy Risk Factor C
Usual Dosage

Adult:
Oral: 4-48 mg/day to start, followed by gradual reduction in dosage to the lowest possible level consistent with maintaining an adequate clinical response

(Continued)

Methylprednisolone *(Continued)*

I.V.: 10-40 mg over a period of several minutes and repeated I.V. or I.M. at intervals depending on clinical response; when high dosages are needed give 30 mg/kg over a period of 10-20 minutes and may be repeated every 4-6 hours for 48 hours

Rectal: 40 mg

Children: Oral:

Anti-inflammatory immunosuppressive: 0.16-0.8/mg/kg/day or 5-25 mg/m^2/24 hours every 6-12 hours

Status asthmaticus: I.V.: Loading: 2 mg/kg/dose; maintenance: 0.5-1 mg/kg/dose every 4-6 hours for up to five days

6-α-Methylprednisolone *see* Methylprednisolone *on previous page*

Methylprednisolone Acetate *see* Methylprednisolone *on previous page*

Methylprednisolone Sodium Succinate *see* Methylprednisolone *on previous page*

Methylrosaniline Chloride *see* Gentian Violet *on page 157*

Methyl Salicylate and Menthol *see* Rubs and Liniments *on page 319*

Methyltestosterone (meth ill tess toss' te rone)

Brand Names Android®; Metandren®; Oreton®; Testred®; Virilon®

Use Males: hypogonadism; delayed puberty; impotence and climacteric symptoms. Females: palliative treatment of metastatic breast cancer; postpartum breast pain and/or engorgement

Pregnancy Risk Factor X

Usual Dosage

Adult male:
Oral: 10-40 mg/day
Buccal: 5-20 mg/day

Adult female:
Breast pain/engorgement: Oral: 80 mg/day for 3-5 days
Buccal: 40 mg/day for 3-5 days
Breast cancer: Oral: 200 mg/day
Buccal: 100 mg/day

Methyprylon (meth i prye' lon)

Brand Names Noludar®

Use Short-term management of insomnia

Restrictions C-III

Pregnancy Risk Factor B

Usual Dosage Oral:

Adult: 200-400 mg at bedtime

Children: > 12 years: 50-200 mg at bedtime

Methysergide Maleate (meth i ser' jide)

Brand Names Sansert®

Use Prophylaxis of vascular headache

Pregnancy Risk Factor X

Usual Dosage Oral: 4-8 mg/day with meals; if no improvement is noted after three weeks, drug is unlikely to be beneficial; must not be given continuously for longer than six months, and a drug-free interval of 3-4 weeks must follow each 6-month course

Meticorten® *see* Prednisone *on page 295*

Metimyd® *see* Sodium Sulfacetamide and Prednisolone Acetate *on page 330*

Metoclopramide (met oh kloe pra' mide)
Brand Names Clopra®; Maxolon®; Octamide®; Reglan®

Use Symptomatic treatment of diabetic gastric stasis, gastroesophageal reflux; prevention of nausea associated with chemotherapy and facilitates intubation of the small intestine

Pregnancy Risk Factor B

Usual Dosage

Adult: Stasis/reflux: Oral, I.M., I.V.: 10-15 mg 30 minutes before meals or food and at bedtime

Gastroesophageal reflux: Oral, I.V.: 0.4-0.8 mg/kg/day in 4 divided doses; efficacy of continuing metoclopramide beyond 12 weeks in reflux has not been determined

Adult and Children: Antiemetic: I.V.: 1-2 mg/kg every 2-4 hours

Children: Facilitate intubation: I.V.:
6-14 years: 2.5-5 mg
< 6 years: 0.1 mg/kg

Metocurine Iodide (met oh kyoor' een)
Brand Names Metubine®

Synonyms Dimethyl Tubocurarine Iodide

Use Adjunct to anesthesia to induce skeletal muscle relaxation

Pregnancy Risk Factor C

Usual Dosage I.V.:

Adult:
Surgery: 0.2-0.4 mg/kg (initial); supplement dose: 0.5-1 mg; use of anesthetics that potentiate effect of neuromuscular blocking drug requires less metocurine
Electric shock therapy: 1.75-5.5 mg

Children:
Chronic respiratory paralysis in neonates: Start 0.25-0.5 mg/kg/dose (repeat once if paralysis is not achieved in three minutes); maintenance: repeat previous dose as soon as movement is observed. The dose should be titrated to achieve a dosage interval of 3-4 hours use, then plateau at 20-30 mg/kg/24 hours
Neuromuscular blockade for surgery: Initial: 0.2-0.4 mg/kg/dose; maintenance: 0.1-0.25 mg/kg/dose every 25-90 minutes

Metolazone (me tole' a zone)
Brand Names Diulo™; Mykrox®; Zaroxolyn®

Use Management of mild to moderate hypertension; treatment of edema in congestive heart failure and nephrotic syndrome; impaired renal function

(Continued)

Metolazone *(Continued)*
Pregnancy Risk Factor D
Usual Dosage

Adult:
Edema: 5-20 mg/dose every 24 hours given daily
Hypertension: 2.5-5 mg/dose every 24 hours given daily

Children: 0.2-0.4 mg/kg/day every 12-24 hours in divided doses

Metopirone® *see Metyrapone Tartrate on next page*

Metoprolol Tartrate *(me toe' proe lole)*
Brand Names Lopressor®
Use Treatment of hypertension and angina pectoris; prevention of myocardial infarction
Pregnancy Risk Factor B
Usual Dosage Adult:
Oral: 100-450 mg/day in 1-2 divided doses
I.V.: 5 mg every two minutes for three doses in early treatment of myocardial infarction

Metric® *see Metronidazole on this page*

Metrizamide *(me tri' za mide)*
Brand Names Amipaque®
Use Parenteral radiopaque agent used in intravascular digital arteriographs of head and neck, adult peripheral arteriograph, pediatric angiocardiograph, and intrathecal myelography
Usual Dosage Varies with procedure

Metrodin® *see Urofollitropin on page 369*

MetroGel® *see Metronidazole on this page*

Metro I.V.® *see Metronidazole on this page*

Metronidazole *(me troe ni' da zole)*
Brand Names Flagyl®; Metric®; MetroGel®; Metro I.V.®; Protostat®
Use Treatment of susceptible infections in the following disease: amebiasis, symptomatic and asymptomatic trichomoniasis; skin and skin structure infections; CNS infections; septicemia; topically for the treatment of acne rosacea
Pregnancy Risk Factor B
Usual Dosage

Adult:
Amebiasis: Oral: 500-750 mg every eight hours
Trichomoniasis: Oral: 250 mg every eight hours or 2 g single dose
Anaerobic infections: Oral: 7.5 mg/kg every six hours; I.V.: 15 mg stat, 15 mg/kg every six hours

Children: Oral:
Amebiasis: 12-17 mg/kg every eight hours
Trichomoniasis: 15 mg/kg/day in three divided doses every eight hours

Metubine® *see* Metocurine Iodide *on page 233*

Metyrapone Tartrate (me teer' a pone)
Brand Names Metopirone®
Use Diagnostic rest for hypothalmic-pituitary ACTH function
Usual Dosage Oral:
Adult: 750 mg every 4 hours for 6 doses
Children: 15 mg/kg every 4 hours for 6 doses

Metyrosine (me tye' roe seen)
Brand Names Demser®
Synonyms AMPT; OGMT
Use Short-term management of pheochromocytoma before surgery, long-term management when surgery is contraindicated or when malignant
Pregnancy Risk Factor C
Usual Dosage Adult and Children: > 12 years of age: Oral: Initially, 250 mg four times a day, increased by 250-500 mg every day up to 4 g/day; maintenance, 2-3 g/day in four divided doses; for preoperative preparation, give optimum effective dosage for 5-7 days

Mevacor® *see* Lovastatin *on page 207*

Mevinolin *see* Lovastatin *on page 207*

Mexate® *see* Methotrexate *on page 227*

Mexiletine (mex' i le teen)
Brand Names Mexitil®
Use Management of serious ventricular arrhythmias
Pregnancy Risk Factor C
Usual Dosage Adult: Oral: 400 mg to start, then 200 mg in eight hours, then 200-400 mg every eight hours

Mexitil® *see* Mexiletine *on this page*

Mezlin® *see* Mezlocillin *on this page*

Mezlocillin (mez loe sill' in)
Brand Names Mezlin®
Use Treatment of susceptible bacterial infections, mainly those of the skin and skin structure, bone and joint, respiratory tract, urinary tract, as well as septicemia
Pregnancy Risk Factor B
Usual Dosage

Adult:
I.M.: 1.5-2 g every six hours
I.V.: 1.5-6 g every six hours

Children: I.M., I.V.: 1 month - 12 years: 50 mg/kg every four hours

Micatin® *see* Miconazole *on next page*

Miconazole (mi kon' a zole)

Brand Names Micatin®; Monistat™; Monistat-Derm™; Monistat iv™

Synonyms Miconazole Nitrate

Use Treatment of vulvovaginal candidiasis, severe systemic fungal infections, and a variety of skin and mucous membrane fungal infections

Pregnancy Risk Factor B

Usual Dosage

Adult:
I.V.: 200-300 mg/day in divided doses every eight hours
Topical: Apply 1-2 times daily
Vaginal: Use once or twice daily

Children:
I.V.: 6.67-13.3 mg/kg every eight hours
Topical: Apply 1-2 times daily
Vaginal: Use once or twice daily

Miconazole Nitrate see Miconazole on this page

MICRhoGAM™ see Rh$_o$(D) Immune Globulin on page 315

Micrin® see Hydrochlorothiazide on page 172

Microfibrillar Collagen Hemostat

Brand Names Avitene®

Synonyms MCH

Use Adjunct to hemostasis when control of bleeding by ligature in ineffective or impractical

Pregnancy Risk Factor C

Usual Dosage Applied dry directly to source of bleeding

Microlipid® [OTC] see Nutritional Formula, Enteral/Oral on page 258

Micronase® see Glyburide on page 159

microNefrin® see Epinephrine on page 131

Microstix-3® [OTC] see Diagnostic Test for Bacteriuria on page 106

Microstix-Nitrite® [OTC] see Diagnostic Test for Bacteriuria on page 106

Microsulfon® see Sulfadiazine on page 336

MicroTrak® see Diagnostic Test for Chlamydia trachomatis on page 107

MicroTrak® HSV 1/HSV 2 Culture see Diagnostic Test for Virus on page 108

Midamor® see Amiloride Hydrochloride on page 17

Midazolam Hydrochloride (mid' ay zoe lam)

Brand Names Versed®

Use Preoperative sedation and provide conscious sedation prior to diagnostic or radiographic procedures

Restrictions C-IV
Pregnancy Risk Factor D
Usual Dosage Adult:

Preoperative sedation: I.M.: 0.07-0.08 mg/kg 1/2-1 hour before surgery

Conscious sedation: I.V.: 0.1-0.15 mg/kg; may give additional dose of 1/4 of initial dose

Midol® 200 [OTC] see Ibuprofen *on page 181*

Midrin® see Acetaminophen and Isometheptene Mucate *on page 5*

Milkinol® [OTC] see Mineral Oil *on this page*

Milk of Magnesia see Magnesium Hydroxide *on page 210*

Milontin® see Phensuximide *on page 280*

Milophene® see Clomiphene Citrate *on page 83*

Miltown® see Meprobamate *on page 220*

Mineral Oil
Brand Names Fleet® Mineral Oil Enema [OTC]; Kondremul® [OTC]; Milkinol® [OTC]
Use Temporary relief of constipation, to relieve fecal impaction, preparation for bowel studies or surgery
Pregnancy Risk Factor C
Usual Dosage

Adult: Kondremul®: Oral: 5-30 mL at bedtime

Children: Oral: 5-20 mL at bedtime

Adult: Mineral Oil
  Oral: 15-30 mL
  Rectal: Retention enema, 90-120 mL

Children: ≥ 6 years of age: 5-15 mL once daily

Mini-Gamulin® Rh see Rh$_o$(D) Immune Globulin *on page 315*

Minipress® see Prazosin Hydrochloride *on page 293*

Minitran® see Nitroglycerin *on page 253*

Minizide® see Prazosin and Polythiazide *on page 290*

Minocin® see Minocycline Hydrochloride *on this page*

Minocin® IV see Minocycline Hydrochloride *on this page*

Minocycline Hydrochloride (mi noe sye' kleen)
Brand Names Minocin®; Minocin® IV
Use Treatment of susceptible bacterial infections of both gram-negative and gram-positive organisms; acne
Pregnancy Risk Factor D
Usual Dosage Adult:

Infection: Oral, I.V.: 200 mg stat, 100 mg every 12 hours

Acne: Oral: 50 mg 1-3 times daily

Minoxidil (mi nox' i dill)
Brand Names Loniten®; Rogaine®
Use Management of severe hypertension; management of alopecia or male pattern alopecia
Pregnancy Risk Factor C
Usual Dosage

Adult:
Hypertension: Oral: 10-40 mg/day
Alopecia: Apply twice daily

Children: < 12 years: Hypertension: Oral: 0.25-1 mg/kg/day in 1-2 divided doses

Mintezol® see Thiabendazole on page 350

Miochol® see Acetylcholine Chloride on page 7

Miostat® see Carbachol on page 57

Misoprostol (mye soe prost' ole)
Brand Names Cytotec®
Use Prevention of NSAID induced gastric ulcers
Pregnancy Risk Factor X
Usual Dosage 200 μg four times a day with food

Mithracin® see Plicamycin on page 288

Mithramycin see Plicamycin on page 288

Mitomycin (mye toe mye' sin)
Brand Names Mutamycin®
Synonyms Mitomycin-C; MTC
Use Therapy of disseminated adenocarcinoma of stomach or pancreas
Pregnancy Risk Factor C
Usual Dosage Adult I.V.: 20 mg/m^2 every 6-8 weeks as platelet and leukocyte levels decrease, decrease the dose. See table.

Nadir After Prior Dose per cu mm		% of Prior Dose to Be Given
Leukocytes	Platelets	
4000	> 100,000	100
3000–3999	75,000–99,999	100
2000–2999	25,000–74,999	70
2000	< 25,000	50

Mitomycin-C see Mitomycin on this page

Mitotane (mye' toe tane)
Brand Names Lysodren®
Synonyms o'-DDD
Use Treatment of inoperable adrenal cortical carcinoma
Pregnancy Risk Factor C
Usual Dosage Adult: Oral: 8-10 g/day in 3-4 divided doses; dose is changed on basis of side effect with aim of giving as high a dose as tolerated

Mitoxantrone Hydrochloride (mye toe zan' trone)
Brand Names Novantrone®
Use Initial therapy of acute nonlymphocytic leukemia
Pregnancy Risk Factor C
Usual Dosage Adult: I.V.: 12 mg/m^2/day on days 1-3

Mitrolan® [OTC] *see* Calcium Polycarbophil *on page 55*

Mixtard® *see* Insulin, Isophane Suspension and Insulin Injection *on page 186*

Mixtard® Human 70/30 *see* Insulin, Isophane Suspension and Insulin Injection *on page 186*

M-M-R® II *see* Measles, Mumps and Rubella Vaccines, Combined *on page 213*

Moban® *see* Molindone Hydrochloride *on this page*

Moctanin® *see* Monoctanoin *on next page*

Modane® [OTC] *see* Phenolphthalein *on page 280*

Modane® Bulk [OTC] *see* Psyllium *on page 308*

Modane® Mild [OTC] *see* Phenolphthalein *on page 280*

Modified Dakin's Solution *see* Sodium Hypochlorite Solution *on page 328*

Modified Shohl's Solution *see* Sodium Citrate and Citric Acid *on page 327*

Moduretic® *see* Amiloride and Hydrochlorothiazide *on page 17*

Moi-Stir® **[OTC]** *see* Saliva Substitute *on page 320*

1/6 Molar Sodium Lactate *see* Sodium Lactate *on page 328*

Molindone Hydrochloride (moe lin' done)
Brand Names Moban®
Use Management of psychotic disorder
Pregnancy Risk Factor C
Usual Dosage 50-75 mg/day; up to 225 mg/day

Molybdenum *see* Trace Metals *on page 358*

Moly-Pak® *see* Trace Metals *on page 358*

Molypen® *see* Trace Metals *on page 358*

MOM *see* Magnesium Hydroxide *on page 210*

MOM/Cascara *see* Cascara Sagrada Fluid Extract and Milk of Magnesia *on page 61*

Monacolin K *see* Lovastatin *on page 207*

***Monilia* Skin Test** *see Candida albicans (Monilia) on page 56*

Monistat™ *see* Miconazole *on page 236*

Monistat-Derm™ *see* Miconazole *on page 236*

Monistat iv™ *see* Miconazole *on page 236*

Mono-Chek® *see* Diagnostic Test for Mononucleosis *on page 107*

Monoclate® *see* Antihemophilic Factor, Human *on page 26*

Monoctanoin (mon oh ock' ta noyn)
Brand Names Moctanin®
Synonyms Monooctanoin
Use To solubilize cholesterol gallstones that are retained in the biliary tract after cholecystectomy
Pregnancy Risk Factor C
Usual Dosage Administer via T-tube into common bile duct at rate of 3-5 mL/hour at pressure of 10 mL water for 7-21 days

Mono-Diff® *see* Diagnostic Test for Mononucleosis *on page 107*

Mono-Gesic® *see* Salsalate *on page 320*

Monooctanoin *see* Monoctanoin *on this page*

Monospot® *see* Diagnostic Test for Mononucleosis *on page 107*

Monosticon® *see* Diagnostic Test for Mononucleosis *on page 107*

Mono-Sure® *see* Diagnostic Test for Mononucleosis *on page 107*

Mono-Test® *see* Diagnostic Test for Mononucleosis *on page 107*

Mono-Vacc® *see* Tuberculin *on page 367*

8-MOP *see* Methoxsalen *on page 228*

More Attenuated Enders Strain *see* Measles Virus Vaccine, Live, Attenuated *on page 214*

More-Dophilus® [OTC] *see Lactobacillus acidophilus* and *Lactobacillus bulgaricus on page 199*

Morphine Sulfate (mor' feen)
Brand Names Astramorph™ PF; Duramorph®; MS Contin®; MSIR®; RMS®; Roxanol™; Roxanol SR™
Synonyms MS

Use Relief of moderate to severe acute and chronic pain after non-narcotic analgesics have failed; preanesthetic medication; pain of myocardial infarction; relieves dyspnea of acute left ventricular failure and pulmonary edema

Restrictions C-II

Pregnancy Risk Factor C

Usual Dosage

Adult and Children: Oral: 10-30 mg every four hours

Adult:

Oral (controlled release): 30 mg every 8-12 hours

I.M., S.C.: 5-20 mg every four hours

I.V.: 2.5-15 mg; continuous I.V.: 0.8-10 mg/hour initially adjusted to maintenance dose of 0.8-80 mg/hour

Rectal: 10-20 mg every four hours

Epidural: Initial, 5 mg in lumbar regional; if inadequate pain relief within one hour, give 1-2 mg with a maximum dose of 10 mg/24 hours

Intrathecal: 1/10 of epidural dose

Children:

I.M., S.C.: 0.1-0.2 mg/kg/dose every four hours

I.V. continuous: 0.04-0.07 mg/kg/hour

Morrhuate Sodium (mor' yoo ate)

Brand Names Scleromate®

Use Treatment of small, uncomplicated varicose veins of the lower extremities

Usual Dosage I.V.: 50-250 mg, repeated at 5-7 day intervals

Motrin® *see* Ibuprofen *on page 181*

Motrin® IB [OTC] *see* Ibuprofen *on page 181*

Moxalactam Disodium (mox' a lak tam)

Brand Names Moxam®

Synonyms Latamoxef Disodium

Use Treatment of serious respiratory, urinary, CNS, intra-abdominal, gynecologic, and skin infections; septicemia, bacteremia, and meningitis; third generation cephalosporin

Pregnancy Risk Factor B

Usual Dosage I.M., I.V.:

Adult: 2-6 g/day in divided doses every 8-12 hours for 5-10 days or up to 14 days; life-threatening infections: 4 g every eight hours

Children: 50 mg/kg every 6-8 hours. **Maximum recommended dose for children and neonates:** 200 mg/kg/day up to 12 g/day

Neonate: 50 mg/kg every 8-12 hours

Moxam® *see* Moxalactam Disodium *on this page*

6-MP *see* Mercaptopurine *on page 220*

MPS® Papers [OTC] *see* Diagnostic Test for Acid Mucopolysaccharides *on page 106*

M-R-VAX® II *see* Measles and Rubella Vaccines, Combined
on page 213

MS *see* Morphine Sulfate *on page 240*

MS Contin® *see* Morphine Sulfate *on page 240*

MSIR® *see* Morphine Sulfate *on page 240*

MSTA *see* Mumps Skin Test Antigen *on this page*

MTC *see* Mitomycin *on page 238*

M.T.E.-4® *see* Trace Metals *on page 358*

M.T.E.-5® *see* Trace Metals *on page 358*

M.T.E.-6® *see* Trace Metals *on page 358*

MTX *see* Methotrexate *on page 227*

Mucomyst® *see* Acetylcysteine *on page 7*

Mucoplex® [OTC] *see* Vitamin B Complex *on page 377*

Multe-Pak-4® *see* Trace Metals *on page 358*

Multiple Sulfonamides *see* Sulfadiazine, Sulfamethazine and
Sulfamerazine *on page 336*

Multitest CMI® *see* Skin Test Antigens, Multiple *on page 325*

Mumps, Measles and Rubella Vaccines, Combines *see*
Measles, Mumps and Rubella Vaccines, Combined
on page 213

Mumps Skin Test Antigen
Synonyms MSTA
Use To assess the status of cell-mediated immunity
Pregnancy Risk Factor C
Usual Dosage Adult and Children: 0.1 mL intradermally into flexor sur-
face of the forearm

Mumpsvax® *see* Mumps Virus Vaccine, Live, Attenuated
on this page

Mumps Virus Vaccine, Live, Attenuated
Brand Names Mumpsvax®
Use Mumps prophylaxis by promoting active immunity
Pregnancy Risk Factor X
Usual Dosage 1 vial (5000 units) S.C. in outer aspect of the upper arm

Mupirocin (myoo peer' oh sin)
Brand Names Bactroban®
Synonyms Pseudomonic Acid A
Use Topical treatment of impetigo
Pregnancy Risk Factor B
Usual Dosage Apply small amount three times a day

Murine® Plus [OTC] *see* Tetrahydrozoline Hydrochloride
on page 347

Muro 128® Ophthalmic [OTC] *see* Sodium Chloride *on page 327*

Murocoll-2® *see* Phenylephrine and Scopolamine *on page 281*

Muromonab-CD3 (myoo roe moe' nab)
Brand Names Orthoclone® OKT3
Use Treatment of acute allograft rejection in kidney transplant patients
Pregnancy Risk Factor C
Usual Dosage Adult: I.V.: 5 mg/day for 10-14 days

Mustargen® *see* Mechlorethamine Hydrochloride *on page 214*

Mustine *see* Mechlorethamine Hydrochloride *on page 214*

Mutamycin® *see* Mitomycin *on page 238*

Myambutol® *see* Ethambutol Hydrochloride *on page 138*

Mycelex® *see* Clotrimazole *on page 84*

Mycifradin® Sulfate *see* Neomycin Sulfate *on page 248*

Mycolog®-II *see* Nystatin and Triamcinolone *on page 258*

Mycostatin® *see* Nystatin *on page 258*

Mydfrin® Ophthalmic Solution *see* Phenylephrine Hydrochloride *on page 282*

Mydriacyl® *see* Tropicamide *on page 367*

Mykinac® *see* Nystatin *on page 258*

Mykrox® *see* Metolazone *on page 233*

Mylanta® [OTC] *see* Aluminum Hydroxide, Magnesium Hydroxide and Simethicone *on page 15*

Mylanta®-II [OTC] *see* Aluminum Hydroxide, Magnesium Hydroxide and Simethicone *on page 15*

Mylaxen® *see* Hexafluorenium *on page 168*

Myleran® *see* Busulfan *on page 50*

Mylicon® [OTC] *see* Simethicone *on page 324*

Myochrysine® *see* Gold Sodium Thiomalate *on page 160*

Myoflex® [OTC] *see* Triethanolamine Salicylate *on page 361*

Myprozine® *see* Natamycin *on page 247*

Mysoline® *see* Primidone *on page 296*

Mytelase® *see* Ambenonium Chloride *on page 16*

Mytrex® F *see* Nystatin and Triamcinolone *on page 258*

Mytussin® [OTC] *see* Guaifenesin *on page 162*

Nabilone (na' bi lone
Brand Names Cesamet®
Use Treat nausea and vomiting associated with cancer chemotherapy
Restrictions C-II
(Continued)

Nabilone *(Continued)*

Pregnancy Risk Factor C

Usual Dosage Adult: Oral: 1-2 mg twice a day beginning 1-3 hours before chemotherapy is administered and continuing around the clock until one dose after chemotherapy is completed; maximum daily dosage is 6 mg divided in three doses

***N*-Acetylcysteine** *see* Acetylcysteine *on page 7*

***N*-Acetyl-L-cysteine** *see* Acetylcysteine *on page 7*

***N*-Acetyl-P-Aminophenol** *see* Acetaminophen *on page 4*

NaCl *see* Sodium Chloride *on page 327*

Nadolol *(nay doe' lole)*

Brand Names Corgard®

Use Treatment of hypertension and angina pectoris; prevention of myocardial infarction

Pregnancy Risk Factor C

Usual Dosage Oral: 40-80 mg/day, up to 240 mg/day

Nafarelin Acetate *(naf' a re lin)*

Brand Names Synarel®

Use Treatment of endometriosis, including pain and reduction of lesions

Usual Dosage Adult: One spray in one nostril each morning and evening

Nafazair® *see* Naphazoline Hydrochloride *on page 246*

Nafcil™ *see* Nafcillin Sodium *on this page*

Nafcillin Sodium *(naf sill' in)*

Brand Names Nafcil™; Nallpen®; Unipen®

Synonyms Ethoxynaphthamido Penicillin Sodium; Sodium Nafcillin

Use Treatment of susceptible bacterial infections; notably penicillinase-producing strains of *Staphylococcus*

Pregnancy Risk Factor B

Usual Dosage

Adult:
I.M.: 500 mg every 4-6 hours
I.V.: 500-1000 mg every 4 hours

Children:
I.M.: 25 mg/kg every 12 hours
I.V.: 50-200 mg/kg/day in divided doses every 4-6 hours

Neonate: I.M.: 10 mg/kg twice daily

Naftifine Hydrochloride *(naf' ti feen)*

Brand Names Naftin®

Use Topical treatment of tinea cruris and tinea corporis

Usual Dosage Apply twice daily

Naftin® *see* Naftifine Hydrochloride *on this page*

NaHCO₃ see Sodium Bicarbonate on page 326

Nalbuphine Hydrochloride (nal' byoo feen)
Brand Names Nubain®
Use Relief of moderate to severe pain
Pregnancy Risk Factor C
Usual Dosage I.M., I.V., S.C.: 10 mg/70 kg every 3-6 hours

Naldecon® see Chlorpheniramine, Phenyltoloxamine, Phenylpropanolamine and Phenylephrine on page 75

Naldecon® Senior EX [OTC] see Guaifenesin on page 162

Nalfon® see Fenoprofen Calcium on page 145

Nalidixic Acid (nal i dix' ik)
Brand Names NegGram®; Wintomylon®
Synonyms Nalidixinic Acid
Use Urinary tract infections
Pregnancy Risk Factor B
Usual Dosage Oral: 1 g four times a day for 2-4 weeks

Nalidixinic Acid see Nalidixic Acid on this page

Nallpen® see Nafcillin Sodium on previous page

Naloxone Hydrochloride (nal ox' one)
Brand Names Narcan®
Use Reverse CNS and respiratory depression in suspected narcotic overdose
Pregnancy Risk Factor B
Usual Dosage

Narcotic overdose:
  Adult: I.V.: 0.6-2 mg (initial); may repeat at 2-3 minute intervals; if no response is observed after 10 mg, question the diagnosis
  Children: I.V.: 0.01 mg/kg followed by 0.2 mg/kg if necessary (may administer I.M. or S.C.)

Postoperative narcotic depressions:
  Adult: I.V.: 0.1-0.2 mg every 2-3 minutes as needed
  Children: I.V.: 0.005-0.01 mg at 2-3 minute intervals, if necessary repeat every 1-2 hours
  Neonates: I.M., I.V., S.C.: 0.01 mg/kg given at 2-3 minute intervals; repeat every 1-2 hours if necessary

Naltrexone Hydrochloride (nal trex' one)
Brand Names Trexan™
Use Adjunct to the maintenance of an opioid-free state in detoxified individual
Pregnancy Risk Factor C
Usual Dosage Adult: Oral: 25 mg; if no withdrawal signs within one hour give another 25 mg; maintenance regimen is flexible, variable and individualized

Nandrobolic® *see* Nandrolone *on this page*

Nandrolone (nan' droe lone)
  Brand Names Anabolin®; Andralone-D®; Androlone®; Deca-Durabolin®; Durabolin®; Hybolin® Decanoate; Hybolin® Improved; Nandrobolic®; Neo-Durabolic®
  Synonyms Nandrolone Decanoate; Nandrolone Phenpropionate
  Use Control of metastatic breast cancer; management of anemia of renal insufficiency
  Pregnancy Risk Factor X
  Usual Dosage I.M.:

  Adult:

  Female: 50-100 mg/week

  Male: 100-200 mg/week

  Children: 2-13 years: 25-50 mg every 3-4 weeks

Nandrolone Decanoate *see* Nandrolone *on this page*

Nandrolone Phenpropionate *see* Nandrolone *on this page*

Naphazoline and Antazoline
  Brand Names Vasocon-A®
  Use Topical ocular congestion, irritation and itching
  Pregnancy Risk Factor C
  Usual Dosage 1-2 drops every 3-4 hours

Naphazoline and Pheniramine
  Brand Names Naphcon-A®
  Synonyms Pheniramine and Naphazoline
  Use Topical ocular vasoconstrictor
  Pregnancy Risk Factor C
  Usual Dosage 1-2 drops every 3-4 hours

Naphazoline Hydrochloride (naf az' oh leen)
  Brand Names AK-Con®; Albalon® Liquifilm®; Allerest® Eye Drops [OTC]; Clear Eyes® [OTC]; Comfort® [OTC]; Degest® 2 [OTC]; Estivin® II [OTC]; I-Naphline®; Nafazair®; Naphcon® [OTC]; Naphcon Forte®; Ocu-Zoline®; Opcon®; Privine® [OTC]; VasoClear® [OTC]; Vasocon Regular®
  Use Topical ocular vasoconstrictor
  Pregnancy Risk Factor C
  Usual Dosage 1-2 drops every 3-4 hours

Naphcon® [OTC] *see* Naphazoline Hydrochloride *on this page*

Naphcon-A® *see* Naphazoline and Pheniramine *on this page*

Naphcon Forte® *see* Naphazoline Hydrochloride *on this page*

Naprosyn® *see* Naproxen *on this page*

Naproxen (na prox' en)
  Brand Names Anaprox®; Naprosyn®
  Synonyms Naproxen Sodium
  Use Treatment of mild to moderate pain; primary dysmenorrhea; acute gout; musculoskeletal or soft tissue irritation; as an antipyretic

Pregnancy Risk Factor B
Usual Dosage Oral:

Adult: (Anaprox®)
Pain, primary dysmenorrhea: 550 mg (two tablets) to start followed by 275 mg every 6-8 hours, up to 1375 mg per day (five tablets)
Gout: 825 mg (three tablets) initially; then 375 mg (one tablet) every eight hours until attack is aborted
Inflammatory diseases: 275 mg twice a day Do not exceed 1.25 g/day

Adult: (Naprosyn®)
Acute gout: 750 mg followed by 250 mg every eight hours until attack subsides
Inflammatory disease: 250-500 mg twice daily
Pain, dysmenorrhea: 500 mg stat, 250 mg every 6-8 hours, up to 1250 mg total daily dose

Children: Inflammatory disease: 10 mg/kg/day in two divided doses

Naproxen Sodium *see* Naproxen *on previous page*

Naqua® *see* Trichlormethiazide *on page 361*

Narcan® *see* Naloxone Hydrochloride *on page 245*

Nardil® *see* Phenelzine Sulfate *on page 278*

Nasahist B® *see* Brompheniramine Maleate *on page 48*

Nasalcrom® *see* Cromolyn Sodium *on page 91*

Nasalide® *see* Flunisolide *on page 149*

Natacyn® *see* Natamycin *on this page*

Natamycin (na ta mye' sin)
Brand Names Myprozine®; Natacyn®
Synonyms Pimaricin
Use Treatment of blepharitis, conjunctivitis, and keratitis caused by susceptible fungi
Pregnancy Risk Factor C
Usual Dosage Adult: One drop in conjunctival sac every 1-2 hours, after 3-4 days dose may be reduced to one drop 6-8 times a day; usual course of therapy is 2-3 weeks

Naturacil® [OTC] *see* Psyllium *on page 308*

Naturetin® *see* Bendroflumethiazide *on page 39*

Navane® *see* Thiothixene *on page 353*

ND-Stat® *see* Brompheniramine Maleate *on page 48*

Nebcin® *see* Tobramycin Sulfate *on page 356*

NegGram® *see* Nalidixic Acid *on page 245*

Nembutal® *see* Pentobarbital *on page 275*

Neo-Calglucon® [OTC] *see* Calcium Glubionate *on page 54*

NeoDecadron® *see* Dexamethasone and Neomycin *on page 102*

Neo-Durabolic® *see* Nandrolone *on page 246*

Neofed® [OTC] *see* Pseudoephedrine *on page 307*

Neo-IM® *see* Neomycin Sulfate *on this page*

Neoloid® [OTC] *see* Castor Oil *on page 61*

Neomycin and Dexamethasone *see* Dexamethasone and Neomycin *on page 102*

Neomycin and Polymyxin

Brand Names Neosporin® Cream [OTC]; Neosporin® G.U. Irrigant

Synonyms Polymyxin and Neomycin

Use To help prevent infection in minor cuts, scrapes and burns

Pregnancy Risk Factor C

Usual Dosage

Topical: Apply cream 2-4 times daily

Bladder irrigation: Add 1 mL irrigant to 1 liter isotonic saline solution and connect container to the inflow of lumen of 3-way catheter; not for injection

Neomycin, Polymyxin and Hydrocortisone

Brand Names Cortisporin® Cream; Cortisporin® Ophthalmic Suspension; Cortisporin® Otic

Use Treatment of topical bacterial infections caused by susceptible bacteria and when the use of an anti-inflammatory is indicated

Pregnancy Risk Factor C

Usual Dosage

Adult and Children:

Ointment: Apply thin layer to affected area 2-4 times/day

Ophthalmic: Ointment: Apply to the affected eye every 3-4 hours

Suspension: One drop every 3-4 hours

Adult: Otic: Solution and suspension: Four drops into affected ear 3-4 times/day

Children: Otic: Solution and suspension: Three drops into affected ear 3-4 times/day

Neomycin, Polymyxin and Prednisolone

Brand Names Poly-Pred® Liquifilm®

Use Treatment of susceptible ophthalmic infections

Pregnancy Risk Factor C

Usual Dosage Instill 1-2 drops in eye(s) 4-6 times daily

Neomycin Sulfate (nee oh mye' sin)

Brand Names Mycifradin® Sulfate; Neo-IM®; Neo-Tabs®

Use Prepare GI tract for surgery; treat diarrhea caused by *E. coli*; treat minor skin infections

Pregnancy Risk Factor C

Usual Dosage

Adult:

Chronic hepatic insufficiency: Oral: 4 g/day for three weeks

Diarrhea: Oral: 50 mg/kg/day in divided doses every six hours
GI surgery: Oral: 1 g 19, 18 and nine hours before surgery hours; then 1 g every four hours
Hepatic coma: Oral: 4-12 g divided into doses for 5-6 days
Topically: Apply 1-3 times daily

Children:
Diarrhea: Oral: 50-100 mg/kg/day every six hours
GI surgery: Oral: 90 mg/kg/day in divided doses every four hours
Hepatic encephalopathy: Oral: Acute 2.5-7 g/m^2/day every six hours for 5-7 days; chronic 2.5 g/m^2/day four times/day
Topically: Apply 1-3 times daily

Premature and neonates: Diarrhea: Oral: 50 mg/kg/day every six hours

Neonatal Trace Metals *see* Trace Metals *on page 358*

Neoquess® *see* Dicyclomine Hydrochloride *on page 111*

Neoquess® *see* Hyoscyamine Sulfate *on page 180*

Neosporin® Cream [OTC] *see* Neomycin and Polymyxin *on previous page*

Neosporin® G.U. Irrigant *see* Neomycin and Polymyxin *on previous page*

Neosporin® Ointment [OTC] *see* Bacitracin, Neomycin and Polymyxin B *on page 36*

Neosporin® Ophthalmic Ointment *see* Bacitracin, Neomycin and Polymyxin B *on page 36*

Neosporin® Ophthalmic Solution *see* Gramicidin, Neomycin and Polymyxin B *on page 161*

Neostigmine (nee oh stig' meen)
Brand Names Prostigmin®
Synonyms Neostigmine Bromide; Neostigmine Methylsulfate
Use Treatment of myasthenia gravis and to prevent and treat postoperative bladder distention and urinary retention; reversal of the effects of nondepolarizing neuromuscular blocking agents after surgery
Pregnancy Risk Factor C
Usual Dosage

Adult:
Myasthenia gravis: Oral: 15-30 mg three times a day to start, increase at daily intervals until response is achieved, up to 375 mg/day; I.M., I.V.: 0.5-2.5 mg every 1-3 hours
Bladder atony prevention: I.M., S.C.: 0.25 mg every 4-6 hours for 2-3 days
Bladder atony treatment: I.M., S.C.: 0.5-1 mg every three hours for five doses after bladder has emptied

Children: Myasthenia gravis: Oral: 7.5-15 mg 3-4 times daily

Neostigmine Bromide *see* Neostigmine *on this page*

Neostigmine Methylsulfate *see* Neostigmine *on previous page*

Neo-Synephrine® 12 Hour Nasal Solution [OTC] *see* Oxymetazoline Hydrochloride *on page 265*

Neo-Synephrine® Nasal Solution [OTC] *see* Phenylephrine Hydrochloride *on page 282*

Neo-Synephrine® Ophthalmic Solution *see* Phenylephrine Hydrochloride *on page 282*

Neo-Tabs® *see* Neomycin Sulfate *on page 248*

Neothylline® *see* Dyphylline *on page 126*

Neotrace-4® *see* Trace Metals *on page 358*

NeoVadrin® B Complex [OTC] *see* Vitamin B Complex *on page 377*

Nephrox Suspension [OTC] *see* Aluminum Hydroxide *on page 15*

Neptazane® *see* Methazolamide *on page 226*

Nesacaine® *see* Chloroprocaine Hydrochloride *on page 70*

Netilmicin Sulfate (ne til mye' sin)

Brand Names Netromycin®

Synonyms I-N-Ethyl Sisomicin

Use Short term treatment of serious or life-threatening infections including septicemia, peritonitis, intra-abdominal abscess, lower respiratory tract infections, urinary tract infections, skin, bone and joint infections caused by sensitive *Pseudomonas aeruginosa*, *Escherichia coli*, *Proteus*, *Klebsiella*, *Serratia*, *Enterobacter*, *Citrobacter*, and *Staphylococcus*

Pregnancy Risk Factor D

Usual Dosage I.M., I.V.:

Adult and Children: > 12 years of age: 3-6.5 mg/kg/day in divided doses normally every 8-12 hours

Children:
6 weeks - 12 years of age: 5.5-8 mg/kg in divided doses every 8-12 hours
< 6 weeks of age: 4-6.5 mg/kg/day in divided doses

Patients with impaired renal function: Doses or frequency of administration should be altered. See Appendix for formula.

Netromycin® *see* Netilmicin Sulfate *on this page*

Neuramate® *see* Meprobamate *on page 220*

Neurosyn® *see* Primidone *on page 296*

Neut® *see* Sodium Bicarbonate *on page 326*

Neutralized Soap, Fatty Acids, Glycerin and Triethanolamine

Brand Names Neutrogena® [OTC]

Use Therapeutic skin cleanser

Neutra-Phos® [OTC] *see* Phosphorus Replacement Products
on page 284

Neutra-Phos®-K [OTC] *see* Phosphorus Replacement Products
on page 284

Neutrogena® [OTC] *see* Neutralized Soap, Fatty Acids, Glycerin
and Triethanolamine *on previous page*

Niac® *see* Niacin *on this page*

Niacin (nye' a sin)
Brand Names Niac®; Nicobid®; Nicolar®
Synonyms Nicotinic Acid
Use Adjunctive treatment of hyperlipidemias; peripheral vascular disease
and circulatory disorders; treatment of pellagra; dietary supplement
Pregnancy Risk Factor A/C
Usual Dosage Oral:

Adult:
Hyperlipidemia: 1.5-3 g/day in three divided doses with or after meals
Vasodilatation: 250-800 mg/day in divided doses
Pellagra: 50 mg 3-10 times a day
Niacin deficiency: 10-20 mg/day

Children: Pellagra: Up to 300 mg/day

Niacinamide (nye a sin' a mide)
Synonyms Nicotinamide; Vitamin B_3
Use Prophylaxis and treatment of pellagra
Pregnancy Risk Factor C
Usual Dosage Oral:

Adult: 50 mg 3-10 times a day
Pellagra: 300-500 mg/day
Hyperlipidemias: 1-2 g three times a day

Children: Pellagra: 100-300 mg/day

Nicardipine Hydrochloride (nye kar' de peen)
Brand Names Cardene®
Use Chronic stable angina; management of essential hypertension
Pregnancy Risk Factor C
Usual Dosage 20 mg three times daily

Niclocide® *see* Niclosamide *on this page*

Niclosamide (ni kloe' sa mide)
Brand Names Niclocide®; Yomesan®
Use Treatment of intestinal beef and fish tapeworm infections and dwarf
tapeworm infections
Pregnancy Risk Factor B
Usual Dosage Oral:

Beef and fish tapeworm:
Adult: 2 g (four tablets) in a single dose
(Continued)
251

Niclosamide *(Continued)*

Children: > 34 kg - 1.5 g (three tablets) in a single dose
Oral: 11-34 kg - 1 g (two tablets) in a single dose

Dwarf tapeworm:
Adult: 2 g (four tablets) daily in a single dose for seven days
Children: > 34 g - 1.5 g (three tablets) daily for six days; 11-34 g - 1 g
(two tablets) chewed thoroughly in a single dose the first day, then
500 mg (one tablet) daily for next six days

Nicobid® *see* Niacin *on previous page*

Nicolar® *see* Niacin *on previous page*

Nicorette® *see* Nicotine Polacrilex *on this page*

Nicotinamide *see* Niacinamide *on previous page*

Nicotine Polacrilex (nik oh teen' pol a krill' ex)
Brand Names Nicorette®
Use Treatment aid to giving up smoking while participating in a behavioral
modification program, under medical supervision
Pregnancy Risk Factor X
Usual Dosage Chew one piece of gum when urge to smoke, up to 30
pieces per day

Nicotinic Acid *see* Niacin *on previous page*

Nifedipine (nye fed' i peen)
Brand Names Adalat®; Procardia®
Use Management of angina pectoris due to coronary insufficiency or vaso-
spasm
Pregnancy Risk Factor C
Usual Dosage Oral: 10-40 mg 3-4 times daily

Niloric® *see* Ergoloid Mesylates *on page 133*

Nilstat® *see* Nystatin *on page 258*

Nimodipine (nye moe' di peen)
Brand Names Nimotop®
Use For improvement of neurological deficits due to spasm following sub-
arachnoid hemorrhage from ruptured congenital intracranial aneurysms
who are in good neurological condition postictus
Pregnancy Risk Factor C
Usual Dosage Adult: Oral: 60 mg every four hours for 21 days

Nimotop® *see* Nimodipine *on this page*

Nipride® *see* Nitroprusside Sodium *on page 254*

Nitrazine® Paper [OTC] *see* Diagnostic Test for pH in Urine
on page 107

Nitro-Bid® *see* Nitroglycerin *on next page*

Nitrocap® TD *see* Nitroglycerin *on next page*

Nitrocine® *see* Nitroglycerin *on this page*

Nitrodisc® *see* Nitroglycerin *on this page*

Nitro-Dur® *see* Nitroglycerin *on this page*

Nitrofural *see* Nitrofurazone *on this page*

Nitrofurantoin (nye troe fyoor an' toyn)
Brand Names Furadantin®; Ivadantin®; Macrodantin®
Use Prevention and treatment of urinary tract infections
Pregnancy Risk Factor B
Usual Dosage

Adult:
  Active infection: Oral: 30-100 mg four times a day; > 55 kg: I.V.: 180 mg
    twice daily; < 55 kg: I.V.: 6.6 mg/kg/day in two divided doses
  Chronic suppression: Oral: 50-100 mg at bedtime

Children: Oral:
  Active infection: 5-7 mg/kg/day in divided doses every six hours
  Chronic suppression: 1 mg/kg/day as single or two divided doses

Nitrofurazone (nye troe fyoor' a zone)
Brand Names Furacin®
Synonyms Nitrofural
Use Antibacterial agent used in second and third degree burns and skin
  grafting
Pregnancy Risk Factor C
Usual Dosage Apply once daily

Nitrogard® *see* Nitroglycerin *on this page*

Nitrogen Mustard *see* Mechlorethamine Hydrochloride
on page 214

Nitroglycerin (nye troe gli' ser in)
Brand Names Deponit®; Minitran®; Nitro-Bid®; Nitrocap® TD; Nitrocine®;
  Nitrodisc®; Nitro-Dur®; Nitrogard®; Nitroglyn®; Nitrol®; Nitrolingual®;
  Nitrong®; Nitrospan®; Nitrostat®; Transdermal-NTG®; Transderm-Nitro®;
  Tridil®
Synonyms Glyceryl Trinitrate; NTG, Nitroglycerol
Use Acute treatment and prophylaxis of angina pectoris; treatment of con-
  gestive heart failure associated with acute myocardial infarction
Pregnancy Risk Factor C
Usual Dosage Adult:
  Oral: 2.5-9 mg 3-4 times daily
  I.V.: 5 μg/minute, increased by 5 μg/minute every 3-5 minutes to 20 μg/
    minute, then increase by 10 μg/minute every 3-5 minutes
  Sublingual: 0.2-0.6 mg every five minutes for three doses
  Ointment: 1-2 inches every eight hours
  Transdermal patch: 2.5-15 mg/24 hours

Nitroglyn® *see* Nitroglycerin *on this page*

Nitrol® *see* Nitroglycerin *on this page*

Nitrolingual® *see* Nitroglycerin *on previous page*

Nitrong® *see* Nitroglycerin *on previous page*

Nitropress® *see* Nitroprusside Sodium *on this page*

Nitroprusside Sodium (nye troe pruss' ide)
Brand Names Nipride®; Nitropress®
Synonyms Sodium Nitroferricyanide; Sodium Nitroprusside
Use Management of hypertensive crises, controlled hypertension during anesthesia
Pregnancy Risk Factor C
Usual Dosage Average dose: 5 μg/kg/minute

Adult and Children: I.V.: 0.5-10 μg/kg/minute

Adult: I.V.: Begin at 5 μg/kg/minute; increase in increments of 5 μg/kg/minute (up to 20 μg/kg/minute), then in increments of 10-20 μg/kg/minute; titrating to the desired hemodynamic effect or the appearance of headache or nausea

Children: Pulmonary hypertension: Initial: 1 μg/kg/minute by continuous I.V. infusion; increment at one μg/kg/minute at intervals of 20-60 minutes; titrating to the desired response; maximum 5 μg/kg/minute

Nitrospan® *see* Nitroglycerin *on previous page*

Nitrostat® *see* Nitroglycerin *on previous page*

Nivea® *see* Emollient Cream *on page 129*

Nix™ *see* Permethrin *on page 277*

Nizatidine (ni za' ti deen)
Brand Names Axid®
Use Treatment and maintenance of duodenal ulcer
Usual Dosage Adult: Oral: 300 mg at bedtime or 150 mg twice daily

Nizoral® *see* Ketoconazole *on page 196*

Noctec® *see* Chloral Hydrate *on page 68*

Noludar® *see* Methyprylon *on page 232*

Nolvadex® *see* Tamoxifen Citrate *on page 341*

Nonoxynol 9 (noe nox' ee nole)
Brand Names Delfen®; Gynol II®
Use As a spermatocide in contraception

Noradrenaline Acid Tartrate *see* Norepinephrine Bitartrate *on next page*

Norcuron® *see* Vecuronium *on page 373*

Nordeoxyguanosine *see* Ganciclovir *on page 155*

Nordette® *see* Ethinyl Estradiol and Levonorgestrel *on page 139*

Norepinephrine Bitartrate (nor ep i nef' rin)

Brand Names Levophed®

Synonyms Levarterenol Bitartrate; Noradrenaline Acid Tartrate

Use Treatment of shock which persists after adequate fluid volume replacement

Pregnancy Risk Factor C

Usual Dosage

Adult: I.V.: Dilute 4 mg in 1000 mL D_5W (4 μg/mL) and infuse at 2-3 mL/minute (8-12 μg/mL/minute); titrate infusion to achieve the desired perfusion

Children: 0.1 μg/kg/minute initially, titrated to attain desired perfusion; the concentration and rate of infusion can be rapidly calculated using the following formulas:

Dilute 0.6 mg x weight (kg) to 100 mL in D_5W or 1.5 mg x weight (kg) to 250 mL in D_5W; then the dose in μg/kg/minute = 0.1 x the infusion rate in mL/hour

Treatment of extravasation: Infiltrate area of extravasation with phentolamine

Norethindrone (nor eth in' drone)

Brand Names Norlutate®; Norlutin®

Synonyms Norethindrone Acetate; Norethisterone

Use Treatment of amenorrhea; abnormal uterine bleeding; endometriosis

Pregnancy Risk Factor X

Usual Dosage Oral:

Adult: (Norlutin®)
Amenorrhea and abnormal uterine bleeding: 5-20 mg on days 5-25 of menstrual cycle
Endometriosis: 10 mg/day for 14 days; increase at increments of 5 mg/day every two weeks up to 30 mg/day

Adult: (Norlutate®)
Amenorrhea and abnormal uterine bleeding: 2.5-10 mg on days 5-25 of menstrual cycle
Endometriosis: 5 mg/day for 14 days; increase at increments of 2.5 mg/day every two weeks up to 15 mg/day

Norethindrone Acetate *see* Norethindrone *on this page*

Norethindrone Acetate and Ethinyl Estradiol *see* Ethinyl Estradiol and Norethindrone Acetate *on page 139*

Norethindrone and Mestranol *see* Mestranol and Norethindrone *on page 222*

Norethisterone *see* Norethindrone *on this page*

Norethynodrel and Mestranol *see* Mestranol and Norethynodrel *on page 222*

Norflex® *see* Orphenadrine Citrate *on page 262*

Norfloxacin (nor flox' a sin)

Brand Names Noroxin®

Use Complicated and uncomplicated urinary tract infections caused by susceptible gram-negative and gram-positive bacteria

(Continued)

Norfloxacin *(Continued)*
Pregnancy Risk Factor C
Usual Dosage Adult: Oral: 400 mg twice a day for 7-21 days depending on infection

Norgesic® *see* Orphenadrine, Aspirin and Caffeine *on page 261*

Norgesic® Forte *see* Orphenadrine, Aspirin and Caffeine *on page 261*

Norgestrel (nor jess' trel)
Brand Names Ovrette®
Use Oral contraceptive
Usual Dosage Administer daily, starting the first day of menstruation, take one tablet at the same time each, every day of the year

Norgestrel and Ethinyl Estradiol *see* Ethinyl Estradiol and Norgestrel *on page 140*

Norinyl® *see* Mestranol and Norethindrone *on page 222*

Norisodrine® *see* Isoproterenol *on page 193*

Norlestrin® 2.5/50 *see* Ethinyl Estradiol and Norethindrone Acetate *on page 139*

Norlutate® *see* Norethindrone *on previous page*

Norlutin® *see* Norethindrone *on previous page*

Normal Human Serum Albumin *see* Albumin Human *on page 10*

Normal Saline *see* Sodium Chloride *on page 327*

Normal Serum Albumin (Human) *see* Albumin Human *on page 10*

Normodyne® *see* Labetalol Hydrochloride *on page 198*

Noroxin® *see* Norfloxacin *on previous page*

Norpace® *see* Disopyramide Phosphate *on page 119*

Norpramin® *see* Desipramine Hydrochloride *on page 100*

Nor-Pred S® *see* Prednisolone *on page 294*

Nor-Pred T.B.A.® *see* Prednisolone *on page 294*

Nor-tet® *see* Tetracycline *on page 346*

North American Coral Snake Antivenin *see* Antivenin (*Micrurus fulvius*) *on page 27*

North and South American Antisnake-bite Serum *see* Antivenin (Crotalidae) Polyvalent *on page 27*

Nortriptyline Hydrochloride (nor trip' ti leen)
Brand Names Aventyl® Hydrochloride; Pamelor®
Use Used in the treatment of various forms of depression, often in conjunction with psychotherapy

Pregnancy Risk Factor D
Usual Dosage Oral:

Adult: 25 mg 3-4 times daily up to 150 mg/day

Elderly and Adolescent: 30-50 mg daily in divided doses

Nortussin® [OTC] *see* Guaifenesin *on page 162*

Norzine® *see* Thiethylperazine Maleate *on page 351*

Nostrilla® Long Acting Nasal Solution [OTC] *see* Oxymetazoline Hydrochloride *on page 265*

Nostril® Nasal Solution [OTC] *see* Phenylephrine Hydrochloride *on page 282*

Novafed® *see* Pseudoephedrine *on page 307*

Novafed® A *see* Chlorpheniramine and Pseudoephedrine *on page 74*

Novahistine® DH *see* Chlorpheniramine, Pseudoephedrine and Codeine *on page 75*

Novahistine® Elixir [OTC] *see* Chlorpheniramine and Phenylephrine *on page 73*

Novantrone® *see* Mitoxantrone Hydrochloride *on page 239*

Novocain® *see* Procaine Hydrochloride *on page 298*

Novolin® 70/30 *see* Insulin, Isophane Suspension and Insulin Injection *on page 186*

Novolin® L *see* Insulin, Zinc Suspension *on page 186*

Novolin® N *see* Insulin, Isophane Suspension *on page 185*

Novolin® R *see* Insulin, Regular *on page 186*

Novolin® R Penfill *see* Insulin, Regular *on page 186*

NP-27® [OTC] *see* Tolnaftate *on page 357*

NPH *see* Insulin, Isophane Suspension *on page 185*

NPH Iletin®I *see* Insulin, Isophane Suspension *on page 185*

NPH Purified Pork *see* Insulin, Isophane Suspension *on page 185*

NSC-102816 *see* Azacitidine *on page 33*

NTG, Nitroglycerol *see* Nitroglycerin *on page 253*

NTZ® Nasal Solution [OTC] *see* Oxymetazoline Hydrochloride *on page 265*

Nubain® *see* Nalbuphine Hydrochloride *on page 245*

Numorphan® *see* Oxymorphone Hydrochloride *on page 265*

Nupercainal® [OTC] *see* Dibucaine *on page 110*

Nuprin® [OTC] *see* Ibuprofen *on page 181*

Nutraplus® [OTC] *see* Urea *on page 369*

Nutrilipid® *see* Fat Emulsion *on page 144*

Nutritional Formula, Enteral/Oral
Brand Names Amin-Aid® [OTC]; Carnation Instant Breakfast® [OTC]; Citrotein® [OTC]; Criticare HN® [OTC]; Ensure® [OTC]; Ensure Plus® [OTC]; Isocal® [OTC]; Magnacal® [OTC]; Microlipid® [OTC]; Osmolite® HN [OTC]; Pedialyte® [OTC]; Polycose® [OTC]; Portagen® [OTC]; Pregestimil® [OTC]; Propac® [OTC]; Soyalac® [OTC]; Vital HN® [OTC]; Vitaneed® [OTC]; Vivonex® [OTC]; Vivonex® T.E.N. [OTC]

Nydrazid® see Isoniazid on page 192

Nylidrin Hydrochloride (nye' li drin)
Brand Names Arlidin®
Use Increases blood supply as to treat peripheral disease and circulatory disturbances of the inner ear
Pregnancy Risk Factor C
Usual Dosage 3-12 mg 3-4 times daily

Nystatin (nye stat' in)
Brand Names Mycostatin®; Mykinac®; Nilstat®; Nystex®; O-V Statin®
Use Treatment of susceptible fungal infections normally caused by the *Candida* species
Pregnancy Risk Factor B
Usual Dosage

Adult:
Intestinal infections: Oral: 500,000-1,000,000 units every eight hours
Mucocutaneous infections: Topical: Apply 3-4 times daily
Oral *Monilia*: Oral: 400,000-600,000 units every 6-8 hours
Vaginal infections: Vaginal tablets: Use 1-2 times daily

Children:
Mucocutaneous infections: Topical: Apply 3-4 times daily
Oral *Monilia*: Oral: 200,000 units every 6-8 hours

Nystatin and Triamcinolone
Brand Names Mycolog®-II; Mytrex® F
Synonyms Triamcinolone and Nystatin
Use Treatment of cutaneous candidiasis
Pregnancy Risk Factor C
Usual Dosage Apply twice a day

Nystex® see Nystatin on this page

Nytilax® [OTC] see Senna on page 322

Occucoat™ see Hydroxypropyl Methylcellulose on page 178

Occult Blood Screening Test see Diagnostic Test for Blood in Feces on page 107

Octamide® see Metoclopramide on page 233

Octreotide Acetate (ok tree' oh tide)
Brand Names Sandostatin®
Use Control of symptoms in patients with metastatic carcinoid and vasoactive intestinal peptide-secreting tumors (VIPomas)

Pregnancy Risk Factor B
Usual Dosage S.C.:

Carcinoid: 100-600 µg/day in 2-4 divided doses

VIPomas: 200-300 µg/day in 2-4 divided doses

Ocu-Carpine® *see* Pilocarpine Hydrochloride *on page 285*

Ocu-Chlor® *see* Chloramphenicol *on page 69*

Ocu-Drop® [OTC] *see* Tetrahydrozoline Hydrochloride *on page 347*

Ocufen® Liquifilm® *see* Flurbiprofen Sodium *on page 153*

Ocugestrin® Ophthalmic Solution *see* Phenylephrine Hydrochloride *on page 282*

Ocular Lubricant
Brand Names Duratears® [OTC]; Lacri-Lube® [OTC]
Use Protection and lubrication of the eye
Usual Dosage Apply small amount as needed

Ocumycin® *see* Gentamicin Sulfate *on page 157*

Ocu-Phrin® Ophthalmic Solution *see* Phenylephrine Hydrochloride *on page 282*

Ocu-Pred® *see* Prednisolone *on page 294*

Ocusert® Pilo *see* Pilocarpine Hydrochloride *on page 285*

Ocu-Tropine® *see* Atropine Sulfate *on page 32*

Ocu-Zoline® *see* Naphazoline Hydrochloride *on page 246*

o'-DDD *see* Mitotane *on page 239*

Ogen® *see* Estropipate *on page 137*

OGMT *see* Metyrosine *on page 235*

Old Tuberculin *see* Tuberculin *on page 367*

Oleovitamin A *see* Vitamin A *on page 376*

Oleum Ricini *see* Castor Oil *on page 61*

Olive Oil
Synonyms Sweet Oil
Use As a pharmaceutical aid in preparing cerates, ointments, liniments, and plasters; as emollient laxative; symptomatic treatment of minor otic irritations
Usual Dosage Oral dose: 30 mL

Omeprazole (oh me' pray zol)
Formerly Known As Losec®
Brand Names Prilosec™
Use Short-term (4-8 weeks) treatment of severe erosive esophagitis (grade 2 or above), diagnosed by endoscopy and short-term treatment of symptomatic gastroesophageal reflux disease (GERD) poorly respon-
(Continued)

Omeprazole *(Continued)*

sible to customary medical treatment; pathological hypersecretory conditions

Pregnancy Risk Factor C

Usual Dosage Adult: Oral:

GERD or severe erosive esophagitis: 20 mg/day for 4-8 weeks

Pathological hypersecretory conditions: 60 mg once a day to start; doses up to 120 mg three times a day have been administered; administer daily doses > 80 mg in divided doses

Omnipaque® *see* Iohexol *on page 189*

Omnipen® *see* Ampicillin *on page 23*

Oncovin® *see* Vincristine Sulfate *on page 376*

OP-CCK *see* Sincalide *on page 325*

Opcon® *see* Naphazoline Hydrochloride *on page 246*

Ophthaine® *see* Proparacaine Hydrochloride *on page 302*

Ophthalgan® *see* Glycerin *on page 159*

Ophthalmic Irrigant Mixture

Ophthetic® *see* Proparacaine Hydrochloride *on page 302*

Ophthochlor® *see* Chloramphenicol *on page 69*

Opium Alkaloids (oh' pee um)

Brand Names Pantopon®

Use For relief of severe pain

Restrictions C-II

Pregnancy Risk Factor B/D

Usual Dosage Adult: I.M., S.C.: 5-20 mg every 4-5 hours

Opium and Belladonna *see* Belladonna and Opium *on page 38*

Opium, Camphorated Tincture of

Synonyms Paregoric

Use Treatment of diarrhea or relief of pain

Restrictions C-III

Pregnancy Risk Factor B/D

Usual Dosage

Adult: 5-10 mL 1-4 times daily

Children: 0.25-0.5 mL/kg 1-4 times daily

Neonatal opiate withdrawal: 3-6 drops every 3-6 hours as needed, or initial dose of 0.2 mL every three hours; increase dosage by approximately 0.05 mL every three hours until withdrawal symptoms are controlled; it is rare to exceed 0.7 mL per dose. After withdrawal symptoms have been stabilized for 3-5 days, dosage should be decreased gradually over a 2-4 week period.

Opium, Tincture of
Synonyms Deodorized Opium Tincture; DTO
Use Treatment of diarrhea or relief of pain
Restrictions C-II
Pregnancy Risk Factor B
Usual Dosage Oral:

Adult: 0.6 mL four times daily

Children:
Diarrhea: 0.005-0.01 mL/kg/dose every 3-4 hours
Analgesia: 0.01-0.02 mL/kg/dose every 3-4 hours

Opticrom® *see* Cromolyn Sodium *on page 91*

Optigene® [OTC] *see* Tetrahydrozoline Hydrochloride *on page 347*

Optimine® *see* Azatadine Maleate *on page 34*

Orabase® Plain [OTC] *see* Gelatin, Pectin and Methylcellulose *on page 156*

Orabase® With Benzocaine [OTC] *see* Benzocaine, Gelatin, Pectin and Sodium Carboxymethylcellulose *on page 41*

Oragrafin® *see* Ipodate Sodium *on page 190*

Oraminic® II *see* Brompheniramine Maleate *on page 48*

Orap™ *see* Pimozide *on page 286*

Orasone® *see* Prednisone *on page 295*

Ora-Testryl® *see* Fluoxymesterone *on page 152*

Orazinc® [OTC] *see* Zinc Sulfate *on page 382*

Orciprenaline Sulfate *see* Metaproterenol Sulfate *on page 223*

Oretic® *see* Hydrochlorothiazide *on page 172*

Oreton® *see* Methyltestosterone *on page 232*

Orex® [OTC] *see* Saliva Substitute *on page 320*

Orexin® [OTC] *see* Vitamin B Complex *on page 377*

Organidin® *see* Iodinated Glycerol *on page 188*

ORG NC 45 *see* Vecuronium *on page 373*

Orimune® Trivalent *see* Poliovirus Vaccine, Live, Trivalent *on page 289*

Orinase® *see* Tolbutamide *on page 357*

Ornade® Spansule® *see* Chlorpheniramine and Phenylpropanolamine *on page 73*

Orphenadrine, Aspirin and Caffeine
Brand Names Norgesic® Forte; Norgesic®
Use Relief of discomfort associated with skeletal muscular conditions
Pregnancy Risk Factor D
Usual Dosage 1-2 tablets 3-4 times daily

Orphenadrine Citrate (or fen' a dreen)
Brand Names Norflex®
Use Treatment of muscle spasm associated with acute painful musculo-skeletal conditions; supportive therapy in tetanus
Pregnancy Risk Factor C
Usual Dosage Adult:
Oral: 100 mg twice daily
I.M., I.V.: 60 mg every 12 hours

Orthoclone® OKT3 see Muromonab-CD3 on page 243

Ortho® Dienestrol see Dienestrol on page 112

Ortho-Novum™ 1/50 see Mestranol and Norethindrone on page 222

Ortho-Novum™ 1/80 see Mestranol and Norethindrone on page 222

Orudis® see Ketoprofen on page 196

Os-Cal® 250 [OTC] see Calcium Carbonate on page 53

Os-Cal® 500 [OTC] see Calcium Carbonate on page 53

Osmitrol® see Mannitol on page 212

Osmoglyn® see Glycerin on page 159

Osmolite® HN [OTC] see Nutritional Formula, Enteral/Oral on page 258

OT see Tuberculin on page 367

Otobiotic® Otic see Hydrocortisone and Polymyxin B on page 175

Otrivin® [OTC] see Xylometazoline Hydrochloride on page 380

Ovide™ see Malathion on page 211

Ovral® see Ethinyl Estradiol and Norgestrel on page 140

Ovrette® see Norgestrel on page 256

O-V Statin® see Nystatin on page 258

Ovulen® see Mestranol and Ethynodiol on page 221

OvuSTICK® [OTC] see Diagnostic Test for Ovulation on page 107

Oxacillin Sodium (ox a sill' in)
Brand Names Prostaphlin®
Use Treatment of susceptible bacterial infections due to penicillinase-producing strains of *Staphylococcus*
Pregnancy Risk Factor B
Usual Dosage I.M., I.V.:

Adult: 250 mg to 2 g/dose every 4-6 hours

Infant and Children: 100-200 mg/kg/day in divided doses every 6 hours

Neonate: Postnatal age < 7 days:
< 2000 g: 50 mg/kg/day in divided doses every 12 hours

> 2000 g: 75 mg/kg/day in divided doses every 8 hours

Neonate: Postnatal age > 7 days:
> < 2000 g: 100 mg/kg/day in divided doses every 8 hours
> > 2000 g: 150 mg/kg/day in divided doses every 6 hours

Oxamniquine (ox am' ni kwin)
Brand Names Vansil™
Use Treat all stages of *Schistosoma mansoni* infection
Pregnancy Risk Factor C
Usual Dosage Oral:

Adult: 12-15 mg/kg as a single dose

Children: < 30 kg: 20 mg/kg in two divided doses of 10 mg/kg at 2-8 hour intervals

Oxazepam (ox a' ze pam)
Brand Names Serax®
Use Treatment of anxiety and management of alcohol withdrawal; may also be used as an anticonvulsant in management of simple partial seizures
Restrictions C-IV
Pregnancy Risk Factor D
Usual Dosage Adult: Oral:

Anxiety: 10-30 mg 3-4 times daily

Alcohol withdrawal: 15-30 mg 3-4 times daily

Oxiconazole Nitrate (ox i kon' a zole)
Brand Names Oxistat®
Use Treatment of tinea pedis, tinea cruris, and tinea corporis
Usual Dosage Apply once daily

Oxilapine Succinate *see* Loxapine *on page 208*

Oxistat® *see* Oxiconazole Nitrate *on this page*

Oxpentifylline *see* Pentoxifylline *on page 276*

Oxsoralen® *see* Methoxsalen *on page 228*

Oxsoralen-Ultra® *see* Methoxsalen *on page 228*

Oxtriphylline (ox trye' fi lin)
Brand Names Choledyl®
Synonyms Choline Theophyllinate
Use Bronchodilator in symptomatic treatment of asthma and reversible bronchospasm
Pregnancy Risk Factor C
Usual Dosage Oral:

Adult: 200 mg four times a day

Children: 2-12 years: 4 mg/kg every six hours

Oxy-5® [OTC] *see* Benzoyl Peroxide *on page 41*

Oxybutynin Chloride (ox i byoo' ti nin)
Brand Names Ditropan®; Dridase®
Use Antispasmodic for neurogenic bladder
Pregnancy Risk Factor C
Usual Dosage Oral:

Adult: 5 mg 2-3 times a day up to 5 mg four times a day maximum

Children: > 5 years of age: 5 mg twice a day, up to 5 mg three times a day

Oxycet® *see* Oxycodone Hydrochloride *on this page*

Oxychlorosene Sodium (ox i klor' oh seen)
Brand Names Chlorpactin® WCS-90
Use Treating localized infections
Usual Dosage Apply by irrigation, instillation, spray, soaks, or wet compresses

Oxycodone and Acetaminophen
Brand Names Percocet®; Tylox®
Synonyms Acetaminophen and Oxycodone
Use Management of moderate to severe pain
Restrictions C-II
Pregnancy Risk Factor C
Usual Dosage Oral:

Adult: 1-2 tablets or capsules every 4-6 hours as needed for pain

Children: Oxycodone: 0.05-0.15 mg/kg/dose to 10 mg/dose every 4-6 hours as needed

Oxycodone and Acetaminophen *see* Oxycodone Hydrochloride *on this page*

Oxycodone and Aspirin
Brand Names Percodan®; Percodan®-Demi
Use Relief of moderate to moderately severe pain
Restrictions C-II
Pregnancy Risk Factor D
Usual Dosage Oral:

Adult:
Percodan®: One tablet every six hours as needed for pain
Percodan®-Demi: 1-2 tablets every six hours as needed for pain

Children:
> 12 years of age: One tablet every six hours as needed for pain
6-12 years: 1/2 tablet every six hours as needed for pain

Oxycodone and Aspirin *see* Oxycodone Hydrochloride *on this page*

Oxycodone Hydrochloride (ox i koe' done)
Brand Names Codoxy®; Oxycet®; Percocet®; Percodan®; Percodan®-Demi; Roxicet®; Roxicodone™; Roxiprin®; Tylox®
Synonyms Dihydrohydroxycodeinone; Oxycodone and Acetaminophen; Oxycodone and Aspirin

Use Management of moderate to severe pain, normally used in combination with non-narcotic analgesics

Restrictions C-II

Pregnancy Risk Factor C

Usual Dosage Oral:

Adult: 5 mg every six hours as needed

Children:
> 12 years: 2.5 mg every six hours as needed
6-12 years: 1.25 mg every six hours as needed

Oxygel® *see* Cellulose, Oxidized *on page 65*

Oxymeta-12® Nasal Solution [OTC] *see* Oxymetazoline Hydrochloride *on this page*

Oxymetazoline Hydrochloride (ox i met az' oh leen)

Brand Names Afrin® Nasal Solution [OTC]; Allerest® 12 Hours Nasal Solution [OTC]; Chlorphed®-LA Nasal Solution [OTC]; Dristan® Long Lasting Nasal Solution [OTC]; Duration® Nasal Solution [OTC]; Genasal® Nasal Solution [OTC]; Neo-Synephrine® 12 Hour Nasal Solution [OTC]; Nōstrilla® Long Acting Nasal Solution [OTC]; NTZ® Nasal Solution [OTC]; Oxymeta-12® Nasal Solution [OTC]; Sinarest® 12 Hour Nasal Solution; Vicks Sinex® Long-Acting Nasal Solution [OTC]; 4-Way® Long Acting Nasal Solution [OTC]

Use Symptomatic relief of nasal mucosal congestion and adjunctive therapy of middle ear infections

Pregnancy Risk Factor C

Usual Dosage

Children and Adults: ≥ 6 years: 0.05% solution: 2-3 drops or 2-3 sprays into each nostril twice/day

Children: 2-5 years of age: 0.025% solution, 2-3 drops in each nostril twice/day

Oxymetholone (ox i meth' oh lone)

Brand Names Anadrol®

Use Anemias caused by the administration of myelotoxic drugs

Pregnancy Risk Factor X

Usual Dosage Erythropoietic effects: 1-5 mg/kg/day in one daily dose up to a maximum of 100 mg/day

Oxymorphone Hydrochloride (ox i mor' fone)

Brand Names Numorphan®

Use Management of moderate to severe pain and preoperatively as a sedative and a supplement to anesthesia

Restrictions C-II

Pregnancy Risk Factor C

Usual Dosage Adult:
I.V.: 5 mg initially
I.M., S.C.: 5 mg initially, 1-1.5 mg every 4-6 hours as needed
Rectal: 5 mg every 4-6 hours

Oxyphenbutazone (ox i fen byoo' ta zone)

Use Management of inflammatory disorders, as an analgesic in the treatment of mild to moderate pain and as an antipyretic; I.V. form used as an alternate to surgery in management of patent ductus arteriosus in premature neonates; acute gouty arthritis

Pregnancy Risk Factor C

Usual Dosage Adult: Oral:

Rheumatoid arthritis: 100-200 mg 3-4 times daily until desired effect, then reduce dose to not exceeding 400 mg/day

Acute gouty arthritis: 400 mg initially, 100 mg every four hours until acute attack subsides

Oxyphencyclimine Hydrochloride (ox i fen sye' kli meen)

Brand Names Daricon®

Use Adjunctive treatment of peptic ulcer

Pregnancy Risk Factor C

Usual Dosage Adult: Oral: 10 mg twice a day or 5 mg three times a day

Oxytetracycline and Polymyxin B

Brand Names Terramycin® Ophthalmic Ointment

Synonyms Polymyxin B and Oxytetracycline

Use Treatment of superficial ocular infections involving the conjunctiva and/or cornea

Pregnancy Risk Factor D

Usual Dosage Apply 1/2 inch of ointment onto the lower lid of affected eye 2-4 times a day

Oxytetracycline Hydrochloride (ox i tet ra sye' kleen)

Brand Names Terramycin® IV

Use Treatment of susceptible bacterial infections; both gram-positive and gram-negative, as well as *Rickettsia* and *Mycoplasma* organisms

Pregnancy Risk Factor D

Usual Dosage I.V.:

Adult: 250-500 mg every 12 hours

Children: > 8 years: 6 mg/kg every 12 hours

Oxytocin (ox i toe' sin)

Brand Names Pitocin®; Syntocinon®

Synonyms Pit

Use Induce labor at term; control postpartum bleeding; nasal preparation used to promote milk letdown in lactating females

Usual Dosage Adult:

Induction of labor: I.V.: 0.001-0.002 unit/minute; increase by 0.001-0.002 every 15-30 minutes until contraction pattern has been established

Postpartum bleeding: I.V.: 0.001-0.002 units/minute as needed

Promotion of milk letdown: Intranasal: One spray or three drops in one or both nostrils 2-3 minutes before breast feeding

P₁E₁® *see* Pilocarpine and Epinephrine *on page 285*

P₂E₁® *see* Pilocarpine and Epinephrine *on page 285*

P₄E₁® *see* Pilocarpine and Epinephrine *on page 285*

P₆E₁® *see* Pilocarpine and Epinephrine *on page 285*

2-PAM *see* Pralidoxime Chloride *on page 292*

Pamelor® *see* Nortriptyline Hydrochloride *on page 256*

Pamine® *see* Methscopolamine Bromide *on page 229*

Pamisyl® *see* Aminosalicylic Acid *on page 19*

Pamprin IB® [OTC] *see* Ibuprofen *on page 181*

Panadol® [OTC] *see* Acetaminophen *on page 4*

Pancrease® *see* Pancrelipase *on this page*

Pancrease® MT *see* Pancrelipase *on this page*

Pancreatin (pan' kree a tin)
Brand Names Creon®; Pancreatin Enseals® [OTC]
Use Replacement therapy in symptomatic treatment of malabsorption syndrome caused by pancreatic insufficiency
Pregnancy Risk Factor C
Usual Dosage Adult: Oral: 1-3 tablets after meals

Pancreatin Enseals® [OTC] *see* Pancreatin *on this page*

Pancrelipase (pan kre li' pase)
Brand Names Cotazym®; Cotazym-S®; Entolase®-HP; Festal®ll [OTC]; Il-ozyme®; Kanular®; Kutrase®; Ku-Zyme®; Pancrease®; Pancrease® MT; Panteric®; Protilase®; Viokase®; Zymase®
Synonyms Lipancreatin
Use Replacement therapy in symptomatic treatment of malabsorption syndrome caused by pancreatic insufficiency
Pregnancy Risk Factor C
Usual Dosage Oral:

Powder: Actual dose depends on the digestive requirements of the patient
Children: < 1 year of age: Start with 1/8 teaspoonful with feedings

Enteric coated microspheres and microtablets: The following dosage recommendations are only an approximation for initial dosages. The actual dosage will depend on the digestive requirements of the individual patient.
Adult: 4,000-16,000 units of lipase with meals and with snacks
Children: < 1 year: 2,000 units of lipase with meals
Children: 1-6 years: 4,000-8,000 units of lipase with meals and 4,000 units with snacks
Children: 7-12 years: 4,000-12,000 units of lipase with meals and snacks

Pancuronium Bromide (pan kyoo roe' nee um)
Brand Names Pavulon®

Use Produce skeletal muscle relaxation during surgery after induction of general anesthesia, increase pulmonary compliance during assisted respiration, facilitate endotracheal intubation

Pregnancy Risk Factor C

Usual Dosage I.V.:

Infants > 1 month, Children and Adult: I.V.: 0.04-0.1 mg/kg; maintenance dose: 0.02-0.1 mg/kg/dose every 30-60 minutes as needed

Neonate: ≤ 1 month: Initial: 0.03 mg/kg/dose repeated twice at 5-10 minute intervals as needed; maintenance: 0.03-0.09 mg/kg/dose every 30 minutes to 4 hours as needed

Panhematin® *see* Hemin *on page 167*

Panmycin® *see* Tetracycline *on page 346*

PanOxyl® [OTC] *see* Benzoyl Peroxide *on page 41*

PanOxyl®-AQ *see* Benzoyl Peroxide *on page 41*

Panteric® *see* Pancrelipase *on previous page*

Panthoderm® *see* Dexpanthenol *on page 103*

Pantopon® *see* Opium Alkaloids *on page 260*

Pantothenic Acid
Synonyms Calcium Pantothenate; Vitamin B_5

Use Pantothenic acid deficiency

Usual Dosage Oral: 4-7 mg/day

Panwarfin® *see* Warfarin Sodium *on page 379*

Papaverine Hydrochloride (pa pav' er een)
Brand Names Cerespan®; Genabid®; Pavabid®; Pavagen®; Pavaspan®; Pavatine® Pavased®; Pavatym®; Paverolan®

Use Relief of cerebral and peripheral ischemia

Pregnancy Risk Factor C

Usual Dosage

Adult:
Oral: 100-300 mg 3-5 times daily
Oral sustained release: 150-300 mg every 12 hours
I.M., I.V.: 30-120 mg every three hours as needed

Children: I.M., I.V.: 1.5 mg/kg four times a day

Para-aminosalicylate Sodium
Synonyms Aminosalicylate Sodium; PAS

Use Adjunctive treatment of tuberculosis

Pregnancy Risk Factor C

Usual Dosage Oral:

Adult: 12-15 g/day in 3-4 divided doses

Children: 240-360 mg/kg/day in 3-4 divided doses

Parabromdylamine *see* Brompheniramine Maleate
on page 48

Paracetaldehyde *see* Paraldehyde *on this page*

Paracetamol *see* Acetaminophen *on page 4*

Parachlorometaxylenol
Brand Names Metasep® [OTC]
Synonyms PCMX
Use An aid in relief of dandruff and associated conditions
Usual Dosage Massage to a foamy lather, allow to remain on hair for five minutes, rinse thoroughly and repeat

Paracort® *see* Prednisone *on page 295*

Paradione® *see* Paramethadione *on this page*

Paraflex® *see* Chlorzoxazone *on page 77*

Parafon Forte™ DSC *see* Chlorzoxazone *on page 77*

Paral® *see* Paraldehyde *on this page*

Paraldehyde (par al' de hyde)
Brand Names Paral®
Synonyms Paracetaldehyde
Use Control convulsions arising from tetanus and status epilepticus; sedative and hypnotic in acute agitation due to alcohol withdrawal; induce basal anesthesia in children
Restrictions C-IV
Pregnancy Risk Factor C
Usual Dosage See table.

Paraldehyde

	Sedative	Hypnotic	Seizures
Adult Oral, rectal	5–10 mL	10–30 mL	
I.M.		5 mL	5–10 mL
I.V.		3–5 mL	0.2–0.4 mL/kg
Children Oral, rectal	0.15 mL/kg	0.3 mL/kg	
I.M.			0.15 mL/kg every 4–6 h
I.V.			5 mL in 95 mL normal saline solution

Paramethad *see* Paramethadione *on this page*

Paramethadione (par a meth a dye' one)
Brand Names Paradione®
Synonyms Isoethadione; Paramethad
Use To control absence (petit mal) seizures refractory to other drugs
(Continued)

269

Paramethadione *(Continued)*

Pregnancy Risk Factor D
Usual Dosage Oral:

Adult: 900 mg-2.4 g/day in 3-4 equally divided doses

Children: 300-900 mg/day in 3-4 equally divided doses

Paramethasone Acetate (par a meth' a sone)

Brand Names Haldrone®; Stemex®
Use Treatment of a variety of diseases including those of hematologic, allergic, inflammatory, neoplastic, and autoimmune in origin
Pregnancy Risk Factor C
Usual Dosage 2-24 mg/day

Paraplatin® *see* Carboplatin *on page 60*

Parathar™ *see* Teriparatide *on page 343*

Paredrine® *see* Hydroxyamphetamine Hydrobromide *on page 177*

Paregoric *see* Opium, Camphorated Tincture of *on page 260*

Parepectolin® *see* Kaolin and Pectin With Opium *on page 195*

Pargyline and Methyclothiazide *see* Methyclothiazide and Pargyline *on page 230*

Pargyline Hydrochloride (par' gi leen)

Brand Names Eutonyl®
Use Treatment of moderate to severe hypertension
Pregnancy Risk Factor C
Usual Dosage Adult: Oral: Initially 25 mg once daily; may be increased once a week by 10 mg increments up to 200 mg/day

Parlodel® *see* Bromocriptine Mesylate *on page 47*

Parnate® *see* Tranylcypromine Sulfate *on page 359*

Paromomycin Sulfate (par oh moe mye' sin)

Brand Names Humatin®
Use Treatment of acute and chronic intestinal amebiasis; preoperatively to suppress intestinal flora; tapeworm infestations; rid bowel of nitrogen forming bacteria in hepatic coma
Pregnancy Risk Factor C
Usual Dosage Oral:

Intestinal amebiasis: Adult and Children: 25-35 mg/kg in three divided doses for 5-10 days

Tapeworm:
Adult: 1 g every 15 minutes for four doses
Children: 11 mg/kg every 15 minutes for four doses

Hepatic coma: Adult: 4 g daily in 2-4 divided doses for 3-5 days

Parsidol® *see* Ethopropazine Hydrochloride *on page 140*

PAS *see* Aminosalicylic Acid *on page 19*

PAS *see* Para-aminosalicylate Sodium *on page 268*

Pathocil® *see* Dicloxacillin Sodium *on page 111*

Pavabid® *see* Papaverine Hydrochloride *on page 268*

Pavagen® *see* Papaverine Hydrochloride *on page 268*

Pavaspan® *see* Papaverine Hydrochloride *on page 268*

Pavatine® Pavased® *see* Papaverine Hydrochloride *on page 268*

Pavatym® *see* Papaverine Hydrochloride *on page 268*

Paverolan® *see* Papaverine Hydrochloride *on page 268*

Pavulon® *see* Pancuronium Bromide *on page 268*

PBZ® *see* Tripelennamine *on page 365*

PBZ-SR® *see* Tripelennamine *on page 365*

PCE® *see* Erythromycin *on page 134*

PCMX *see* Parachlorometaxylenol *on page 269*

Pectin and Kaolin *see* Kaolin and Pectin *on page 195*

Pedameth® *see* Methionine *on page 227*

PedavaxHIB® *see* Haemophilus b Vaccine *on page 165*

Pediaflor® *see* Fluoride *on page 150*

Pedialyte® *see* Infant Nutritional Formulas *on page 184*

Pedialyte® [OTC] *see* Nutritional Formula, Enteral/Oral *on page 258*

Pediamycin® *see* Erythromycin *on page 134*

Pediapred® *see* Prednisolone *on page 294*

PediaProfen™ *see* Ibuprofen *on page 181*

Pediazole® *see* Erythromycin and Sulfisoxazole *on page 134*

Pedi-Dri *see* Zinc Undecylenate *on page 382*

Pedte-Pak-5® *see* Trace Metals *on page 358*

Pedtrace-4® *see* Trace Metals *on page 358*

Peganone® *see* Ethotoin *on page 141*

Pemoline (pem' oh leen)
  Brand Names Cylert®
  Synonyms Phenylisohydantoin; PIO
  Use Treatment of attention deficit disorder with hyperactivity (ADDH); narcolepsy
  Restrictions C-IV
  Pregnancy Risk Factor B
  Usual Dosage Oral: Children: ≥ 6 years: 37.5 mg to start in the morning, increase by 18.75 mg at weekly intervals; effective dose range is 56.25-75 mg/day; maximum is 112.5 mg/day

Penamp® *see* Ampicillin *on page 23*

Penicillamine (pen i sill' a meen)
Brand Names Cuprimine®; Depen®
Synonyms D-3-Mercaptovaline; β,β-Dimethylcysteine; D-Penicillamine
Use Treatment of Wilson's disease, cystinuria, adjunct in the treatment of rheumatoid arthritis; lead poisoning, primary biliary cirrhosis
Pregnancy Risk Factor C
Usual Dosage Oral:

Rheumatoid arthritis:
Adult: 125-250 mg/day, may increase dose at 1-3 month intervals up to 1-1.5 g/day
Children: Initially: 3 mg/kg/day ($\leq$ 250 mg/day) for three months, then 6 mg/kg/day ($\leq$ 500 mg/day) in divided doses twice a day for 3 months to a maximum of 10 mg/kg/day in 3-4 divided doses

Wilson's disease:
Adult: 1 g/day in four divided doses
Children: 20 mg/kg/day in four divided doses

Cystinuria:
Adult: 500 mg four times a day
Children: 30 mg/kg/day in four divided doses

Lead poisoning:
Adult: 1-1.5 g/day for 1-2 months
Children: 25-40 mg/kg/day in 2-3 divided doses

Primary biliary cirrhosis: 250 mg/day to start, increase by 250 mg every two weeks up to a maintenance dose of 1 g/day, usually given 250 mg four times a day

Penicillin G Benzathine and Procaine Combined
Brand Names Bicillin® C-R; Bicillin® C-R 900/300
Synonyms Penicillin G Procaine and Benzathine Combined
Use Active against most gram-negative organisms; some gram-negative such as *Neisseria gonorrhoeae* and some anaerobes and spirochetes
Pregnancy Risk Factor B
Usual Dosage I.M.:

Adult and Children > 60 lbs: 2.4 million units in a single dose

Children 30-60 lbs: 900,000-1.2 million units in a single dose

Children < 30 lbs: 600,000 units in a single dose

Penicillin G Benzathine, Oral (pen i sill' in)
Synonyms Benzathine Benzylpenicillin; Benzathine Penicillin G
Use Active against most gram-positive organisms; some gram-negative such as *Neisseria gonorrhoeae* and some anaerobes and spirochetes
Usual Dosage Oral: 400,000-600,000 units every 4-6 hours

Penicillin G Benzathine, Parenteral
Brand Names Bicillin®; Bicillin® L-A; Megacillin®; Permapen®
Synonyms Benzathine Benzylpenicillin; Benzathine Penicillin G
Use Active against most gram-positive organisms; some gram-negative such as *Neisseria gonorrhoeae* and some anaerobes and spirochetes

Pregnancy Risk Factor B

Usual Dosage I.M.: Give undiluted injection, very slowly released from site of injection, providing uniform levels over 2-4 weeks; higher doses result in more sustained rather than higher levels. Use a penicillin G benzathine-penicillin G procaine combination to achieve early peak levels in acute infections

Adult: 0.6-2.4 million units x 1

Children and Infants: 50,000 units/kg/dose x 1 up to a maximum of 2.4 million units/dose

Newborns: 50,000 units/kg x 1

Penicillin G, Parenteral

Brand Names Cilloral®; Liquapen®; Pentids®; Pfizerpen®

Synonyms Benzylpenicillin Potassium; Benzylpenicillin Sodium; Crystalline Penicillin; Penicillin G Potassium; Penicillin G Sodium

Use Active against most gram-positive organisms; some gram-negative such as *Neisseria gonorrhoeae* and some anaerobes and spirochetes

Pregnancy Risk Factor B

Usual Dosage I.M,: Give undiluted injection, very slowly released from site of injection, providing uniform levels over 2-4 weeks; higher doses result in more sustained rather than higher levels. Use a penicillin G benzathine-penicillin G procaine combination to achieve early peak levels in acute infections

Adult: 0.6-2.4 million units x 1

Children and Infants: 50,000 units/kg/dose x 1 up to a maximum of 2.4 million units/dose

Newborns: 50,000 units/kg x 1

Penicillin G Potassium *see* Penicillin G, Parenteral *on this page*

Penicillin G Potassium, Oral

Brand Names Pentids®

Use Treatment of susceptible bacterial infections including most gram-positive organisms and some gram-negative organisms

Pregnancy Risk Factor B

Usual Dosage Oral:

Adult: 250-500 mg every six hours

Children: 25,000-90,000 units/kg/day in divided doses every 4-6 hours

Penicillin G Procaine and Benzathine Combined *see* Penicillin G Benzathine and Procaine Combined *on previous page*

Penicillin G Procaine, Aqueous

Brand Names Crysticillin® A.S.; Duracillin® A.S.; Pfizerpen®-AS; Wycillin®

Synonyms APPG; Aqueous Procaine Penicillin G; Procaine Benzylpenicillin; Procaine Penicillin G

Use Moderately severe infections due to penicillin G-sensitive microorganisms that are susceptible to low but prolonged serum penicillin concentrations

(Continued)

Penicillin G Procaine, Aqueous *(Continued)*
Pregnancy Risk Factor B
Usual Dosage I.M.:

Adult and Children: > 12 years of age:
Uncomplicated gonorrhea: > 12 years of age: 1 g probenecid, then 30 minutes later 4.8 million units divided into two injection sites
Pneumococcal pneumonia: 300,000-600,000 units daily every 6-12 hours

Adult: 0.3-1.2 million units/24 hours divided 1-2 times a day; doses up to 4.8 million units/24 hours may be used for serious infections

Children: 25,000-50,000 units/kg/24 hours, up to a maximum of 4.8 million until/24 hours, divided 1-2 times a day

Newborn: 50,000 units/kg/24 hours given daily; avoid use in this age group; sterile abscesses and procaine toxicity are of much greater concern than in older patients

Penicillin G Sodium *see* Penicillin G, Parenteral *on previous page*

Penicillin V Potassium
Brand Names Beepen-VK®; Betapen®-VK; Ledercillin® VK; Pen.Vee® K; Robicillin® VK; V-Cillin K®; Veetids®; Wincillin®-VK
Synonyms Phenoxymethyl Penicillin
Use Treatment of moderate to severe susceptible bacterial infections; endocarditis prophylaxis for dental surgery; prophylaxis in rheumatic fever
Pregnancy Risk Factor B
Usual Dosage Oral:

Adult and Children: > 12 years of age:
Systemic infections: 125-500 mg every 6-8 hours
Dental prophylaxis: 2 g 1/2-1 hour prior to procedure, then 500 mg every six hours in eight doses

Children: < 12 years:
Systemic infections: 15-50 mg/kg/day in 3-6 divided doses
Dental prophylaxis: < 30 kg: 1/2 adult dose

Pentaerythritol Tetranitrate *(pen ta er ith' ri tole)*
Brand Names Duotrate®; Peritrate®; Peritrate® SA
Synonyms PETN
Use Prophylactic long-term management of angina pectoris
Pregnancy Risk Factor C
Usual Dosage Adult: Oral: 10-20 mg four times a day up to 40 mg four times daily before or after meals and at bedtime; sustained release preparation 80 mg twice a day

Pentagastrin *(pen ta gas' trin)*
Brand Names Peptavlon®
Use To evaluate gastric acid secretory function in pernicious anemia, gastric carcinoma; in suspected duodenal ulcer or Zollinger-Ellison tumor
Usual Dosage Adult: S.C.: 6 µg/kg

Pentam-300® *see* Pentamidine Isethionate *on this page*

Pentamidine Isethionate (pen tam' i deen)
Brand Names Pentam-300®
Use Treatment and prevention of pneumonia caused by *Pneumocystis carinii*
Pregnancy Risk Factor C
Usual Dosage

Adult:
Treatment: I.M., I.V.: 4 mg/kg/day for 14 days
Prevention: Inhalation: 300 mg every four weeks via Respiragard® II nebulizer

Children: Treatment: I.M., I.V.: 4 mg/kg/day for 14 days

Pentazocine (pen taz' oh seen)
Brand Names Fortal®; Talwin®; Talwin® NX
Synonyms Pentazocine Hydrochloride; Pentazocine Lactate
Use Relief of moderate to severe pain; has also been used as a sedative prior to surgery and as a supplement to surgical anesthesia
Restrictions C-IV
Pregnancy Risk Factor C
Usual Dosage Adult:
Oral: 50-100 mg every 3-4 hours; total oral dose should not exceed 600 mg/day
I.M., S.C.: 30-60 mg every 3-4 hours
I.V.: 30 mg every 3-4 hours

Pentazocine and Aspirin
Brand Names Talwin® Compound
Use Relief of moderate to severe pain; has also been used as a sedative prior to surgery and as a supplement to surgical anesthesia
Pregnancy Risk Factor D
Usual Dosage Adult: Oral: Two tablets 3-4 times daily

Pentazocine Hydrochloride *see* Pentazocine *on this page*

Pentazocine Lactate *see* Pentazocine *on this page*

Penthrane® *see* Methoxyflurane *on page 229*

Pentids® *see* Penicillin G, Parenteral *on page 273*

Pentids® *see* Penicillin G Potassium, Oral *on page 273*

Pentobarbital (pen toe bar' bi tal)
Brand Names Nembutal®
Synonyms Pentobarbital Sodium
Use Short-term treatment of insomnia; preoperative sedation
Restrictions C-II
Pregnancy Risk Factor D

(Continued)

Pentobarbital *(Continued)*
Usual Dosage
Adult:
  Insomnia: Oral: 100-200 mg at bedtime; I.M.: 150-200 mg at bedtime;
    I.V.: 100 mg initially, up to 500 mg; rectal: 120-200 mg at bedtime
  Preoperative sedation: Oral, I.M.: 150-200 mg
Children: Insomnia:
  I.M.: 3-5 mg/kg at bedtime
  Rectal: 12-14 years: 60-120 mg at bedtime; 5-12 years: 60 mg at bed-
    time; 1-4 years: 30-60 mg at bedtime

Pentobarbital Sodium *see* Pentobarbital *on previous page*

Pentothal® Sodium *see* Thiopental Sodium *on page 352*

Pentoxifylline *(pen tox i' fi leen)*
Brand Names Trental®
Synonyms Oxpentifylline
Use Symptomatic management of peripheral vascular disease, mainly in-
termittent claudication
Pregnancy Risk Factor C
Usual Dosage Adult: Oral: 400 mg three times a day

Pentrax® [OTC] *see* Coal Tar *on page 85*

Pen.Vee® K *see* Penicillin V Potassium *on page 274*

Pepcid® *see* Famotidine *on page 144*

Peptavlon® *see* Pentagastrin *on page 274*

Pepto-Bismol® [OTC] *see* Bismuth *on page 45*

Percocet® *see* Oxycodone and Acetaminophen *on page 264*

Percocet® *see* Oxycodone Hydrochloride *on page 264*

Percodan® *see* Oxycodone and Aspirin *on page 264*

Percodan® *see* Oxycodone Hydrochloride *on page 264*

Percodan®-Demi *see* Oxycodone and Aspirin *on page 264*

Percodan®-Demi *see* Oxycodone Hydrochloride *on page 264*

Percogesic® [OTC] *see* Acetaminophen and Phenyltoloxamine
on page 5

Perdiem® Plain [OTC] *see* Psyllium *on page 308*

Pergolide Mesylate *(per' go lide)*
Brand Names Permax®
Use Adjunctive treatment to levodopa/carbidopa in the management of
Parkinson's Disease
Pregnancy Risk Factor B
Usual Dosage Adult: Oral: Start with 0.05 mg/daily for two days, then in-
crease dosage by 0.1 or 0.15 mg/day every three days over next 12
days, increase dose by 0.25 mg/day every three days until optimal thera-
peutic dose is achieved

Pergonal® *see* Menotropins *on page 218*

Periactin® *see* Cyproheptadine Hydrochloride *on page 95*

Peri-Colace® [OTC] *see* Docusate and Casanthranol
on page 121

Peridex® *see* Chlorhexidine Gluconate *on page 70*

Peritrate® *see* Pentaerythritol Tetranitrate *on page 274*

Peritrate® SA *see* Pentaerythritol Tetranitrate *on page 274*

Permapen® *see* Penicillin G Benzathine, Parenteral
on page 272

Permax® *see* Pergolide Mesylate *on previous page*

Permethrin (per meth' rin)
Brand Names Elemite®; Nix™
Use Single application treatment of infestation with *Pediculus humanus*
(head louse) and its nits or *Sarcoptes scabiei* (scabies)
Usual Dosage
Nix™ (head louse): After hair has been washed with shampoo, rinsed
with water and towel dried, apply a sufficient volume to saturate the
hair and scalp. Leave on hair for 10 minutes before rinsing off with
water; remove remaining nits
Elemite® (scabies): Single application topically: Thoroughly massage
into skin from the head to the soles of the feet; wash off after 8-14
hours; infants require scalp application

Perphenazine (per fen' a zeen)
Brand Names Trilafon®
Use Symptomatic management of psychotic disorders, as well as severe
nausea and vomiting
Pregnancy Risk Factor C
Usual Dosage

Adult:
Psychoses: Oral: 4-16 mg 2-4 times daily; I.M.: 5 mg every six hours
Nausea/vomiting: Oral: 8-16 mg/day in divided doses; I.M.: 5-10 mg; I.V.
(severe): 1 mg at 1-2 minute intervals up to a total of 5 mg

Children: > 12 years: Psychoses: Oral: 4-16 mg 2-4 times daily; I.M.: 5 mg
every six hours

Perphenazine and Amitriptyline *see* Amitriptyline and
Perphenazine *on page 20*

Persa-Gel® *see* Benzoyl Peroxide *on page 41*

Persantine® *see* Dipyridamole *on page 119*

Pertofrane® *see* Desipramine Hydrochloride *on page 100*

Pethidine Hydrochloride *see* Meperidine Hydrochloride
on page 218

PETN *see* Pentaerythritol Tetranitrate *on page 274*

Petroleum Jelly *see* White Petrolatum *on page 379*

Pfizerpen® *see* Penicillin G, Parenteral *on page 273*

Pfizerpen® A *see* Ampicillin *on page 23*

Pfizerpen®-AS *see* Penicillin G Procaine, Aqueous
on page 273

PGE₁ *see* Alprostadil *on page 14*

PGE₂ *see* Dinoprostone *on page 117*

PGF₂ₐ *see* Dinoprost Tromethamine *on page 117*

Phazyme® [OTC] *see* Simethicone *on page 324*

Phenantoin *see* Mephenytoin *on page 219*

Phenaphen® #3 *see* Acetaminophen and Codeine
on page 5

Phenazine® *see* Promethazine Hydrochloride *on page 301*

Phenazopyridine Hydrochloride (fen az oh peer' i deen)
Brand Names Azo-Standard®; Geridium®; Phenzodine®; Pyridiate®; Pyridium®; Urodine®
Use Symptomatic relief of urinary burning, itching, frequency and urgency in association with urinary tract infection or following urologic procedures
Pregnancy Risk Factor B
Usual Dosage Oral:

Adult: 200 mg three times a day

Children: 4 mg/kg three times a day

Phencen® *see* Promethazine Hydrochloride *on page 301*

Phenelzine Sulfate (fen' el zeen)
Brand Names Nardil®
Use Symptomatic treatment of atypical, nonendogenous or neurotic depression
Pregnancy Risk Factor C
Usual Dosage Adult: Oral: 15 mg three times a day

Phenergan® *see* Promethazine Hydrochloride *on page 301*

Phenergan® VC *see* Promethazine and Phenylephrine
on page 300

Phenergan® VC With Codeine *see* Promethazine, Phenylephrine and Codeine *on page 301*

Phenergan® with Codeine *see* Promethazine and Codeine
on page 300

Pheniramine and Naphazoline *see* Naphazoline and
Pheniramine *on page 246*

Pheniramine, Phenylpropanolamine and Pyrilamine
Brand Names Triaminic® Oral Infant Drops
Use Symptomatic relief of nasal congestion and postnasal drip as well as allergic rhinitis

Pregnancy Risk Factor C
Usual Dosage

Children: Syrup:
    < 1 year of age: 0.4 mL/kg/dose four times a day
    1-6 years: 2.5 mL/dose every four hours
    6-12 years: 5 mL dose every four hours

Infants: Drops: < 1 year: 0.05 mL/kg/dose four times a day

Phenistix® *see* Diagnostic Test for Phenylketonuria
on page 107

Phenmetrazine Hydrochloride (fen met' ra zeen)
Brand Names Preludin®
Use Short-term adjunct in exogenous obesity
Restrictions C-II
Pregnancy Risk Factor C
Usual Dosage Adult: Oral: 75 mg mid-morning

Phenobarbital (fee noe bar' bi tal)
Brand Names Barbita®; Luminal®; Solfoton®
Synonyms Phenobarbital Sodium; Phenobarbitone; Phenylethylmalony-
lurea
Use Management of grand mal and partial seizures and febrile seizures in
children; also used as a preoperative sedative and other situations when
sedation is needed, and as a hypnotic; may also be used for prevention
and treatment of neonatal hyperbilirubinemia and lowering of bilirubin in
chronic cholestasis
Restrictions C-IV
Pregnancy Risk Factor D
Usual Dosage

Adult:
    Anticonvulsant: Oral: 50-100 mg 2-3 times daily; I.V.: 100-300 mg, re-
    peated as necessary up to 600 mg/day
    Sedation: Oral, I.M.: 30-120 mg/day in 2-3 divided doses
    Hypnotic: Oral: 100-300 mg at bedtime; I.M., I.V., S.C.: 100-325 mg at
    bedtime
    Hyperbilirubinemia: Oral: 30-60 mg three times a day
    Preoperative sedation: I.M.: 130-200 mg 1-1 1/2 hours before proce-
    dure

Children:
    Anticonvulsant: Oral: 3-5 mg/kg/day; I.V.: 10-20 mg kg initially, followed
    by 1-6 mg/kg/day maintenance dose
    Sedation: Oral: 2 mg/kg three times a day
    Hypnotic: I.M., I.V., S.C.: 3-5 mg/kg at bedtime
    Hyperbilirubinemia: Oral, up to 12 years: 1-4 mg/kg three times a day
    Preoperative sedation: Oral, I.M., I.V.: 1-3 mg/kg 1-1 1/2 hours before
    procedure

Phenobarbital Sodium *see* Phenobarbital *on this page*

Phenobarbitone *see* Phenobarbital *on previous page*

Phenolax® [OTC] *see* Phenolphthalein *on this page*

Phenolphthalein (fee nole thay' leen)
Brand Names Alophen Pills® [OTC]; Evac-U-Gen® [OTC]; Evac-U-Lax® [OTC]; Ex-Lax® [OTC]; Feen-A-Mint® [OTC]; Lax-Pills® [OTC]; Medilax® [OTC]; Modane® [OTC]; Modane® Mild [OTC]; Phenolax® [OTC]; Pru-let® [OTC]
Synonyms Phenolphthalein, White; Phenolphthalein, Yellow
Use Stimulant laxative
Pregnancy Risk Factor C
Usual Dosage Adult: Oral: 60-200 mg preferably at bedtime

Phenolphthalein, White *see* Phenolphthalein *on this page*

Phenolphthalein, Yellow *see* Phenolphthalein *on this page*

Phenol Red *see* Phenolsulfonphthalein *on this page*

Phenolsulfonphthalein (fee nole sul fon thay' leen)
Synonyms Phenol Red; PSP
Use Evaluation of renal blood flow to aid in the determination of renal function
Pregnancy Risk Factor C
Usual Dosage I.M. or I.V. 6 mg

Phenoxybenzamine Hydrochloride (fen ox ee ben' za meen)
Brand Names Dibenzyline®
Use Symptomatic management of pheochromocytoma; treatment of hypertensive crisis caused by sympathomimetic amines
Pregnancy Risk Factor C
Usual Dosage Oral:

Adult: 20-40 mg 2-3 times daily

Children: 0.4-1.2 mg/kg/day

Phenoxymethyl Penicillin *see* Penicillin V Potassium
on page 274

Phensuximide (fen sux' i mide)
Brand Names Milontin®
Use Control of absence (petit mal) seizures
Pregnancy Risk Factor D
Usual Dosage Adult and Children: Oral: 0.5-1 g 2-3 times daily

Phentermine Hydrochloride (fen' ter meen)
Brand Names Adipex-P®; Fastin®; Ionamin®
Use Short term adjunct in exogenous obesity
Restrictions C-IV
Pregnancy Risk Factor C
Usual Dosage Adult and Children: Oral: 8 mg three times a day 1/2 hour before meals or food or 15-37.5 mg daily before breakfast

Phentolamine Mesylate (fen tole' a meen)
Brand Names Regitine®

Use Diagnosis of pheochromocytoma, and treatment of hypertension associated with pheochromocytoma or other caused by excess sympathomimetic amines; also used as prevention and treatment of dermal necrosis

Pregnancy Risk Factor C

Usual Dosage

Prevention of necrosis: Add 10 mg to every 1000 mL of fluid containing norepinephrine

Treatment of alpha-adrenergic drug extravasation: S.C.: 0.1-0.2 mg/kg up to 10 mg maximum, infiltrated into area of extravasation within 12 hours

Diagnosis of pheochromocytoma:
Adult: I.M., I.V.: 5 mg
Children: I.M.: 3 mg; I.V.: 3 mg/m^2 or 0.1 mg/kg

Hypertension:
Adult: I.M., I.V.: 5 mg given 1-2 hours before procedure
Children: I.M., I.V.: 1 mg or 0.1 mg/kg or 3 mg/m^2 given 1-2 hours before procedure

Phenylalanine Mustard *see* Melphalan *on page 217*

Phenylbutazone (fen ill byoo' ta zone)
Brand Names Azolid®; Butazolidin®

Use Management of inflammatory disorders, as an analgesic in the treatment of mild to moderate pain and as an antipyretic; I.V. form used as an alternate to surgery in management of patent ductus arteriosus in premature neonates; acute gouty arthritis

Pregnancy Risk Factor C

Usual Dosage Adult: Oral:

Rheumatoid arthritis: 100-200 mg 3-4 times daily until desired effect, then reduce dose to not exceeding 400 mg/day

Acute gouty arthritis: 400 mg initially, 100 mg every four hours until acute attack subsides

Phenylephrine and Chlorpheniramine *see* Chlorpheniramine and Phenylephrine *on page 73*

Phenylephrine and Cyclopentolate *see* Cyclopentolate and Phenylephrine *on page 93*

Phenylephrine and Scopolamine
Brand Names Murocoll-2®

Synonyms Scopolamine and Phenylephrine

Use For mydriasis, cycloplegia and to break posterior synechiae in iritis

Pregnancy Risk Factor C

Usual Dosage 1-2 drops into eye(s); repeat in five minutes

Phenylephrine Hydrochloride (fen ill ef' rin)

Brand Names AK-Dilate® Ophthalmic Solution; AK-Nefrin® Ophthalmic Solution; Alconefrin® Nasal Solution [OTC]; Dilatair® Ophthalmic Solution; Doktors® Nasal Solution [OTC]; I-Phrine® Ophthalmic Solution; Isopto® Frin Ophthalmic Solution; I-White® Ophthalmic Solution; Mydfrin® Ophthalmic Solution; Neo-Synephrine® Nasal Solution [OTC]; Neo-Synephrine® Ophthalmic Solution; Nostril® Nasal Solution [OTC]; Ocugestrin® Ophthalmic Solution; Ocu-Phrin® Ophthalmic Solution; Prefrin™ Ophthalmic Solution; Relief® Ophthalmic Solution; Rhinall® Nasal Solution [OTC]; Sinarest® Nasal Solution [OTC]; St. Joseph® Measured Dose Nasal Solution [OTC]; Vicks Sinex® Nasal Solution [OTC]

Use Treatment of vascular failure in shock; as a vasoconstrictor in regional analgesia; symptomatic relief of nasal and nasopharyngeal mucosal congestion; as a mydriatic in ophthalmic procedures and treatment of wide-angle glaucoma

Pregnancy Risk Factor C

Usual Dosage

Ophthalmic procedures: Adult:

Ophthalmic: One drop of 2.5% or 10% solution, 15-30 minutes prior to desired time of examination

Decongestant: Nasal: 2-3 drops or sprays every four hours of 0.25% or 1% solution

Ophthalmic procedures: Children: Decongestant: Nasal:

6-12 years: 2-3 drops or sprays every four hours of 0.25% solution

< 6 years: 2-3 drops or sprays every four hours of 0.125% solution

Hypotension: Adult:

I.M., S.C.: 2-5 mg/dose every 1-2 hours as needed; the initial dose should not exceed 5 mg

I.V. bolus: 0.1-0.5 mg/dose every 10-15 minutes as needed; the initial dose should not exceed 0.5 mg

I.V. infusion: 1-4 μg/kg/minute; dilute 10 mg to 500 mL (20 μg/mL); then infuse at 2-5 mL/minute; titrate the rate to achieve desired effect

Hypotension: Children:

I.M., S.C.: 0.1 mg/kg/dose every 102 hours as needed

I.V. bolus: 5-20 μg/kg/dose every 10-15 minutes as needed

I.V. infusion: 0.1-0.5 μg/kg/minute; the concentration and rate of infusion can be calculated using the following formulas: Dilute 0.3 mg x weight (kg) to 50 mL or 1.5 mg x weight/kg to 250 mL; then the dose in μg/kg/minute = 0.1 x the infusion rate in mL/hour

Paroxysmal supraventricular tachycardia: I.V.:
Adult: 0.25-0.5 mg/dose over 20-30 seconds
Children: 5-10 μg/kg/dose over 20-30 seconds

Phenylethylmalonylurea *see* Phenobarbital *on page 279*

Phenylisohydantoin *see* Pemoline *on page 271*

Phenylpropanolamine and Brompheniramine *see*
Brompheniramine and Phenylpropanolamine *on page 48*

Phenylpropanolamine and Caramiphen *see* Caramiphen and Phenylpropanolamine *on page 57*

Phenylpropanolamine and Chlorpheniramine *see* Chlorpheniramine and Phenylpropanolamine *on page 73*

Phenylpropanolamine and Guaifenesin *see* Guaifenesin and Phenylpropanolamine *on page 163*

Phenylpropanolamine and Hydrocodone *see* Hydrocodone and Phenylpropanolamine *on page 174*

Phenylpropanolamine Hydrochloride
(fen ill proe pa nole' a meen)

Brand Names Acutrim® Precision Release® [OTC]; Control® [OTC]; Dex-A-Diet® [OTC]; Dexatrim® [OTC]; Maigret-50®; Prolamine® [OTC]; Propadrine; Propagest® [OTC]; Rhindecon®; Stay Trim® Diet Gum [OTC]; Westrim® LA [OTC]

Synonyms *dl*-Norephedrine Hydrochloride; PPA

Use As an oral decongestant and anorexiant; nasal decongestant; appetite control

Pregnancy Risk Factor C

Usual Dosage Oral:

Adult:
Decongestant: 25 mg every 4 hour or 50 mg every 8 hours
Anorexic: 25 mg 3 times daily 30 minutes before meals or 75 mg (timed release) once daily in the morning

Children: Decongestant:
6-12 years: 12.5 mg every 4 hours
2-6 years: 6.25 mg every 4 hours

Phenyltoloxamine, Phenylpropanolamine and Acetaminophen

Brand Names Sinubid®

Use Intermittent symptomatic treatment of nasal congestion in sinus or other frontal headache; allergic rhinitis, vasomotor rhinitis, coryza; facial pain and pressure of acute and chronic sinusitis

Pregnancy Risk Factor C

Usual Dosage Oral:

Adult: One tablet every 12 hours (twice a day)

Children: 6-12 years of age: 1/2 tablet every 12 hours (twice a day)

Phenytoin (fen' i toyn)

Brand Names Dilantin®; Diphenylan Sodium®

Synonyms Diphenylhydantoin; DPH; Phenytoin Sodium, Extended; Phenytoin Sodium, Prompt

Use Treatment and prevention of grand mal and complex partial seizures; arrhythmias associated with digitalis toxicity

Pregnancy Risk Factor D

Usual Dosage

Adult:
Status epilepticus (treatment): I.V.: 150-250 mg stat, 100-150 mg after 30 minutes

(Continued)

Phenytoin *(Continued)*

Anticonvulsant (prevention): Oral: 10-15 mg/kg loading dose, then 300-400 mg/day; maximum dose is 600 mg/day

Antiarrhythmic: Oral: 100 mg 2-4 times daily; I.V.: 100 mg every five minutes until arrhythmia is aborted

Children:

Status epilepticus (treatment): I.V.: 10-15 mg/kg at rate of 0.5-1.5 mg/kg/minute

Anticonvulsant (prevention): Oral: 5 mg/kg loading dose, 4-8 mg/kg/day in divided doses every 8-12 hours

Phenytoin Sodium, Extended *see* Phenytoin *on previous page*

Phenytoin Sodium, Prompt *see* Phenytoin *on previous page*

Phenzodine® *see* Phenazopyridine Hydrochloride *on page 278*

Pheryl-E® [OTC] *see* Vitamin E *on page 378*

pHisoAc BP® [OTC] *see* Benzoyl Peroxide *on page 41*

pHisoHex® *see* Hexachlorophene *on page 168*

pHiso® Scrub *see* Hexachlorophene *on page 168*

Phosphaljel® [OTC] *see* Aluminum Phosphate *on page 15*

Phospholine Iodide® *see* Echothiophate Iodide *on page 126*

Phosphoric Acid, Levulose and Dextrose *see* Levulose, Dextrose and Phosphoric Acid *on page 203*

Phosphorus Replacement Products

Brand Names K-PHOS® Neutral [OTC]; Neutra-Phos® [OTC]; Neutra-Phos®-K [OTC]; Uro-KP-Neutral® [OTC]

Synonyms Potassium Phosphate; Sodium Phosphate

Use Dietary supplements of phosphorus

Usual Dosage Oral:

Adult: 800 mg/day recommended daily allowance

Children:

11-18 years: 1200 mg/day recommended daily allowance

1-10 years: 800 mg/day recommended daily allowance

1/2-1 year: 360 mg/day recommended daily allowance

0-1/2 year: 240 mg/day recommended daily allowance

p-Hydroxyampicillin *see* Amoxicillin *on page 21*

Phyllocontin® *see* Aminophylline *on page 18*

Phylloquinone *see* Phytonadione *on next page*

Physostigmine Salicylate *(fye zoe stig' meen)*

Brand Names Antilirium®; Isopto® Eserine

Synonyms Eserine Salicylate

Use Reverse toxic CNS effects caused by anticholinergic drugs; used as miotic in treatment of glaucoma

Pregnancy Risk Factor C
Usual Dosage

Postoperative reversal of anticholinergic effects: (ie, scopolamine or atropine): Give twice as much (on a weight basis) physostigmine (I.M. or I.V.) as anticholinergic given

Anticholinergic drug overdose:

Adult: I.M., I.V., S.C.: 0.5-2 mg to start; with no response: repeat every 20 minutes until response occurs or cholinergic effects occur; with response: repeat 1-4 mg every 30-60 minutes as life-threatening signs (arrhythmias, seizures, deep coma) recur; maximum I.V. rate: 1 mg/minute

Children (reserve for life-threatening situations only): I.M., I.V.: 0.02 mg/kg; may repeat at 5-10 minute intervals until response occurs, adverse cholinergic effects occur, or a total dose of 2 mg has been received; maximum I.V. rate: 0.5 mg/minute (or 0.01 mg/kg/minute) whichever is slower

Phytomenadione *see* Phytonadione *on this page*

Phytonadione (fye toe na dye' one)
Brand Names AquaMEPHYTON®; Konakion®; Mephyton®
Synonyms Methylphytyl Napthoquinone; Phylloquinone; Phytomenadione; Vitamin K_1
Use Prevention and treatment of hypoprothrombinemia
Pregnancy Risk Factor C/X
Usual Dosage

Neonatal hemorrhagic disease:
Prophylaxis: I.M.: 0.5-1 mg/dose x 1
Treatment: I.M., S.C.: 1-2 mg/dose daily

Oral anticoagulant overdose:
Adult and Children: I.M., S.C.: 5-10 mg/dose
Infant: I.M., S.C.: 1-2 mg/dose every 4-8 hours

Vitamin K deficiency:
Adult: Oral: 5-25 mg/24 hours
Children and Infants: I.V.: 1-2 mg/dose x 1; Oral: 2-5 mg/24 hours

Pilocar® *see* Pilocarpine Hydrochloride *on this page*

Pilocarpine and Epinephrine
Brand Names P_1E_1®; P_2E_1®; P_4E_1®; P_6E_1®
Use Treatment of glaucoma; counter effect of cycloplegics
Pregnancy Risk Factor C
Usual Dosage 1-2 drops up to six times daily

Pilocarpine Hydrochloride (pye loe kar' peen)
Brand Names Adsorbocarpine®; Akarpine®; I-Pilocarpine®; Isopto® Carpine®; Ocu-Carpine®; Ocusert® Pilo; Pilocar®; Pilokair®; Pilopine HS®; Piloptic®; Pilostat®
Use Management of chronic simple glaucoma, chronic and acute angle-closure glaucoma; counter effects of cycloplegics
(Continued)

Pilocarpine Hydrochloride *(Continued)*
Pregnancy Risk Factor C
Usual Dosage
1-2 drops up to six times daily; adjust the concentration and frequency as required to control elevated intraocular pressure
To counteract the mydriatic effects of sympathomimetic agents: 1 drop of a 1% solution in the affected eye

Pilokair® *see Pilocarpine Hydrochloride on previous page*

Pilopine HS® *see Pilocarpine Hydrochloride on previous page*

Piloptic® *see Pilocarpine Hydrochloride on previous page*

Pilostat® *see Pilocarpine Hydrochloride on previous page*

Pima® *see Potassium Iodide on page 291*

Pimaricin *see Natamycin on page 247*

Pimozide (pi' moe zide)
Brand Names Orap™
Use Suppression of severe motor and phonic tics in patients with Tourette's disorder
Pregnancy Risk Factor C
Usual Dosage Adult and Children: > 12 years of age: Initially, 1-2 mg/day, then increase dosage as needed every other day; range is usually 7-16 mg/day, maximum dose is 20 mg/day

Pindolol (pin' doe lole)
Brand Names Visken®
Use Management of hypertension
Pregnancy Risk Factor B
Usual Dosage 5 mg twice daily

PIO *see Pemoline on page 271*

Piperacillin Sodium (pi per' a sill in)
Brand Names Pipracil®
Use Treatment of susceptible bacterial infections including gram-positive and gram-negative and anaerobic strains
Pregnancy Risk Factor B
Usual Dosage Not approved for children < 12 years old; cystic fibrosis patients may require higher doses

Adult:
I.V.: 3-4 g/dose every 4-6 hours
I.M.: 2-3 g/dose every 6-12 hours
Maximum: 24 g/24 hours

Children: 200-300 mg/kg/24 hours divided every 4-6 hours; maximum 24 g/24 hours

Neonate: 100 mg/kg/dose every 12 hours

Piperazine Citrate (pi' per a zeen)
Brand Names Antepar®; Bryrel®
Use Treatment of pinworm and roundworm infections
Pregnancy Risk Factor B

Usual Dosage Oral:

Pinworms: Adult and Children: 65 mg/kg for seven days; severe: repeat course, after a one week interval

Roundworms:
Adult: 3.5 g/day for two days
Children: 75 mg/kg for two days

Piperazine Estrone Sulfate see Estropipate on page 137

Pipobroman (pi poe broe' man)
Brand Names Vercyte®
Use To treat polycythemia vera; chronic myelocytic leukemia
Pregnancy Risk Factor D
Usual Dosage Adult and Children: > 15 years of age: Oral:

Polycythemia: 1 mg/kg/day for 30 days; may increase to 1.5-3 mg/kg until hematocrit reduced to 50-55%, then 0.1 to 0.2 mg/kg daily maintenance

Myelocytic leukemia: 1.5-2.5 mg/kg/day until WBC drops to 10,000 mm^3 then start maintenance 7-175 mg/day; stop if WBC falls below 3000/mm^3 or platelets fall below 150,000/mm^3

Pipracil® see Piperacillin Sodium on previous page

Pirbuterol Acetate (peer byoo' ter ole)
Use Prevention and treatment of reversible bronchospasm
Usual Dosage Two inhalations every 8 hours for prevention; two inhalations at an interval of at least 1-3 minutes, followed by a third inhalation in treatment of bronchospasm

Piroxicam (peer ox' i kam)
Brand Names Feldene®
Use Management of inflammatory disorders; symptomatic treatment of acute and chronic rheumatoid arthritis, osteoarthritis, and ankylosing spondylitis
Pregnancy Risk Factor D
Usual Dosage Adult: Oral: 10-20 mg/day

p-Isobutylhydratropic Acid see Ibuprofen on page 181

Pit see Oxytocin on page 266

Pitocin® see Oxytocin on page 266

Pitressin® see Vasopressin on page 373

Pitressin® Tannate in Oil see Vasopressin on page 373

Pituitary Hormones, Posterior
Brand Names Pituitrin® (5)
Use Induce peristalsis by directly stimulating smooth muscle contraction to relieve postoperative abdominal distention and abdominal radiographic procedures; to control or prevent enuresis in diabetes insipidus
Pregnancy Risk Factor C
Usual Dosage Adult: I.M., S.C.: 10 units (usual range 5-20 units)

Pituitrin® (5) *see* Pituitary Hormones, Posterior *on previous page*

Placidyl® *see* Ethchlorvynol *on page 138*

Plague Vaccine
Use For vaccination of persons at high risk exposure to plaque
Pregnancy Risk Factor C
Usual Dosage Adult: I.M.: Series of 2 injections followed by a third in 3-6 months

Plantago Seed *see* Psyllium *on page 308*

Plantain Seed *see* Psyllium *on page 308*

Plaquenil® *see* Hydroxychloroquine Sulfate *on page 177*

Plasmanate® *see* Plasma Protein Fraction *on this page*

Plasma Protein Fraction
Brand Names Plasmanate®; Plasmatein®; Protemate®
Use Plasma volume expansion and maintenance of cardiac output in the treatment of certain types of shock or impending shock
Pregnancy Risk Factor C
Usual Dosage I.V.: 250-1500 mL/day

Plasmatein® *see* Plasma Protein Fraction *on this page*

Platinol® *see* Cisplatin *on page 80*

Platinol®-AQ *see* Cisplatin *on page 80*

Plicamycin (plye kay mye' sin)
Brand Names Mithracin®
Synonyms Mithramycin
Use Malignant testicular tumors
Pregnancy Risk Factor C
Usual Dosage Adult I.V.: 25-30 μg/kg/day for 8-10 days

Pneumococcal Vaccine, Polyvalent
Brand Names Pneumovax® 23
Use Immunization against diseases caused by pneumococci included in the vaccine
Pregnancy Risk Factor C
Usual Dosage Adult and Children: > 2 years: I.M., S.C.: 0.5 mL

Pneumovax® 23 *see* Pneumococcal Vaccine, Polyvalent *on this page*

Podophyllin and Salicylic Acid
Brand Names Verrex-C&M®
Synonyms Salicylic Acid and Podophyllin
Use Topical treatment of benign growths including external genital and perianal warts, papillomas, fibroids
Usual Dosage Apply daily with applicator, allow to dry; remove necrotic tissue before each application

Podophyllin Resin

Use Topical treatment of benign growths including external genital and perianal warts, papillomas, fibroids

Usual Dosage 10-25% solution in compound benzoin tincture; apply drug to dry surface, use one drop at a time allowing drying between drops until area is covered; total volume should be limited to less than 0.5 mL per treatment session

Polaramine® *see* Dexchlorpheniramine Maleate *on page 103*

Poliomyelitis Vaccine *see* Poliovirus Vaccine, Inactivated *on this page*

Poliovirus Vaccine, Inactivated (poe lee oh vye' russ)

Synonyms IPV; Poliomyelitis Vaccine; Salk

Use Active immunization for the prevention of poliomyelitis

Pregnancy Risk Factor C

Usual Dosage S.C.:

Three doses of 0.5 mL; the first two doses should be administered at an interval of eight weeks; the third dose should be given at least six and preferably 12 months after the second dose

Booster dose: All children who have received the three dose primary series in infancy and early childhood should receive a booster dose of 0.5 mL before entering school. However, if the third dose of the primary series is administered on or after the fourth birthday, a fourth (booster) dose is not required at school entry.

Poliovirus Vaccine, Live, Trivalent

Brand Names Diplovax®; Orimune® Trivalent

Synonyms Sabin; TOPV

Use Poliovirus immunization

Pregnancy Risk Factor C

Usual Dosage Oral:

Adult (adolescents through age 18), and older Children: 2-0.5 mL doses eight weeks apart; third dose of 0.5 mL 6-12 months after second dose; a reinforcing dose of 0.5 mL should be given before entry to school, in children who received the third primary dose before their fourth birthday

Infants: 0.5 mL dose at age two months, four months, and 18 months; optional dose may be given at six months in areas where poliomyelitis is endemic

Polocaine® *see* Mepivacaine Hydrochloride *on page 219*

Polycillin® *see* Ampicillin *on page 23*

Polycitra® *see* Sodium Citrate and Potassium Citrate Mixture *on page 327*

Polycose® [OTC] *see* Nutritional Formula, Enteral/Oral *on page 258*

Polyestradiol Phosphate (pol ee ess tra dye' ole)
Brand Names Estradurin®

Use Palliative treatment of advanced, inoperable carcinoma of the prostate

Usual Dosage Adult: I.M.: 40 mg every 2-4 weeks or less frequently

Polyethylene Glycol-Electrolyte Solution (pol ee eth' i leen)
Brand Names CoLyte®; GoLYTELY®

Use Bowel cleansing prior to colonoscopy and barium enema x-ray examination

Usual Dosage The recommended dose for adults is four liters of solution prior to gastrointestinal examination, as ingestion of this dose produces a satisfactory preparation in over 95% of patients. Ideally the patient should fast for approximately three or four hours prior to administration, but in no case should solid food be given for at least two hours before the solution is given. The solution is usually administered orally, but may be given via nasogastric tube to patients who are unwilling or unable to drink the solution.

Oral administration: At a rate of 240 mL (eight ounces) every 10 minutes, until four liters are consumed or the rectal effluent is clear; rapid drinking of each portion is preferred to drinking small amounts continuously

Nasogastric tube administration: At the rate of 20-30 mL per minute (1.2-1.8 liters per hour); the first bowel movement should occur approximately one hour after the start of administration

Polymox® *see* Amoxicillin *on page 21*

Polymyxin and Neomycin *see* Neomycin and Polymyxin *on page 248*

Polymyxin B and Oxytetracycline *see* Oxytetracycline and Polymyxin B *on page 266*

Polymyxin B Sulfate (pol i mix' in)
Brand Names Aerosporin®

Use Acute systemic or ophthalmic infections caused by susceptible strain of *Pseudomonas aeruginosa*; may also be used for meningitis caused by *P. aeruginosa* or *H. influenzae* when other antibiotics are contraindicated or ineffective

Pregnancy Risk Factor B

Usual Dosage

Continuous I.V. Drip:
 Adult and Children: 15,000-25,000 units/kg/day
 Infants: Up to 40,000 units/kg/day

Intramuscular: not recommended (severe pain):
 Adult and Children: 25,000-30,000 units/kg/day every 4-6 hours
 Infants: Up to 40,000 units/kg/day
 Reduce dose in renal impairment

Intrathecal: (*P. aeruginosa* meningitis):
 Adult and Children: 50,000 units every day for 3-4 days, then 50,000 units once every other day for at least two weeks after CSF cultures are negative and glucose content returned to normal

Children: < 2 years of age: 20,000 units every day for 3-4 days or 25,000 units once every other day for at least two weeks after CSF cultures are negative and glucose content returned to normal

Polymyxin E *see* Colistin Sulfate *on page 88*

Poly-Pred® Liquifilm® *see* Neomycin, Polymyxin and Prednisolone *on page 248*

Polysporin® *see* Bacitracin and Polymyxin B *on page 36*

Polytar® [OTC] *see* Coal Tar *on page 85*

Polytrim® *see* Trimethoprim and Polymyxin B *on page 364*

Pondimin® *see* Fenfluramine Hydrochloride *on page 145*

Ponstel® *see* Mefenamic Acid *on page 216*

Pontocaine® *see* Tetracaine Hydrochloride *on page 346*

Pontocaine® With Dextrose *see* Tetracaine With Dextrose *on page 346*

Pork NPH Iletin® II *see* Insulin, Isophane Suspension *on page 185*

Pork Regular Iletin® II *see* Insulin, Regular *on page 186*

Portagen® [OTC] *see* Nutritional Formula, Enteral/Oral *on page 258*

Potassium Acid Phosphate
Brand Names K-Phos® Modified Formula

Potassium Chloride
Brand Names Kaochlor® S-F; Kato®; K-Dur® 20; K-Lor™; K-Lyte/CL®; Rum-K®; Slow-K®
Use Potassium deficiency, hypopotassemia
Pregnancy Risk Factor A

Potassium Chloride, Sodium Chloride and Dextrose *see* Dextrose and Sodium Chloride with Potassium Chloride *on page 105*

Potassium Gluconate
Brand Names Kaon®
Use Potassium deficiency, hypopotassemia

Potassium Iodide
Brand Names Iosat®; Pima®; Potassium Iodide Enseals®; Thyro-Block®
Synonyms KI; Lugol's Solution; SSKI®; Strong Iodine Solution
Use To facilitate bronchial drainage and cough; to reduce thyroid vascularity prior to thyroidectomy and management of thyrotoxic crisis; block thyroidal uptake of radioactive isotopes of iodine in a radiation emergency
Pregnancy Risk Factor D
(Continued)

Potassium Iodide *(Continued)*

Usual Dosage Oral:

Expectorant:
 Adult: 300-650 mg 3-4 times a day
 Children: 60-250 mg four times a day

Preoperative thyroidectomy:
 Adult and Children: 50-250 mg three times a day (1-5 drops SSKI®); give for 10 days before surgery

Thyrotoxic crisis:
 Adult and Children: 300 mg = six drops SSKI® every 8 hours
 Infants: < 1 year: 1/2 adult dosage

Graves' disease in neonates: 1 drop of Lugol's solution every 8 hours

Potassium Iodide Enseals® *see* Potassium Iodide
 on previous page

Potassium Permanganate

Synonyms $KMnO_4$
Use Disinfectant and oxidizing agent

Potassium Phosphate *see* Phosphorus Replacement Products
 on page 284

Potassium Phosphate and Sodium Phosphate

Brand Names K-Phos® Neutral
Synonyms Sodium Phosphate and Potassium Phosphate
Use Treatment of conditions associated with excessive renal phosphate loss or inadequate GI absorption of phosphate
Usual Dosage

Adult: 100-150 mmol/24 hours in divided doses after meals and at bedtime

Children: 2-3 mmol/kg/24 hours given four times daily

Povidone-Iodine *(poe' vi done)*

Brand Names Betadine® [OTC]; Efodine® [OTC]; Isodine® [OTC]
Use External antiseptic with broad microbicidal spectrum against bacteria, fungi, viruses, protozoa, and yeasts
Usual Dosage Apply as needed for treatment and prevention of susceptible microbicidal infections

PPA *see* Phenylpropanolamine Hydrochloride *on page 283*

PPD *see* Tuberculin *on page 367*

Pralidoxime Chloride *(pra li dox' eem)*

Brand Names Protopam®
Synonyms 2-PAM; 2-Pyridine Aldoxime Methochloride
Use To reverse muscle paralysis with toxic exposure to organophosphate anticholinesterase pesticides and chemicals; control of overdose drugs used to treat myasthenia gravis
Pregnancy Risk Factor C

Usual Dosage I.V.:

Adult:

Overdosage: 1-2 g; Stat: 250 mg every five minutes

Poisoning: 1-2 g

Children: Poisoning: 20-40 mg/kg/dose

Pramosone® *see* Hydrocortisone and Pramoxine *on page 175*

Pramoxine and Hydrocortisone *see* Hydrocortisone and Pramoxine *on page 175*

Pramoxine Hydrochloride (pra mox' een)

Brand Names Prax® [OTC]; Proctofoam® [OTC]; Tronolane® [OTC]

Use For temporary relief of pain and itching associated with anogenital pruritus or irritation; dermatosis, minor burns or hemorrhoids

Pregnancy Risk Factor C

Usual Dosage Apply as directed, usually every 3-4 hours

Prax® [OTC] *see* Pramoxine Hydrochloride *on this page*

Prazepam (pra' ze pam)

Brand Names Centrax®

Use Treatment of anxiety and management of alcohol withdrawal; may also be used as an anticonvulsant in management of simple partial seizures

Restrictions C-IV

Pregnancy Risk Factor D

Usual Dosage Adult: Oral: 30 mg/day in divided doses

Praziquantel (pray zi kwon' tel)

Brand Names Biltricide®; Droncit®

Use Treatment of all stages of schistosomiasis caused by all*Schistosoma* species pathogenic to humans

Pregnancy Risk Factor B

Usual Dosage Adult and Children: > 4 years of age: 20 mg/kg three times a day every 4-6 hours

Prazosin and Polythiazide

Brand Names Minizide®

Use Management of mild to moderate hypertension

Pregnancy Risk Factor C

Usual Dosage Adult: Oral: 1 mg 2-3 times daily; usual maintenance dose is 2-20 mg/day in 2-3 divided doses

Prazosin Hydrochloride (pra' zoe sin)

Brand Names Minipress®

Synonyms Furazosin

Use Management of mild to moderate hypertension; used in conjunction with cardiac glycosides and diuretics for the management of severe congestive heart failure

Pregnancy Risk Factor C

(Continued)

Prazosin Hydrochloride *(Continued)*

Usual Dosage Oral:

Adult: 1 mg 2-3 times daily; usual maintenance dose is 2-20 mg/day in 2-3 divided doses

Children: Initial: 5 µg/kg as a total dose (to assess hypotensive effects); maintenance: 25-150 µg/kg/24 hours divided every 6 hours

Predair® *see Prednisolone on this page*

Predaject® *see Prednisolone on this page*

Predalone T.B.A.® *see Prednisolone on this page*

Predate® S *see Prednisolone on this page*

Predate® TBA *see Prednisolone on this page*

Predcor® *see Prednisolone on this page*

Predcor-TBA® *see Prednisolone on this page*

Pred Forte® *see Prednisolone on this page*

Pred-G® *see Prednisolone and Gentamicin on next page*

Pred Mild® *see Prednisolone on this page*

Prednicen-M® *see Prednisone on next page*

Prednisolone *(pred niss' oh lone)*

Brand Names AK-Pred®; AK-Tate®; Cortalone®; Delta-Cortef®; Econopred®; Econopred® Plus; Hydeltrasol®; Hydeltra-T.B.A.®; Inflamase®; Inflamase® Mild; I-Pred®; Key-Pred®; Key-Pred-SP®; Nor-Pred S®; Nor-Pred T.B.A.®; Ocu-Pred®; Pediapred®; Predair®; Predaject®; Predalone T.B.A.®; Predate® S; Predate® TBA; Predcor®; Predcor-TBA®; Pred Forte®; Pred Mild®; Prelone®

Synonyms Deltahydrocortisone; Metacortandralone; Prednisolone Acetate; Prednisolone Acetate, Ophthalmic; Prednisolone Sodium Phosphate; Prednisolone Sodium Phosphate, Ophthalmic; Prednisolone Tebutate

Use Treatment of palpebral and bulbar conjunctivitis; corneal injury from chemical, radiation, thermal burns, or foreign body penetration; in endocrine disorders, rheumatic disorders, collagen diseases, dermatologic diseases, allergic states, ophthalmic diseases, respiratory diseases, hematologic disorders, neoplastic diseases, edematous states, and gastrointestinal diseases

Pregnancy Risk Factor C

Usual Dosage

Acute asthma: 1-2 mg/kg/24 hours divided 1-2 times/day

Anti-inflammatory or immunosuppressive: 02.-1 mg/kg/24 hours or 6-30 mg/m²/24 hours divided every 6-12 hours

Nephrotic syndrome:

Initial: 2 mg/kg/24 hours (maximum = 80 mg/24 hours) divided 3-4 times/day until urine is protein-free for five days; if urine is not protein-free within 28 days, the dose may be changed to 4 mg/kg/dose (maximum = 120 mg/24 hours); give on alternate days for up to 28 additional days

Maintenance: 2 mg/kg/dose (maximum = 80 mg/dose) every other morning for 28 days; then taper by 10 mg/dose at intervals of 2-3 weeks to 30 mg/dose; then by 5 mg/dose at intervals of 2-3 weeks until discontinued

Prednisolone Acetate *see* Prednisolone *on previous page*

Prednisolone Acetate, Ophthalmic *see* Prednisolone *on previous page*

Prednisolone and Gentamicin
Brand Names Pred-G®
Synonyms Gentamicin and Prednisolone
Use Treatment of steroid responsive inflammatory conditions and superficial ocular infections due to strains of microorganisms susceptible to gentamicin
Pregnancy Risk Factor C
Usual Dosage 1-2 drops in affected eye(s) every 3-4 hours

Prednisolone Sodium Phosphate *see* Prednisolone *on previous page*

Prednisolone Sodium Phosphate, Ophthalmic *see* Prednisolone *on previous page*

Prednisolone Tebutate *see* Prednisolone *on previous page*

Prednisone (pred' ni sone)
Brand Names Cortran®; Deltasone®; Meticorten®; Orasone®; Paracort®; Prednicen-M®; Sterapred®
Synonyms Deltacortisone; Deltadehydrocortisone
Use Management of adrenocortical insufficiency
Pregnancy Risk Factor C
Usual Dosage Dose depends upon condition being treated and response of patient; dosage for infants and children should be based on severity of the disease and response of the patient rather than on strict adherence to dosage indicated by age, weight, or body surface area. Consider alternate day therapy for long term therapy. Discontinuation of long term therapy requires gradual withdrawal by tapering the dose.

Adult: 5-60 mg/day depending upon disease, given in 2-4 divided doses

Children:
  Acute asthma: 1-2 mg/kg/day given 1-2 times a day (transfer to inhaled steroids, while tapering the dose of oral product, as soon as possible)
  Anti-inflammatory or immunosuppressive: 0.14-2 mg/kg/day in four divided doses
  Nephrotic syndrome: Initial dose: 2 mg/kg/day (maximum: 80 mg/day) given 3-4 times/day until urine is protein-free for five days (maximum of 28 days). If urine is not protein-free within 28 days, change dose to 4 mg/kg/day (maximum: 120 mg/day) given with breakfast on alternate days for up to an additional 28 days. Maintenance: 2 mg/kg/dose (maximum: 80 mg/dose) every other day for 28 days; taper dose over 4-6 weeks

Prefrin™ Ophthalmic Solution *see* Phenylephrine Hydrochloride
  on page 282

Pregestimil® [OTC] *see* Nutritional Formula, Enteral/Oral
  on page 258

Pregnenedione *see* Progesterone *on page 299*

Pregnyl® *see* Chorionic Gonadotropin *on page 78*

Prelone® *see* Prednisolone *on page 294*

Preludin® *see* Phenmetrazine Hydrochloride *on page 279*

Premarin® *see* Estrogen, Conjugated *on page 136*

Premarin® With Methyltestosterone *see* Estrogens With
  Methyltestosterone *on page 137*

Pre-Par® *see* Ritodrine Hydrochloride *on page 317*

Pre-Pen® *see* Benzylpenicilloyl-polylysine *on page 42*

Prilosec™ *see* Omeprazole *on page 259*

Primaclone *see* Primidone *on this page*

Primaderm® [OTC] *see* Vitamin A and Vitamin D *on page 377*

Primaquine and Chloroquine *see* Chloroquine and Primaquine
  on page 70

Primaquine Phosphate (prim' a kween)
  Use Provide radical cure of *P. vivax* or *P. ovale* malaria after a clinical at-
    tack has been confirmed by blood smear or serologic titer and postexpo-
    sure prophylaxis
  Pregnancy Risk Factor C
  Usual Dosage Oral:

  Adult: 15 mg (base) every day for 14 days or 45 mg base once weekly for
    8 weeks

  Children: 0.3 mg base/kg/day every day for 14 days not to exceed 15
    mg/day or 0.9 mg base/kg once weekly for 8 weeks not to exceed 45
    mg base per week

Primatene® Mist *see* Epinephrine *on page 131*

Primaxin® *see* Imipenem/Cilastatin *on page 182*

Primidone (pri' mi done)
  Brand Names Mysoline®; Neurosyn®
  Synonyms Desoxyphenobarbital; Primaclone
  Use Management of grand mal, complex partial, and focal seizures
  Pregnancy Risk Factor D
  Usual Dosage Oral:

  Adult and Children: > 8 years of age: Initial dose: 250 mg/day given
    daily; increase by 250 mg/day at one week intervals; maintenance
    dose: 750-1500 mg/day given 3-4 times/day

  Children: < 8 years: Initial dose: 125 mg/day given daily; increase by 125
    mg/day at one week intervals; maintenance dose: 10-20 mg/kg/day
    given 3-4 times/day

Neonate: Loading dose: 15-25 mg/kg/dose x 1; maintenance dose: 12-20 mg/kg/day divided 2-4 times/day

Principen® *see* Ampicillin *on page 23*

Prinivil® *see* Lisinopril *on page 205*

Priscoline® *see* Tolazoline Hydrochloride *on page 357*

Privine® [OTC] *see* Naphazoline Hydrochloride *on page 246*

Probalan® *see* Probenecid *on this page*

Pro-Banthine® *see* Propantheline Bromide *on page 302*

Probenecid (proe ben' e sid)
Brand Names Benemid®; Probalan®
Use Prevention of gouty arthritis; hyperuricemia; prolonged serum levels of penicillin/cephalosporin
Pregnancy Risk Factor B
Usual Dosage Oral:

Adult:
Hyperuricemia with gout: 250 mg twice daily for one week; increase to 500 mg twice daily; may increase by 500 mg/month, if needed, to maximum of 2-3 g/day (dosages may be increased by 500 mg every six months if serum urate concentrations are controlled)
Prolong penicillin serum levels: 500 mg four times a day
Gonorrhea: 1 g 30 minutes before penicillin, ampicillin or amoxicillin

Children:
Prolong penicillin serum levels: 25 mg/kg starting dose, then 40 mg/kg/day given four times/day
Gonorrhea: < 45 kg: 25 mg/kg x 1 (maximum: 1 g/dose) 30 minute before penicillin, ampicillin or amoxicillin

Probenecid and Colchicine *see* Colchicine and Probenecid *on page 87*

Probucol (proe' byoo kole)
Brand Names Lorelco®
Synonyms Biphenabid
Use Adjunct to dietary therapy to decrease elevated serum total and LDL cholesterol concentrations in primary hypercholesterolemia
Pregnancy Risk Factor B
Usual Dosage Adult: Oral: 500 mg twice daily

Procainamide Hydrochloride (proe kane a' mide)
Brand Names Procan® SR; Pronestyl®
Synonyms Procaine Amide Hydrochloride
Use Ventricular arrhythmias, atrial fibrillation or flutter (maintain sinus rhythm after conversion by other methods), prevent recurrence of paroxysmal atrial fibrillation, paroxysmal atrial tachycardia, paroxysmal A-V junctional rhythm, ventricular tachycardia and/or atrial or ventricular premature contractions
(Continued)

Procainamide Hydrochloride *(Continued)*

Pregnancy Risk Factor C

Usual Dosage I.M. is the preferred parenteral route (peak effect in one hour)

Adult (parenteral):

Oral: 15-50 mg/kg/24 hours every 4-8 hours in divided doses; maximum 4 g/24 hours

I.M.: 500-1000 mg every 4-8 hours (100-500 mg I.M. for arrhythmias associated with anesthesia/surgery)

I.V.: Loading dose: 500-600 mg at a constant rate over 25-30 minutes (maximum 1 g, however, unusual to need more than 600 mg)

Maintenance dose: 1-6 mg/minute

Children (parenteral): Consult specialized references

Oral: 250-500 mg/dose every 3-6 hours; usual dose 50 mg/kg/24 hours or 2-4 g/24 hours

I.M.: 20-30 mg/kg/day given every six hours

I.V.: Loading dose: 3-6 mg/kg/dose over five minutes (maximum: 100 mg/dose)

Maintenance dose: 0.02-0.08 mg/kg/minute (maximum 2 g/day)

Procaine Amide Hydrochloride *see* Procainamide Hydrochloride *on previous page*

Procaine Benzylpenicillin *see* Penicillin G Procaine, Aqueous *on page 273*

Procaine Hydrochloride (proe' kane)

Brand Names Durathesia®; Novocain®

Use To produce spinal anesthesia and epidural and peripheral nerve block by injection and infiltration methods

Pregnancy Risk Factor C

Usual Dosage Dose varies with procedure, desired depth, and duration of anesthesia, desired muscle relaxation, vascularity of tissues, physical condition, and age of patient

Procaine Penicillin G *see* Penicillin G Procaine, Aqueous *on page 273*

Procan® SR *see* Procainamide Hydrochloride *on previous page*

Procarbazine Hydrochloride (proe kar' ba zeen)

Brand Names Matulane®

Synonyms Ibenzmethyzin

Use Treatment of Hodgkin's disease

Pregnancy Risk Factor D

Usual Dosage Oral:

Adult: 50-100 mg/m^2/day for 7-14 days as per protocol

Children: 50-100 mg/m^2/day as per protocol

BMT aplastic anemia conditioning regimen: 12.5 mg/kg/dose every other day for 4 doses

Investigational doses: 100-200 mg/m^2/day as per protocol

Procardia® *see* Nifedipine *on page 252*

Prochlorperazine (proe klor per' a zeen)
Brand Names Compazine®
Synonyms Prochlorperazine Edisylate; Prochlorperazine Maleate
Use Management of nausea and vomiting, as well as acute and chronic psychosis
Pregnancy Risk Factor C
Usual Dosage

Adult:
Oral: 5-10 mg 3-4 times daily or 10 mg twice daily sustained release
I.M.: 5-10 mg every 3-4 hours; maximum 40 mg/24 hours
I.V.: 5-10 mg 15-30 minutes before induction of anesthesia for postoperative nausea and vomiting, may repeat one time
Rectal: 25 mg twice daily

Children:
Oral, Rectal: > 10 kg: 0.4 mg/kg/24 hours divided 3-4 times/day
I.M.: > 10 kg: 0.1-0.15 mg/kg in single dose
I.V.: **Do not use by this route**

Prochlorperazine Edisylate *see* Prochlorperazine *on this page*

Prochlorperazine Maleate *see* Prochlorperazine *on this page*

Proctofoam® [OTC] *see* Pramoxine Hydrochloride *on page 293*

Proctofoam®-HC *see* Hydrocortisone and Pramoxine *on page 175*

Procyclidine Hydrochloride (proe sye' kli deen)
Brand Names Kemadrin®
Use Relieve symptoms of Parkinsonian syndrome and drug-induced extrapyramidal symptoms
Pregnancy Risk Factor C
Usual Dosage Adult: Oral: 2-2.5 mg three times a day after meals; if tolerated, gradually increase dose to 4-5 mg three times daily

Profasi® HP *see* Chorionic Gonadotropin *on page 78*

Profenal® *see* Suprofen *on page 340*

Profilate® HP *see* Antihemophilic Factor, Human *on page 26*

Profilnine® Heat-Treated *see* Factor IX Complex (Human) *on page 143*

Progestaject® *see* Progesterone *on this page*

Progesterone (proe jess' ter one)
Brand Names Gesterol®; Progestaject®
Synonyms Pregnenedione; Progestin
Use Endometrial carcinoma or renal carcinoma as well as secondary amenorrhea or abnormal uterine bleeding due to hormonal imbalance
(Continued)

Progesterone *(Continued)*
Pregnancy Risk Factor X
Usual Dosage Adult: I.M.: 5-10 mg/day for 6-8 days

Progestin *see* Progesterone *on previous page*

ProHIBiT® *see Haemophilus* b Conjugate Vaccine *on page 165*

ProHIBiT® *see Haemophilus* b Vaccine *on page 165*

Prolamine® [OTC] *see* Phenylpropanolamine Hydrochloride *on page 283*

Prolifate® SD *see* Antihemophilic Factor, Human *on page 26*

Prolixin® *see* Fluphenazine *on page 152*

Prolixin Decanoate® *see* Fluphenazine *on page 152*

Prolixin Enanthate® *see* Fluphenazine *on page 152*

Proloid® *see* Thyroglobulin *on page 354*

Proloprim® *see* Trimethoprim *on page 364*

Promazine Hydrochloride (proe' ma zeen)
Brand Names Sparine®
Use Treatment of psychoses
Pregnancy Risk Factor C
Usual Dosage Oral, I.M.:

Adult: 10-200 mg every 4-6 hours

Children: > 12 years of age: 10-25 mg every 4-6 hours

Prometh® *see* Promethazine Hydrochloride *on next page*

Promethazine and Codeine
Brand Names Phenergan® with Codeine
Use Temporary relief of coughs and upper respiratory symptoms associated with allergy or the common cold
Restrictions C-V
Pregnancy Risk Factor C
Usual Dosage Oral:

Adult: 5 mL every 4-6 hours up to 30 mL in 24 hours

Children:
6-12 years of age: 2.5-5 mL every 4-6 hours up to 20 mL in 24 hours
2-6 years of age: 1.25-2.5 mL every 4-6 hours up to 10 mL in 24 hours

Promethazine and Phenylephrine
Brand Names Phenergan® VC
Use Temporary relief of upper respiratory symptoms associated with allergy or the common cold
Pregnancy Risk Factor C
Usual Dosage Oral:

Adult: 5 mL every 4-6 hours, not to exceed 30 mL in 24 hours

Children:

6-12 years of age: 2.5-5 mL every 4-6 hours, not to exceed 30 mL in 24 hours

2-6 years: 1.25-2.5 mL every 4-6 hours, not to exceed 30 mL in 24 hours

Promethazine Hydrochloride (proe meth' a zeen)

Brand Names Anergan®; Phenazine®; Phencen®; Phenergan®; Prometh®; Prorex®; V-Gan®

Use Symptomatic treatment of various allergic conditions, antiemetic, motion sickness, and as a sedative

Pregnancy Risk Factor C

Usual Dosage

Adult:

Antihistamine (including allergic reactions to blood or plasma): Oral: 12.5 mg three times/day and 25 mg at bedtime; I.M., I.V., rectal: 25 mg, may repeat in two hours when necessary; switch to oral route as soon as feasible

Motion sickness: Oral, rectal: 25 mg twice a day; initial dose 1/2 to one hour before travel

Nausea/vomiting: Oral, rectal, I.M., I.V.: 12.5-25 mg every 4-6 hours as needed

Preoperative or sedative: Oral, rectal, I.M., I.V.: 25-50 mg/dose

Children:

Antihistamine (including reactions to blood or plasma): Oral: 0.1 mg/kg/dose every six hours during the day nd 0.5 mg/kg/dose at bedtime and as needed

Motion sickness: Oral, rectal: 0.5 mg/kg/dose every 12 hours as needed

Nausea/vomiting: Oral, rectal, I.M., I.V.: 0.25-0.5 mg/kg/dose every 4-6 hours as needed

Preoperative or sedative: Oral, rectal, I.M., I.V.: 0.5-1 mg/kg/dose every six hours as needed

Promethazine, Phenylephrine and Codeine

Brand Names Phenergan® VC With Codeine

Use Temporary relief of coughs and upper respiratory symptoms including nasal congestion

Restrictions C-V

Pregnancy Risk Factor C

Usual Dosage

Adult: 5 mL every 4-6 hours, not to exceed 30 mL in 24 hours

Children:

6-12 years of age: 2.5-5 mL every 4-6 hours, not to exceed 30 mL in 24 hours

< 6 years, weight 40 pounds: 1.25-2.5 mL every 4-6 hours, not to exceed 9 mL in 24 hours

< 6 years, weight 35 pounds: 1.25-2.5 mL every 4-6 hours, not to exceed 8 mL in 24 hours

< 6 years, weight 30 pounds: 1.25-2.5 mL every 4-6 hours, not to exceed 7 mL in 24 hours

< 6 years, weight 25 pounds: 1.25-2.5 mL every 4-6 hours, not to exceed 6 mL in 24 hours

(Continued)

Promethazine, Phenylephrine and Codeine (Continued)

Not recommended for children < 2 years of age

Promethazine With Dextromethorphan

Use Temporary relief of coughs and upper respiratory symptoms associated with allergy or the common cold

Usual Dosage Oral:

Adult: 5 mL every 4-6 hours up to 30 mL in 24 hours

Children:
6-12 years: 2.5-5 mL every 4-6 hours up to 20 mL in 24 hours
2-6 years: 1.25-2.5 mL every 4-6 hours up to 10 mL in 24 hours

Promit® see Dextran 1 on page 104

Pronestyl® see Procainamide Hydrochloride on page 297

Propac® [OTC] see Nutritional Formula, Enteral/Oral on page 258

Propacet® see Propoxyphene and Acetaminophen on page 304

Propadrine see Phenylpropanolamine Hydrochloride on page 283

Propagest® [OTC] see Phenylpropanolamine Hydrochloride on page 283

Propantheline Bromide (proe pan' the leen)

Brand Names Pro-Banthine®

Use Adjunctive treatment of peptic ulcer, irritable bowel syndrome, pancreatitis, ureteral and urinary bladder spasm; to reduce duodenal motility during diagnostic radiologic procedures

Pregnancy Risk Factor C

Usual Dosage Oral:

Elderly patients: 7.5 mg three times a day before meals or food

Adult: 15 mg three times a day before meals or food and 30 mg at bedtime, up to 60 mg three times a day

Children: 2-3 mg/kg/day in divided doses every 4-6 hours and at bedtime

Proparacaine Hydrochloride (proe par' a kane)

Brand Names Alcaine®; Ophthaine®; Ophthetic®

Synonyms Proxymetacaine

Use Anesthesia for tonometry, gonioscopy; suture removal from cornea; removal of corneal foreign body; cataract extraction, glaucoma surgery

Pregnancy Risk Factor C

Usual Dosage

Tonometry, gonioscopy, suture removal: Adult: 1-2 drops 0.5% solution in eye just prior to procedure

Ophthalmic surgery: Adult and Children: 1 drop of 0.5% solution in eye every 5-10 minutes for 5-7 doses

Proparacaine With Fluorescein

Brand Names Fluoracaine®

Use Anesthesia for tonometry, gonioscopy; suture removal from cornea; removal of corneal foreign body; cataract extraction, glaucoma surgery

Pregnancy Risk Factor C

Usual Dosage

Tonometry, gonioscopy, suture removal: Adult: 1-2 drops 0.5% solution in eye just prior to procedure

Ophthalmic surgery: Adult and Children: One drop of 0.5% solution in eye every 5-10 minutes for 5-7 doses

Propine® *see* Dipivefrin *on page 119*

Proplex® SX-T *see* Factor IX Complex (Human) *on page 143*

Proplex® T *see* Factor IX Complex (Human) *on page 143*

Propofol (proe' po fole)

Brand Names Diprivan®

Use Induction or maintenance of anesthesia for inpatient or outpatient surgery

Pregnancy Risk Factor B

Usual Dosage Dosage must be individualized and titrated to the desired clinical effect; however, as a general guideline:

Induction:

Adults up to 55 years of age, and or ASA I or II patients: I.V.: 2.0-2.5 mg/kg of body weight (approximately 40 mg every 10 seconds until onset of induction)

Elderly, debilitated, hypovolemic, and/or ASA III or IV patients: I.V.: 1.0-1.5 mg/kg of body weight (approximately 20 mg every 10 seconds until onset of induction)

Maintenance: I.V. infusion:

Adults up to 55 years of age, and/or ASA I or II patients: 0.1-0.2 mg/kg of body weight per minute (6-12 mg per kg of body weight per hour)

Elderly, debilitated, hypovolemic, and/or ASA III or IV patients: 0.05-0.1 mg/kg of body weight per minute (3-6 mg per kg of body weight per hour)

I.V. intermittent: 25-50 mg increments, as needed

No pediatric dose has been established

Propoxyphene (proe pox' i kane)

Brand Names Darvon®; Darvon-N®

Synonyms Dextropropoxyphene; Propoxyphene Hydrochloride; Propoxyphene Napsylate

Use Management of mild to moderate pain

Restrictions C-IV

Pregnancy Risk Factor C

Usual Dosage 1-2 capsules or tablets every four hours as needed

Propoxyphene and Acetaminophen

Brand Names Darvocet-N®; Darvocet-N® 100; Dolene® AP-65; Genagesic®; Propacet®; Wygesic®

Synonyms Propoxyphene Hydrochloride and Acetaminophen; Propoxyphene Napsylate and Acetaminophen

Use Management of mild to moderate pain

Restrictions C-IV

Pregnancy Risk Factor C

Usual Dosage One tablet every four hours as needed

Propoxyphene and Aspirin

Brand Names Darvon® Compound-65 Pulvules®; Darvon® Compound Pulvules®; Darvon-N® With A.S.A.®; Darvon® With A.S.A.® Pulvules®

Synonyms Propoxyphene Hydrochloride and Aspirin; Propoxyphene Napsylate and Aspirin

Use Management of mild to moderate pain

Restrictions C-IV

Pregnancy Risk Factor D

Usual Dosage 1-2 capsules every four hours as needed

Propoxyphene Hydrochloride *see* Propoxyphene *on previous page*

Propoxyphene Hydrochloride and Acetaminophen *see* Propoxyphene and Acetaminophen *on this page*

Propoxyphene Hydrochloride and Aspirin *see* Propoxyphene and Aspirin *on this page*

Propoxyphene Napsylate *see* Propoxyphene *on previous page*

Propoxyphene Napsylate and Acetaminophen *see* Propoxyphene and Acetaminophen *on this page*

Propoxyphene Napsylate and Aspirin *see* Propoxyphene and Aspirin *on this page*

Propranolol and Hydrochlorothiazide

Brand Names Inderide®

Use Management of hypertension, angina pectoris, pheochromocytoma, and arrhythmias; prevention of myocardial infarction, migraine headache; symptomatic treatment of hypertrophic subaortic stenosis

Pregnancy Risk Factor C

Usual Dosage Dose is individualized

Propranolol Hydrochloride (proe pran' oh lole)

Brand Names Betachron®; Inderal®; Inderal® LA

Use Management of hypertension, angina pectoris, pheochromocytoma, and arrhythmias. Prevention of myocardial infarction, migraine headache; symptomatic treatment of hypertrophic subaortic stenosis

Pregnancy Risk Factor C

Usual Dosage

Adult and Adolescent: Thyrotoxicosis: Oral: 10-40 mg every six hours; I.V.: 1-3 mg/dose one (1) time over 10 minutes

Adult:

Hypertension: Oral: Initial: 10 mg/dose four times/day; Maintenance: 160-480 mg/day in 2-3 divided doses

Angina: Oral: Initial: 10-20 mg 3-4 times daily; Maintenance: 160-240 mg/day

Pheochromocytoma: Oral: 30-60 mg/day in 2-4 divided doses

Tachyarrhythmias: Oral: 30-120 mg/24 hours, 3-4 times daily; I.V.: 0.5-3 mg; may repeat in two minutes, then use every four hours

Myocardial infarction prophylaxis: Oral: 180-240 mg/day in 2-4 divided doses

Migraine prophylaxis: Oral: 160-240 mg/day

Hypertrophic subaortic stenosis: Oral: 20-40 mg 3-4 times daily

Children:

Arrhythmias: Oral: 0.5-4 mg/kg/24 hours divided every 6-8 hours, maximum: 60 mg/24 hours; I.V.: 0.01-0.1 mg/kg/dose, maximum: 1 mg/dose

Hypertension: Oral: Initial: 0.5-1 mg/kg/24 hours divided every 6-12 hours; increase slowly at 3-5 day intervals, to a maximum of 2 mg/kg/24 hours

Thyrotoxicosis: Neonatal: Oral: 2 mg/kg/24 hours divided every 6 hours

Propylene Glycol (proe' pi leen)
Brand Names Sirlene®
Use Solvent, extractant, preservative, and demulcent

Propylene Glycol and Salicylic Acid see Salicylic Acid and Propylene Glycol on page 320

Propyliodone (proe pill eye' oh done)
Brand Names Dionosil Oily®
Use Contrast medium for bronchography

2-Propylpentanoic Acid see Valproic Acid and Derivatives on page 371

Propylthiouracil (proe pill thye oh yoor' a sill)
Synonyms PTU
Use Treatment of hyperthyroidism
Pregnancy Risk Factor D
Usual Dosage Oral:

Adult: Initial: 300-450 mg/day in divided doses every 8 hours; maintenance: 100-150 mg/day in divided doses every 8-12 hours

Children: Initial: 5-7 mg/kg/day in divided doses every 8 hours or
6-10 years: 50-150 mg/day
> 10 years: 150-300 mg/day
Maintenance: 1/3 - 2/3 of the initial dose

Neonates: 5-10 mg/kg/day in divided doses every 8 hours

2-Propylvaleric Acid see Valproic Acid and Derivatives on page 371

Prorex® *see* Promethazine Hydrochloride *on page 301*

Prostaglandin E₁ *see* Alprostadil *on page 14*

Prostaglandin E₂ *see* Dinoprostone *on page 117*

Prostaglandin F₂ Alpha *see* Dinoprost Tromethamine *on page 117*

Prostaphlin® *see* Oxacillin Sodium *on page 262*

Prostigmin® *see* Neostigmine *on page 249*

Prostin E₂® *see* Dinoprostone *on page 117*

Prostin F₂ Alpha® *see* Dinoprost Tromethamine *on page 117*

Prostin VR Pediatric® *see* Alprostadil *on page 14*

Protamine Sulfate (proe' ta meen)
  Use Treatment of heparin overdosage
  Pregnancy Risk Factor C
  Usual Dosage 1 mg of protamine neutralizers, 90 USP units of heparin (lung), and 115 USP units of heparin (intestinal)

Protamine, Zinc and Iletin®I *see* Insulin, Protamine Zinc Suspension *on page 186*

Protamine, Zinc and Iletin® II (Beef) *see* Insulin, Protamine Zinc Suspension *on page 186*

Protamine, Zinc and Iletin® II (Pork) *see* Insulin, Protamine Zinc Suspension *on page 186*

Protemate® *see* Plasma Protein Fraction *on page 288*

Protilase® *see* Pancrelipase *on page 267*

Protirelin (proe tye' re lin)
  Brand Names Thypinone®
  Synonyms Lopremone
  Use Adjunct in the diagnostic assessment of thyroid function; an adjunct may yield useful information in patients with pituitary or hypothalamic dysfunction
  Usual Dosage I.V.:

  Adult: 500 μg (range 200-500 μg)

  Children: 6-16 years of age: 7 μg/kg up to 500 μ/g

  Infants and Children: < 6 years of age: Experience limited, but doses of 7 μg/kg have been administered

Protopam® *see* Pralidoxime Chloride *on page 292*

Protostat® *see* Metronidazole *on page 234*

Protriptyline Hydrochloride (proe trip' ti leen)
  Brand Names Vivactil®
  Use Treatment of various forms of depression, often in conjunction with psychotherapy

Pregnancy Risk Factor C
Usual Dosage Oral:

Adult: 15-60 mg in 3-4 divided doses

Adolescent and Elderly: 15-20 mg/day

Protropin® *see* Somatrem-Human Growth Hormone
on page 331

Proventil® *see* Albuterol *on page 10*

Provera® *see* Medroxyprogesterone Acetate *on page 216*

Provocholine® *see* Methacholine Chloride *on page 224*

Proxymetacaine *see* Proparacaine Hydrochloride *on page 302*

Prozac® *see* Fluoxetine Hydrochloride *on page 151*

PRP-D *see* Haemophilus b Vaccine *on page 165*

Prulet® [OTC] *see* Phenolphthalein *on page 280*

Pseudoephedrine (soo doe e fed' rin)
Brand Names Afrinol® [OTC]; Cenafed® Syrup [OTC]; Decofed® Syrup [OTC]; Neofed® [OTC]; Novafed®; Sudafed® [OTC]; Sudafed® 12 Hour [OTC]; Sudafed® Tablet [OTC]; Sufedrin® [OTC]
Synonyms *d*-Isoephedrine Hydrochloride; Pseudoephedrine Hydrochloride; Pseudoephedrine Sulfate
Use Temporary symptomatic relief of nasal congestion due to common cold, upper respiratory allergies, and sinusitis; also promotes nasal or sinus drainage
Pregnancy Risk Factor B
Usual Dosage Oral:

Adult: 30-60 mg every 4-6 hours; maximum 240 mg/24 hours

Children:
2-5 years: 15 mg every six hours; maximum 60 mg/24 hours
6-12 years: 30 mg every six hours; maximum 120 mg/24 hours or 4 mg/kg/24 hours divided four times/day

Pseudoephedrine and Azatadine *see* Azatadine and
Pseudoephedrine *on page 34*

Pseudoephedrine and Carbinoxamine *see* Carbinoxamine and
Pseudoephedrine *on page 59*

Pseudoephedrine and Chlorpheniramine *see* Chlorpheniramine
and Pseudoephedrine *on page 74*

Pseudoephedrine and Dexbrompheniramine *see*
Dexbrompheniramine and Pseudoephedrine *on page 103*

Pseudoephedrine and Guaifenesin *see* Guaifenesin and
Pseudoephedrine *on page 163*

Pseudoephedrine and Triprolidine *see* Triprolidine and
Pseudoephedrine *on page 365*

Pseudoephedrine Hydrochloride see Pseudoephedrine
on previous page

Pseudoephedrine Sulfate see Pseudoephedrine *on previous page*

Pseudomonic Acid A see Mupirocin *on page 242*

PSP see Phenolsulfonphthalein *on page 280*

Psyllium (sill' i yum)
Brand Names Effer-Syllium® [OTC]; Hydrocil® [OTC]; Konsyl® [OTC]; Konsyl-D® [OTC]; Metamucil® [OTC]; Metamucil® Instant Mix [OTC]; Modane® Bulk [OTC]; Naturacil® [OTC]; Perdiem® Plain [OTC]; Reguloid® [OTC]; Serutan® [OTC]; Siblin® [OTC]; Syllact® [OTC]; V-Lax® [OTC]
Synonyms Plantago Seed; Plantain Seed; Psyllium Hydrophilic Mucilloid
Use Treatment of chronic atonic or spastic constipation and in constipation associated with rectal disorders; manage irritable bowel syndrome
Pregnancy Risk Factor C
Usual Dosage
> Adult (Perdiem®): 1-2 rounded teaspoonfuls in the evening and/or before breakfast

> Adult (Metamucil®): 1-2 rounded teaspoonfuls or one packet in full (8 ounce) glass of liquid 2-3 times a day

> Children: > 6 years of age: One (1) level teaspoonful in 4 ounces of liquid at bedtime

Psyllium Hydrophilic Mucilloid see Psyllium *on this page*

P.T.E.-4® see Trace Metals *on page 358*

P.T.E.-5® see Trace Metals *on page 358*

Pteroylglutamic Acid see Folic Acid *on page 153*

PTU see Propylthiouracil *on page 305*

Purge® [OTC] see Castor Oil *on page 61*

Purified Protein Derivative see Tuberculin *on page 367*

Purinethol® see Mercaptopurine *on page 220*

Purodigin® see Digitoxin *on page 113*

Pyopen® see Carbenicillin *on page 58*

Pyrantel Pamoate (pi ran' tel)
Brand Names Antiminth®; Reese's® Pinworm Medicine [OTC]
Use Roundworm and pinworm infestations
Pregnancy Risk Factor C
Usual Dosage Oral: Adult and Children: 11 mg/kg (5 mg/lb) body weight administered in a single dose; maximum dose is 1 g; pinworm dosage should be repeated in two weeks; treat all family members

Pyrazinamide (peer a zin' a mide)
Synonyms Pyrazinoic Acid Amide
Use Adjunctive treatment of tuberculosis when primary and secondary agents cannot be used or have failed

Pregnancy Risk Factor C
Usual Dosage Adult: Oral: 20-35 mg/kg/day in 3-4 divided doses up to 3 g/day maximum daily dose

Pyrazinoic Acid Amide *see* Pyrazinamide *on previous page*

Pyrethrins (peer' e thrins)
Brand Names A-200™ Pyrinate [OTC]; RID® [OTC]; Tisit® [OTC]
Use Treatment of *Pediculus humanus* infestations
Pregnancy Risk Factor C
Usual Dosage

Application of pyrethins:
    Apply enough solution to completely wet infested area, including hair
    Allow to remain on area for 10 minutes
    Wash and rinse with large amounts of warm water
    Use fine-toothed comb to remove lice and eggs from hair
    Shampoo hair to restore body and luster
    Treatment may be repeated if necessary once in a 24-hours period
    Repeat treatment in 7-10 days to kill newly hatched lice

Pyribenzamine® *see* Tripelennamine *on page 365*

Pyridiate® *see* Phenazopyridine Hydrochloride *on page 278*

2-Pyridine Aldoxime Methochloride *see* Pralidoxime Chloride *on page 292*

Pyridium® *see* Phenazopyridine Hydrochloride *on page 278*

Pyridostigmine Bromide (peer id oh stig' meen)
Brand Names Mestinon®; Regonol®
Use Symptomatic treatment of myasthenia gravis; also used as an antidote for nondepolarizing neuromuscular blockers
Pregnancy Risk Factor C
Usual Dosage

Adult:
    Myasthenia gravis: Oral: 60-180 mg 2-4 times daily; I.M., I.V.: 2 mg every 2-3 hours
    Antidote for nondepolarizing neuromuscular blockers: I.V.: 10-20 mg

Children: Myasthenia gravis: Oral: 7 mg/kg/day in 5-6 divided doses

Pyridoxine Hydrochloride (peer i dox' een)
Brand Names Beesix®; Hexa-Betalin®; Rodex®
Synonyms Vitamin B_6
Use Prevent and treat vitamin B_6 deficiency
Pregnancy Risk Factor A/C
Usual Dosage Adult:

Dietary deficiency: Oral: 10-20 mg every day for three weeks

Pyridoxine-dependent infants:
    Oral: 2-100 mg every day
    I.M., I.V.: 50-100 mg
(Continued)

Pyridoxine Hydrochloride *(Continued)*

Drug-induced neuritis:
    Prophylaxis: 2 mg/kg/24 hours
    Treatment: 10-50 mg/24 hours

Pyrimethamine (peer i meth' a meen)

Brand Names Daraprim®

Use Prophylaxis of malaria due to susceptible strains of plasmodia; conjointly with fast-acting schizonticide to initiate transmission control and suppression cure; synergistic combination with sulfonamide in treatment of toxoplasmosis

Pregnancy Risk Factor C

Usual Dosage Oral:

Malaria chemoprophylaxis:
    Adult and Children: 7-10 years: 25 mg once weekly or 0.5 mg/kg once weekly to maximum of 25 mg
    Children: 4-10 years of age: 12.5 mg once weekly; < 4 years of age: 6.25 mg once weekly
    Dosage should be continued for all age groups for at least 10 weeks after leaving endemic areas

Toxoplasmosis:
    Adult: 50-75 mg daily together with 1-4 g of a sulfonamide for 1-3 weeks depending on patients tolerance and response
    Children: 1 mg/kg/day divided into two equal daily doses; decrease dose after 2-4 days by 1/2, continue for about one month; used with 100 mg sulfadiazine kg/day divided every six hours

Pyrithione Zinc (peer i thye' one)

Brand Names Zincon® Shampoo [OTC]

Use Relieves the itching, irritation and scalp flaking associated with dandruff and/or seborrheal dermatitis of the scalp

Usual Dosage Shampoo hair twice weekly, wet hair, apply to scalp and massage vigorously, rinse and repeat

PZI *see* Insulin, Protamine Zinc Suspension *on page 186*

Quazepam (kwa' ze pam)

Brand Names Dormalin®

Use Treatment of insomnia

Restrictions C-IV

Pregnancy Risk Factor C

Usual Dosage Adult: Oral: 15-30 mg at bedtime

Quelicin® *see* Succinylcholine Chloride *on page 334*

Quemid® *see* Cholestyramine Resin *on page 78*

Questran® *see* Cholestyramine Resin *on page 78*

Quibron®-T *see* Theophylline *on page 348*

Quibron®-T/SR *see* Theophylline *on page 348*

Quiess® *see* Hydroxyzine *on page 178*

Quinacrine Hydrochloride (kwin' a kreen)

Brand Names Atabrine®

Synonyms Mepacrine Hydrochloride

Use Treatment of giardiasis and cestodiasis (tapeworm); suppression and chemoprophylaxis of malaria

Pregnancy Risk Factor C

Usual Dosage Oral:

Adult:

Dwarf tapeworm: 900 mg in three portions 20 minutes apart, then 100 mg three times a day for three days

Tapeworm (beef, pork, or fish): 200 mg every 10 minutes for four doses

Giardiasis: 100 mg three times/day for 5-7 days

Children:

Dwarf tapeworm: 4-8 years: 200 mg stat, 100 mg before breakfast for three days; 8-10 years: 300 mg stat, 100 mg twice daily for three days; 11-14 years: 400 mg stat, 100 mg three times a day for three days

Tapeworm (beef, pork, or fish): 5-10 years: 100 mg every 10 minutes for four doses; 11-14 years: 200 mg every 10 minutes for three doses

Giardiasis: 6 mg/kg/day in three divided doses for 5-7 days

Quinaglute® Dura-Tabs® *see* Quinidine *on this page*

Quinalan® *see* Quinidine *on this page*

Quinalbarbitone Sodium *see* Secobarbital Sodium *on page 321*

Quin-Amino® *see* Quinine Sulfate *on next page*

Quinaminoph® *see* Quinine Sulfate *on next page*

Quinamm® *see* Quinine Sulfate *on next page*

Quinatime® *see* Quinidine *on this page*

Quindan® *see* Quinine Sulfate *on next page*

Quine® [OTC] *see* Quinine Sulfate *on next page*

Quinestrol (kwin ess' trole)

Brand Names Estrovis®

Use Atrophic vaginitis; hypogonadism; primary ovarian failure; vasomotor symptoms of menopause; prostatic carcinoma; osteoporosis prophylactic

Pregnancy Risk Factor X

Usual Dosage Adult: Oral: 100 μg once daily for seven days; followed by 100 μg weekly beginning two weeks after inception of treatment; may increase to 200 μg/week if necessary

Quinidex® Extentabs® *see* Quinidine *on this page*

Quinidine (kwin' i deen)

Brand Names Cardioquin®; Cin-Quin®; Duraquin®; Quinaglute® Dura-Tabs®; Quinalan®; Quinatime®; Quinidex® Extentabs®; Quinora®

Synonyms Quinidine Gluconate; Quinidine Polygalacturonate; Quinidine Sulfate

(Continued)

Quinidine *(Continued)*

Use Prophylaxis after cardioversion of atrial fibrillation and/or flutter to maintain normal sinus rhythm. The drug is also used to prevent reoccurrence of paroxysmal atrial fibrillation, paroxysmal atrial tachycardia, paroxysmal A-V junctional rhythm, paroxysmal ventricular tachycardia, and atrial or ventricular premature contractions; also effective in the treatment of *Plasmodium falciparum* malaria

Pregnancy Risk Factor C

Usual Dosage Note: Dosage expressed in terms of the salt: approximately 267 mg of quinidine gluconate or 275 mg of quinidine polygalacturonate is equivalent to 200 mg of quinidine sulfate

Adult: Test dose: 200 mg administered several hours before full dosage (to determine possible idiosyncrasy)
Oral (sulfate or gluconate): 100-600 mg/dose every 4-6 hours; begin at 200 mg/dose and titrate to desired effect
I.M. (gluconate): 400 mg/dose every 4-6 hours
I.V. (gluconate): 200-400 mg/dose

Children: Test dose: 2 mg/kg or 60 mg/m^2
Oral (quinidine sulfate): 30 mg/kg/24 hours or 900 mg/m^2/24 hours in five divided doses or 6 mg/kg every 2-4 hours, 3-5 times daily
I.V. (quinidine gluconate): 2-10 mg/kg/dose every 3-6 hours as needed (**not** recommended)

Quinidine Gluconate *see* Quinidine *on previous page*

Quinidine Polygalacturonate *see* Quinidine *on previous page*

Quinidine Sulfate *see* Quinidine *on previous page*

Quinine Sulfate *(kwye' nine)*

Brand Names Legatrin® [OTC]; Quin-Amino®; Quinaminoph®; Quinamm®; Quindan®; Quine® [OTC]; Quiphile®

Use Suppression or prophylaxis of malaria; prevention and treatment of recumbency leg muscle cramps

Pregnancy Risk Factor X

Usual Dosage Oral:

Adult:
Malaria: 650 mg every eight hours for 10-14 days
Leg cramps: 260-300 mg at bedtime

Children:
Malaria: 25 mg/kg/day in divided doses every eight hours for 10-14 days
Babesia: 25 mg/kg/24 hours, up to a maximum of 650 mg/dose, three times a day for seven days

Quinora® *see* Quinidine *on previous page*

Quinsana® Plus [OTC] *see* Zinc Undecylenate *on page 382*

Quiphile® *see* Quinine Sulfate *on this page*

Rabies Immune Globulin, Human (ray' beez)

Brand Names Hyperab®

Synonyms RIG

Use Passive immunity to rabies for postexposure prophylaxis of individuals exposed to the virus

Pregnancy Risk Factor C

Usual Dosage Adult and Children: I.M.: 20 IU/kg in a single dose (RIG should always be administered in conjunction with rabies vaccine (HDCV)) (Infiltrate 1/2 of the dose locally around the wound; give the remainder I.M.)

Rabies Virus Vaccine, Human Diploid

Brand Names Imovax®

Synonyms HDCV

Use Pre-exposure rabies immunization for high risk persons; postexposure antirabies immunization along with local treatment and immune globulin

Pregnancy Risk Factor C

Usual Dosage I.M.:

Pre-exposure: 1 mL on days 0, 7, 21, or 28; booster doses given every 2 years after initial immunization

Postexposure: 1 mL on days 0, 3, 7, 14, and 28 with rabies immune globulin on day 0

Racemic Amphetamine Sulfate *see* Amphetamine Sulfate *on page 22*

Racemic Epinephrine *see* Epinephrine *on page 131*

Ranitidine Hydrochloride (ra nye' te deen)

Brand Names Zantac®

Use Short-term treatment of active duodenal ulcers and benign gastric ulcers; long-term prophylaxis of duodenal ulcer and gastric hypersecretory states

Pregnancy Risk Factor B

Usual Dosage

Adult:

Short-term management of ulcers: Oral: 150 mg twice daily or 300 mg at bedtime; I.M., I.V.: 50 mg every 6-8 hours

Gastric hypersecretory conditions: Oral: 150 mg twice daily, up to 6 g/day

Children: 2-18 years of age:

Oral: 1.25-2 mg/kg/dose every 12 hours

I.V.: 0.1-0.8 mg/kg/dose every 6-8 hours

RapidTest® Strep *see* Diagnostic Test for Streptococci *on page 108*

Rea-Lo® [OTC] *see* Urea *on page 369*

Recombivax HB® *see* Hepatitis B Vaccine *on page 168*

Redisol® *see* Cyanocobalamin *on page 92*

Reese's® Pinworm Medicine [OTC] *see* Pyrantel Pamoate *on page 308*

Refined Wool Fat *see* Lanolin *on page 199*

Regitine® *see* Phentolamine Mesylate *on page 281*

Reglan® *see* Metoclopramide *on page 233*

Regonol® *see* Pyridostigmine Bromide *on page 309*

Regular Iletin® I *see* Insulin, Regular *on page 186*

Regular Purified Pork *see* Insulin, Regular *on page 186*

Reguloid® [OTC] *see* Psyllium *on page 308*

Rela® *see* Carisoprodol *on page 61*

Relief® Ophthalmic Solution *see* Phenylephrine Hydrochloride *on page 282*

Renacidin® *see* Citric Acid Bladder Mixture *on page 80*

Renografin® *see* Diatrizoate Meglumine and Diatrizoate Sodium *on page 109*

Renografin®-60 *see* Sodium Diatrizoate and Meglumine Diatrizoate *on page 328*

Renografin®-76 *see* Sodium Diatrizoate and Meglumine Diatrizoate *on page 328*

Renoquid® *see* Sulfacytine *on page 336*

Reserpine (re ser' peen)
Brand Names Serpalan®; Serpasil®
Use Management of mild to moderate hypertension
Pregnancy Risk Factor C
Usual Dosage Adult: Oral: 0.1-0.5 mg/day in 1-2 doses

Reserpine and Chlorothiazide *see* Chlorothiazide and Reserpine *on page 72*

Reserpine and Hydrochlorothiazide *see* Hydrochlorothiazide and Reserpine *on page 172*

Respbid® *see* Theophylline *on page 348*

Respiralex® *see* Diagnostic Test for Streptococci *on page 108*

Respirastick® *see* Diagnostic Test for Streptococci *on page 108*

Restoril® *see* Temazepam *on page 342*

Retin-A™ *see* Tretinoin *on page 359*

Retinoic Acid *see* Tretinoin *on page 359*

Retrovir® *see* Zidovudine *on page 381*

Reversol® *see* Edrophonium Chloride *on page 128*

R-Gen® *see* Iodinated Glycerol *on page 188*

R-Gene® *see* Arginine Hydrochloride *on page 28*

R-Gene® 10 *see* Arginine Hydrochloride *on page 28*

Rheaban® [OTC] *see* Attapulgite *on page 32*

Rheomacrodex® *see* Dextran *on page 103*

Rhesonativ® *see* Rh₀(D) Immune Globulin *on this page*

Rheumanosticon® Dri-Dot® *see* Diagnostic Test for Rheumatoid Factor *on page 108*

Rheumatrex® *see* Methotrexate *on page 227*

Rhinall® Nasal Solution [OTC] *see* Phenylephrine Hydrochloride *on page 282*

Rhindecon® *see* Phenylpropanolamine Hydrochloride *on page 283*

Rh₀(D) Immune Globulin
Brand Names Gamulin® Rh; HypRho®-D; MICRhoGAM™; Mini-Gamulin® Rh; Rhesonativ®; RhoGAM™
Use To prevent isoimmunization in Rh-negative individuals exposed to Rh-positive RBC in pregnancy or in female of childbearing age; in termination of pregnancy (spontaneous or induced abortion or ectopic pregnancy) up to 13 weeks gestation unless father is conclusively shown to be Rh-negative; transfusion accident
Pregnancy Risk Factor C
Usual Dosage Adult: I.M.:

Obstetrical usage: 1 vial (300 μg) prevents maternal sensitization if fetal packed red blood cell volume is < 15 mL, if it is more, give another vial

Postpartum prophylaxis: 200 μg within 72 hours of delivery

Antepartum prophylaxis: 300 μg at approximately 26-28 weeks gestation; followed by 300 μg within 72 hours of delivery if infant is Rh-positive

Following miscarriage, abortion, ectopic pregnancy: 50 μg ideally within three hours, but may be given up to 72 hours after

RhoGAM™ *see* Rh₀(D) Immune Globulin *on this page*

Rhulicaine® [OTC] *see* Benzocaine *on page 40*

Ribavirin (rye ba vye' rin)
Brand Names Virazole®
Synonyms RTCA; Tribavirin
Use Treatment of patients with respiratory syncytial virus (RSV) infections; may also be used in other viral infections including influenza A and B and adenovirus; specially indicated for treatment of RSV infections in patients with underlying cardiopulmonary and immunodeficiency syndromes
Pregnancy Risk Factor X
Usual Dosage

Use with Viratek® small particle aerosol generator (SPAG-2) at a concentration of 20 mg/mL

(Continued)

Ribavirin (Continued)

Aerosol only: 12-18 hours daily for three days, up to seven days in length

Riboflavin (rye' boe flay vin)
Synonyms Lactoflavin; Vitamin B_2; Vitamin G
Use Prevent riboflavin deficiency and treat ariboflavinosis
Pregnancy Risk Factor A/C
Usual Dosage Riboflavin deficiency: Oral:

Adult: 5-30 mg/day in divided doses

Children: 2.5-10 mg/day

RID® [OTC] see Pyrethrins on page 309

Ridaura® see Auranofin on page 33

Rifadin® see Rifampin on this page

Rifampicin see Rifampin on this page

Rifampin (rif' am pin)
Brand Names Rifadin®; Rimactane®
Synonyms Rifampicin
Use Management of active tuberculosis; eliminate meningococci from asymptomatic carriers; prophylaxis of Haemophilus influenzae type B infection
Pregnancy Risk Factor C
Usual Dosage Oral:

Adult:
Active TB: 10 mg/kg/day; maximum: 600 mg/day
Asymptomatic meningococcus carriers: 600 mg twice daily for two days
Prophylaxis Haemophilus influenzae Type B: 20 mg/kg/day single dose for four days; maximum: 600 mg every day for four days

Children:
Active TB: 10-20 mg/kg/day; maximum: 600 mg/day
Asymptomatic meningococcus carriers: 1-12 years: 10 mg/kg twice daily for two days; 3 months - 1 year: 5 mg/kg twice daily for two days
Prophylaxis Haemophilus influenzae Type B: 20 mg/kg/day single dose for four days; maximum: 600 mg every day for four days

rIFN-A see Interferon Alfa-2a on page 187

RIG see Rabies Immune Globulin, Human on page 313

Rimactane® see Rifampin on this page

Rimso®-50 see Dimethyl Sulfoxide on page 117

Ringer's Injection, Lactated
Synonyms Hartmann's Solution; Lactated Ringer's
Pregnancy Risk Factor C

Riopan® [OTC] see Magaldrate on page 209

Riopan Plus® [OTC] *see* Magaldrate and Simethicone *on page 209*

Ritalin® *see* Methylphenidate Hydrochloride *on page 231*

Ritodrine Hydrochloride (ri' toe dreen)
Brand Names Pre-Par®; Yutopar®
Use To inhibit uterine contraction in preterm labor
Pregnancy Risk Factor B
Usual Dosage Adult:
Oral: Start 1/2 hour before stopping I.V. infusion; 10 mg every two hours for 24 hours, then 10-20 mg every 4-6 hours up to 120 mg/day
I.V.: 50-100 μg/minute; increase by 50 μg/minute every 10 minutes; continue for 12 hours after contractions have stopped

rLFN-α2 *see* Interferon Alfa-2b *on page 187*

RMS® *see* Morphine Sulfate *on page 240*

Robafen® [OTC] *see* Guaifenesin *on page 162*

Robaxin® *see* Methocarbamol *on page 227*

Robicillin® VK *see* Penicillin V Potassium *on page 274*

Robimycin® *see* Erythromycin *on page 134*

Robinul® *see* Glycopyrrolate *on page 160*

Robitet® *see* Tetracycline *on page 346*

Robitussin® [OTC] *see* Guaifenesin *on page 162*

Robitussin® A-C *see* Guaifenesin and Codeine *on page 162*

Robitussin-CF® [OTC] *see* Guaifenesin, Phenylpropanolamine and Dextromethorphan *on page 163*

Robitussin®-DAC *see* Guaifenesin, Pseudoephedrine and Codeine *on page 164*

Robitussin-DM® [OTC] *see* Guaifenesin and Dextromethorphan *on page 162*

Robitussin-PE® [OTC] *see* Guaifenesin and Pseudoephedrine *on page 163*

Robomol® *see* Methocarbamol *on page 227*

Rocaltrol® *see* Calcitriol *on page 53*

Ro-Ceph® *see* Cephradine *on page 67*

Rocephin® *see* Ceftriaxone Sodium *on page 65*

Rodex® *see* Pyridoxine Hydrochloride *on page 309*

Roferon-A® *see* Interferon Alfa-2a *on page 187*

Rogaine® *see* Minoxidil *on page 238*

Ronase® *see* Tolazamide *on page 357*

Rondec® *see* Carbinoxamine and Pseudoephedrine *on page 59*

Rondec®-DM *see* Carbinoxamine, Pseudoephedrine and Dextromethorphan *on page 59*

Rondec® Drops *see* Carbinoxamine Maleate *on page 59*

Rondec® Filmtab® *see* Carbinoxamine Maleate *on page 59*

Rondec® Syrup *see* Carbinoxamine Maleate *on page 59*

Rondec-TR® *see* Carbinoxamine Maleate *on page 59*

Rondomycin® *see* Methacycline Hydrochloride *on page 224*

Rose Bengal
Use Diagnostic agent for routine ocular exams or when superficial corneal or conjunctival tissue change is suspected
Usual Dosage 1-2 drops in conjunctival sac before exam

Rotalex® Rubacell II® *see* Diagnostic Test for Virus *on page 108*

Rowasa® *see* Mesalamine *on page 220*

Roxanol™ *see* Morphine Sulfate *on page 240*

Roxanol SR™ *see* Morphine Sulfate *on page 240*

Roxicet® *see* Oxycodone Hydrochloride *on page 264*

Roxicodone™ *see* Oxycodone Hydrochloride *on page 264*

Roxiprin® *see* Oxycodone Hydrochloride *on page 264*

RTCA *see* Ribavirin *on page 315*

Rubella and Measles Vaccines, Combined *see* Measles and Rubella Vaccines, Combined *on page 213*

Rubella and Mumps Vaccines, Combined (rue bell' a)
Brand Names Biavax®ₗₗ
Use Promote active immunity to rubella and mumps by inducing production of antibodies
Pregnancy Risk Factor X
Usual Dosage Adult and Children: S.C.: > 12 months of age: One vial in outer aspect of the upper arm

Rubella, Measles and Mumps Vaccines, Combined *see* Measles, Mumps and Rubella Vaccines, Combined *on page 213*

Rubella Virus Vaccine, Live
Brand Names Meruvax® II
Use Provide vaccine-induced immunity to rubella
Pregnancy Risk Factor X
Usual Dosage S.C.: 1000 $TCID_{50}$ of rubella

Rubeola vaccine *see* Measles Virus Vaccine, Live, Attentuated *on page 214*

Rubramin-PC® *see* Cyanocobalamin *on page 92*

Rubs and Liniments

Brand Names Mentholatum® [OTC]; Mentholatum® Deep Heating Rub [OTC]

Synonyms Analgesic Balm; Boric Acid, Menthol and Camphor; Camphor, Menthol and Boric Acid; Methyl Salicylate and Menthol

Ru-Est-Span® *see* Estradiol *on page 135*

Rufen® *see* Ibuprofen *on page 181*

Rum-K® *see* Potassium Chloride *on page 291*

Ru-Tuss® Liquid *see* Chlorpheniramine and Phenylephrine *on page 73*

Ru-Vert-M® *see* Meclizine Hydrochloride *on page 215*

Rynatan® Pediatric Suspension *see* Chlorpheniramine, Pyrilamine and Phenylephrine *on page 76*

Rynatuss® Pediatric Suspension *see* Chlorpheniramine, Ephedrine, Phenylephrine and Carbetapentane *on page 74*

Sabin *see* Poliovirus Vaccine, Live, Trivalent *on page 289*

Salbutamol *see* Albuterol *on page 10*

Saleto-200® [OTC] *see* Ibuprofen *on page 181*

Saleto-400® *see* Ibuprofen *on page 181*

Salflex® *see* Salsalate *on next page*

Salgesic® *see* Salsalate *on next page*

Salicylazosulfapyridine *see* Sulfasalazine *on page 338*

Salicylic Acid (sal i sill' ik)

Brand Names Ionil® [OTC]

Use Use topically for its keratolytic effect in controlling seborrheic dermatitis or psoriasis of body and scalp, dandruff, and other scaling dermatoses. Also used to remove warts, corns and calluses

Pregnancy Risk Factor C

Usual Dosage May be used daily in place of shampoo

Salicylic Acid and Benzoic Acid *see* Benzoic Acid and Salicylic Acid *on page 41*

Salicylic Acid and Lactic Acid

Brand Names Duofilm®

Synonyms Lactic Acid and Salicylic Acid

Use Treatment of benign epithelial tumors such as warts

Pregnancy Risk Factor C

Usual Dosage Apply a thin layer directly to wart once daily (may be useful to apply at bedtime and wash off in morning)

Salicylic Acid and Podophyllin *see* Podophyllin and Salicylic Acid *on page 288*

Salicylic Acid and Propylene Glycol
Brand Names Keralyt®

Synonyms Propylene Glycol and Salicylic Acid

Use Removal of excessive keratin in hyperkeratotic skin disorders, including various ichthyosis, keratosis palmaris and plantaris and psoriasis; may be used to remove excessive keratin in dorsal and plantar hyperkeratotic lesions

Pregnancy Risk Factor C

Usual Dosage Apply to area at night after soaking region for at least five minutes to hydrate area, and place under occlusion; medication is washed off in morning

Salicylic Acid and Sulfur see Sulfur and Salicylic Acid on page 339

Salicylsalicylic Acid see Salsalate on this page

Salivart® [OTC] see Saliva Substitute on this page

Saliva Substitute
Brand Names Moi-Stir® [OTC]; Orex® [OTC]; Salivart® [OTC]; Xero-Lube® [OTC]

Use For relief of dry mouth and throat in xerostomia

Usual Dosage Use as needed

Salk see Poliovirus Vaccine, Inactivated on page 289

Salsalate (sal' sa late)
Brand Names Argesic®-SA; Artha-G®; Disalcid®; Mono-Gesic®; Salflex®; Salgesic®; Salsitab®

Synonyms Disalicylic Acid; Salicylsalicylic Acid

Use Treatment of minor pain or fever; arthritis

Pregnancy Risk Factor C

Usual Dosage Adult: Oral: 1 g 2-4 times daily

Salsitab® see Salsalate on this page

Salt see Sodium Chloride on page 327

Saluron® see Hydroflumethiazide on page 176

Salutensin® see Hydroflumethiazide and Reserpine on page 176

Sandimmune® see Cyclosporine on page 94

Sandoglobulin® see Immune Globulin on page 183

Sandostatin® see Octreotide Acetate on page 258

Sansert® see Methysergide Maleate on page 232

Santyl® see Collagenase on page 88

Sarna [OTC] see Camphor, Menthol and Phenol on page 55

SclavoTest®-PPD see Tuberculin on page 367

Scleromate® see Morrhuate Sodium on page 241

Scopolamine (skoe pol' a meen)
Brand Names Isopto® Hyoscine; Transderm Scop®
Synonyms Hyoscine Hydrobromide; Scopolamine Hydrobromide
Use Preoperative medication to produce amnesia and decrease salivation and respiratory secretions; producing cycloplegia and mydriasis; treatment of iridocyclitis
Pregnancy Risk Factor C
Usual Dosage

Adult:
I.M., I.V., S.C.: 0.3-0.65 mg 3-4 times daily
Ophthalmic: Iritis: 1-2 drops of 0.1% solution; refraction: 1-2 drops of 0.25% solution

Children: Refraction: One drop of 0.2% solution

Scopolamine and Phenylephrine see Phenylephrine and Scopolamine on page 281

Scopolamine Hydrobromide see Scopolamine on this page

Scott's® Emulsion [OTC] see Vitamin A and Vitamin D on page 377

Sebulex® [OTC] see Sulfur and Salicylic Acid on page 339

Secobarbital and Amobarbital see Amobarbital and Secobarbital on page 21

Secobarbital Sodium (see koe bar' bi tal)
Brand Names Seconal™
Synonyms Quinalbarbitone Sodium
Use Short-term treatment of insomnia and as preanesthetic agent
Restrictions C-II
Pregnancy Risk Factor D
Usual Dosage

Adult:
Hypnotic: Oral, I.M.: 100-200 mg/ dose; I.V.: 50-250 mg/dose
Preoperative sedation: Oral: 100-300 mg 1-2 hours before procedure
Sedation: Oral: 20-40 mg/dose 2-3 times/day

Children:
Hypnotic: I.M.: 3-5 mg/kg/dose; maximum: 100 mg/dose
Preoperative sedation: Oral: 50-100 mg 1-2 hours before procedure
Sedation: Oral: 6 mg/kg/day divided every 8 hours

Seconal™ see Secobarbital Sodium on this page

Secretin
Brand Names Secretin-Kabi
Use Diagnosis of Zollinger-Ellison syndrome and pancreatic exocrine disease
Usual Dosage I.V.:

Pancreatic function: 1 CU/kg

Zollinger-Ellison: 2 CU/kg

Secretin-Kabi *see* Secretin *on previous page*

Sectral® *see* Acebutolol Hydrochloride *on page 4*

Seldane® *see* Terfenadine *on page 343*

Selegiline Hydrochloride (se lej' a leen)
Brand Names Eldepryl®
Synonyms Deprenyl; L-Deprenyl
Use Adjunct in the management of Parkinsonian patients in which levodopa/carbidopa therapy is deteriorating
Pregnancy Risk Factor C
Usual Dosage Adult: Oral: 5 mg twice a day

Selenium (se lee' nee um)
Brand Names Selsun®
Use To treat itching and flaking of the scalp associated with dandruff, to control scalp seborrheic dermatitis; treatment of tinea versicolor
Usual Dosage

Seborrheic dermatitis: Massage 5-10 mL into wet scalp, leave on scalp 2-3 minutes, rinse thoroughly and repeat application. Initially: apply two times per week; later: apply weekly, biweekly, or monthly depending upon control

Tinea versicolor: Apply to affected area and lather with small amounts of water, leave on skin for 10 minutes, then rinse thoroughly; use every day for seven days

Selenium *see* Trace Metals *on page 358*

Sele-Pak® *see* Trace Metals *on page 358*

Selepen® *see* Trace Metals *on page 358*

Selestoject® *see* Betamethasone *on page 43*

Selsun® *see* Selenium *on this page*

Semilente® *see* Insulin, Zinc Suspension, Prompt *on page 187*

Semilente® Iletin®I *see* Insulin, Zinc Suspension, Prompt *on page 187*

Semilente® Purified Pork *see* Insulin, Zinc Suspension, Prompt *on page 187*

Senna
Brand Names Black Draught® [OTC]; Gentle Nature® [OTC]; Nytilax® [OTC]; Senna-Gen® [OTC]; Senokot® [OTC]; Senokot® S [OTC]; Senolax® [OTC]; X-Prep® Liquid [OTC]
Use Short-term treatment of constipation; evacuate the colon for bowel or rectal examinations
Pregnancy Risk Factor C
Usual Dosage Oral:

Adult:
Granules: 1 teaspoonful at bedtime, not to exceed 2 teaspoonfuls twice a day

Syrup: 10-15 mL at bedtime, not to exceed 15 mL twice a day
Tablet: 2 tablets at bedtime, not to exceed 4 tablets twice a day

Children:
Granules: > 27 kg: 1/2 teaspoonful at bedtime, not to exceed 1 teaspoonful twice a day
Syrup: 1-5 years: 2.5-5 mL at bedtime, not to exceed 5 mL twice a day; 5-15 years: 5-10 mL at bedtime, not to exceed 10 mL twice a day
Tablet: > 27 kg: 1 tablet at bedtime, not to exceed 2 tablets twice a day

Infant: 1 month - 1 year: Syrup: 1.25-2.5 mL at bedtime, not to exceed 2.5 mL twice a day

Senna-Gen® [OTC] *see* Senna *on previous page*

Senokot® [OTC] *see* Senna *on previous page*

Senokot® S [OTC] *see* Senna *on previous page*

Senolax® [OTC] *see* Senna *on previous page*

Sensorcaine® *see* Bupivacaine Hydrochloride *on page 49*

Septisol® *see* Hexachlorophene *on page 168*

Septra® *see* Sulfamethoxazole and Trimethoprim *on page 338*

Septra® DS *see* Sulfamethoxazole and Trimethoprim *on page 338*

Ser-Ap-Es® *see* Hydralazine, Hydrochlorothiazide, and Reserpine *on page 172*

Serax® *see* Oxazepam *on page 263*

Serentil® *see* Mesoridazine Besylate *on page 221*

Seromycin® Pulvules® *see* Cycloserine *on page 94*

Serophene® *see* Clomiphene Citrate *on page 83*

Serpalan® *see* Reserpine *on page 314*

Serpasil® *see* Reserpine *on page 314*

Serpasil®-Apresoline® *see* Hydralazine and Reserpine *on page 171*

Serutan® [OTC] *see* Psyllium *on page 308*

Siblin® [OTC] *see* Psyllium *on page 308*

Sickledex™ *see* Diagnostic Test for Sickle Cell *on page 108*

Silain® [OTC] *see* Simethicone *on next page*

Silvadene® *see* Silver Sulfadiazine *on next page*

Silver Nitrate

Use Prevention of gonorrheal ophthalmia neonatorum; treat indolent wounds; freshen ulcer and fissure edges; plantar warts; impetigo vulgaris; burns

Pregnancy Risk Factor C

(Continued)

Silver Nitrate *(Continued)*

Usual Dosage Adult:
Solution: Use as directed on burns
Sticks: Apply directly to mucous membranes and other moist surfaces.
Dry skin therapy: Applicator tip should be dipped in water immediately before use

Silver Protein, Mild

Brand Names Argyrol® S.S. 20% [OTC]
Use In eye surgery to stain and coagulate mucus which is then removed by irrigation; eye infections
Pregnancy Risk Factor C
Usual Dosage
Preop in eye surgery: 20%, place 2-3 drops into eye(s), then rinse out with sterile irrigating solution
Eye infections: 20%, 1-3 drops into the affected eye(s) every 3-4 hours for several days

Silver Sulfadiazine

Brand Names Flint SSD®; Silvadene®; Thermazene®
Use Prevention and treatment of infection in second and third degree burns
Pregnancy Risk Factor C
Usual Dosage Apply once or twice daily with a sterile gloved hand; apply to a thickness of 1/16"; burned area should be covered with cream at all times

Simethicone (sye meth' i kone)

Brand Names Gas-X® [OTC]; Mylicon® [OTC]; Phazyme® [OTC]; Silain® [OTC]
Synonyms Activated Dimethicone; Methylpolysiloxane
Use For the relief of the painful symptoms of excess gas in the digestive tract
Pregnancy Risk Factor C
Usual Dosage Oral:
Adult: 150-400 mg/day, usually given four times/day after meals and at bedtime as needed
Children: 2-12 years of age: Reduce adult dose as needed (pediatric dose should be based on severity of condition; AHFS recommends using BSA rather than weight, but provides no guidelines)

Simethicone and Calcium Carbonate *see* Calcium Carbonate and Simethicone *on page 53*

Simethicone and Magaldrate *see* Magaldrate and Simethicone *on page 209*

Sinarest® 12 Hour Nasal Solution *see* Oxymetazoline Hydrochloride *on page 265*

Sinarest® Nasal Solution [OTC] *see* Phenylephrine Hydrochloride *on page 282*

Sincalide (sin' ka lide)
Brand Names Kinevac®
Synonyms C8-CCK; OP-CCK
Use Postevacuation cholecystography; gallbladder bile sampling; stimulate pancreatic secretion for analysis
Usual Dosage Adult: I.V.:

Contraction of gallbladder: 0.02 μg/kg over 1/2-1 minute, may repeat in 15 minutes a 0.04 μg/kg dose

Pancreatic function: 0.02 μg/kg over 30 minutes

Sinemet® *see* Levodopa and Carbidopa *on page 202*

Sinequan® *see* Doxepin Hydrochloride *on page 122*

Sinografin® *see* Diatrizoate Meglumine and Iodipamide Meglumine *on page 109*

Sinubid® *see* Phenyltoloxamine, Phenylpropanolamine and Acetaminophen *on page 283*

Sinusol-B® *see* Brompheniramine Maleate *on page 48*

Sinutab® [OTC] *see* Acetaminophen, Chlorpheniramine and Pseudoephedrine *on page 5*

Sirlene® *see* Propylene Glycol *on page 305*

Skelaxin® *see* Metaxalone *on page 224*

Skin Test Antigens, Multiple
Brand Names Multitest CMI®
Use Detection of nonresponsiveness to antigens by means of delayed hypersensitivity skin testing
Pregnancy Risk Factor C
Usual Dosage Select only test sites that permit sufficient surface area and subcutaneous tissue to allow adequate penetration of all 8 points, avoid hairy areas

Slo-bid™ *see* Theophylline *on page 348*

Slo-Phyllin® *see* Theophylline *on page 348*

Slow-K® *see* Potassium Chloride *on page 291*

SMX-TMP *see* Sulfamethoxazole and Trimethoprim *on page 338*

Snake (Pit Vipers) Antivenin *see* Antivenin (Crotalidae) Polyvalent *on page 27*

Sodium Acetate
Use As a sodium source in large volume I.V. fluids to prevent or correct hyponatremia in patients with restricted intake; used to counter acidosis
Usual Dosage To be determined

Sodium Acid Carbonate *see* Sodium Bicarbonate *on next page*

Sodium Ascorbate (a skor' bate)

Brand Names Cenolate®

Use Prevention and treatment of scurvy and to acidify the urine; large doses may decrease the severity of "colds"

Pregnancy Risk Factor C

Usual Dosage Oral:

Adult:
Scurvy: 100-250 mg 1-2 times daily
Urinary acidification: 4-12 g/day in divided doses
Dietary supplement: 45-60 mg/day
Prevention and treatment of cold: 1-3 g/day

Children: Scurvy: 100-300 mg/day in divided doses

Sodium Benzoate and Caffeine *see* Caffeine and Sodium
Benzoate *on page 52*

Sodium Bicarbonate

Brand Names Neut®

Synonyms Baking Soda; NaHCO$_3$; Sodium Acid Carbonate; Sodium Hydrogen Carbonate

Use Management of metabolic acidosis; antacid; alkalinize urine

Pregnancy Risk Factor C

Usual Dosage Neonates and children < 2 years of age should receive 4.2% (0.5 mEq/mL) solution

Cardiac arrest: (Routine use of NaHCO$_3$ not recommended; should only be given after adequate alveolar ventilation has been established and effective cardiac compressions are provided)
Adult: I.V.: Initial: 1 mEq/kg/dose one time; maintenance: 0.5 mEq/kg/dose every 10 minutes or as indicated by arterial blood gases
Children and Infants: I.V.: 0.5-1 mEq/kg/dose repeated every 10 minutes or as indicated by arterial blood gases

Metabolic acidosis:
Adult and older children: I.V.: 2-5 mEq/kg/dose over 4-8 hours infusion or calculate dose based on base deficit (re-evaluate acid-base status frequently)
Neonate: I.V.: 1-3 mEq/kg/dose slowly (usually over 20-60 minutes)

Chronic renal failure:
Adult: Oral: Start with 20-36 mEq/day in divided doses; titrate to bicarbonate level of 18-20 mEq/L
Children: Oral: 1-3 mEq/kg/day

Renal tubular acidosis:
Distal: Oral: Adult: 1 mEq/kg/day; infant: 2-3 mEq/kg/day; divided into 4-5 doses
Proximal: Initial: 5-10 mEq/kg/day given in divided doses
Titrate dosage to maintain bicarbonate levels in normal range

Antacid: Adult: Oral: 325-1950 mg, 1-4 times/day; maximum: 7.8 g/day

Urine alkalinization:
Adult: Oral: 48 mEq initially, then 12-24 mEq every 4 hours; maximum dose: < 60 years of age: 192 mEq, > 60 years: 100 mEq

Children: Oral: 1-10 mEq/kg/day (ie, 2 mEq/kg every 4-6 hours to titrate urine pH)

Sodium Cellulose Phosphate *see* Cellulose Sodium Phosphate *on page 66*

Sodium Chloride

Brand Names Adsorbonac® [OTC] Ophthalmic; Ayr®; Muro 128® Ophthalmic [OTC]

Synonyms NaCl; Normal Saline; Salt

Use Prevention of muscle cramps and heat prostration; restoration of sodium ion in hyponatremia; induce abortion; restore moisture to nasal membranes; GU irrigant; reduction of corneal edema

Pregnancy Risk Factor C

Usual Dosage

Adult:

Heat cramps: Oral: 0.5-1 g with full glass of water, up to 4.8 g/day

Replacement: Determined by laboratory determinations

Abortion: Up to 250 mL of 20%

Nasal: Use as often as needed

GI irrigant: 1-3 L/day by intermittent irrigation

Ophthalmic: Solution: 1-2 drops in eye(s) every 3-4 hours; ointment: Apply once a day or more often

Children:

Replacement: Determined by laboratory determinations

Nasal: Use as often as needed

Sodium Chloride and Dextrose *see* Dextrose and Sodium Chloride *on page 105*

Sodium Chloride, Dextrose and Potassium Chloride *see* Dextrose and Sodium Chloride with Potassium Chloride *on page 105*

Sodium Citrate and Citric Acid

Brand Names Bicitra®

Synonyms Modified Shohl's Solution

Use Treatment of metabolic acidosis; alkalinizing in conditions; agent where long-term maintenance of an alkaline urine is desirable

Usual Dosage

Alkalinization:

Adult: Oral: 10-30 mL with water after meals and at bedtime

Children: Oral: 5-15 mL with water after meals and at bedtime

Gastric antacid:

Adult: > 60 years of age: 200 mEq/day divided 3-4 times/day; > 60 years: 100 mEq/day divided 3-4 times/day

Children and Infants: 2-3 mEq/kg/day divided 3-4 times/day

Sodium Citrate and Potassium Citrate Mixture

Brand Names Polycitra®

Use For conditions where long term maintenance of an alkaline urine is desirable as in control and dissolution of uric acid and cystine calculi of the urinary tract

(Continued)

Sodium Citrate and Potassium Citrate Mixture
(Continued)
Usual Dosage Oral:

Adult: 15-30 mL diluted in water after meals and at bedtime

Children: 5-15 mL diluted in water after meals and at bedtime

Sodium Diatrizoate and Meglumine Diatrizoate
Brand Names Gastrografin®; Hypaque®-M; Renografin®-60; Renografin®-76

Usual Dosage Dose varies with procedure

Sodium Edetate *see* Edetate Disodium *on page 127*

Sodium Etidronate *see* Etidronate Disodium *on page 142*

Sodium Hyaluronate
Brand Names Amvisc®; Healon®

Use Surgical aid in cataract extraction, intraocular implantation, corneal transplant, glaucoma filtration, and retinal attachment surgery

Usual Dosage Depends upon procedure (slowly introduce a sufficient quantity into eye)

Sodium Hyaluronate-Chrondroitin Sulfate *see* Chondroitin Sulfate-Sodium Hyaluronate *on page 78*

Sodium Hydrogen Carbonate *see* Sodium Bicarbonate *on page 326*

Sodium Hypochlorite Solution (hye poe klor' ite)
Synonyms Modified Dakin's Solution

Use Treatment of athlete's foot (0.5%); wound irrigation (0.5%); to disinfect utensils and equipment (5%)

Sodium Iodide I 131
Use Treat hyperthyroidism and thyrotoxicosis and selected cases of thyroid carcinoma; as a diagnostic aid in thyroid function studies in suspected hyperthyroidism and to visualize thyroid malignancy and metastasis

Pregnancy Risk Factor X

Usual Dosage Oral:

Hyperthyroidism: 4-10 millicuries (mCi) in single dose; repeat in six weeks, if needed

Thyroid carcinoma: 50 mCi; subsequent dose is 100-150 mCi, if necessary

Sodium Iothalamate *see* Iothalamate Sodium *on page 190*

Sodium Lactate (lak' tate)
Synonyms 1/6 Molar Sodium Lactate

Use Source of bicarbonate for prevention and treatment of mild to moderate metabolic acidosis

Pregnancy Risk Factor C
Usual Dosage Dosage depends on degree of acidosis

Sodium *L*-Tri-iodothyronine *see* Liothyronine Sodium
on page 205

Sodium Methicillin *see* Methicillin Sodium *on page 226*

Sodium Nafcillin *see* Nafcillin Sodium *on page 244*

Sodium Nitroferricyanide *see* Nitroprusside Sodium
on page 254

Sodium Nitroprusside *see* Nitroprusside Sodium *on page 254*

Sodium-PCA and Lactic Acid *see* Lactic Acid and Sodium-PCA
on page 198

Sodium Phosphate
Brand Names Fleet® Enema [OTC]; Fleet® Phospho®-Soda [OTC]
Use Source of phosphate in large volume I.V. fluids; short-term treatment
of constipation and to evacuate the colon for rectal and bowel exams;
source of sodium and phosphorus in parenteral nutrition
Pregnancy Risk Factor C
Usual Dosage

Adult: I.V.: Bolus situations: Maximum infusion concentration: 0.855 mEq
Na^+/mL; maximum infusion rate: 0.05 mmol/kg/hour

Fleet® enema:
Adult: > 12 years of age: 118 mL
Children: 2-12 years: 67.5 mL (pediatric)

Fleet® Phospho®-Soda: Oral:
Adult: 20-30 mL mixed with 120 mL cold water
Children: 5-15 mL

Na phosphorus injection: General maintenance requirement (non-
newborn) (based on phosphorus) 2 mmol/kg/day; maximum: 15-30
mmol/day; dose may vary widely based upon clinical condition

Sodium Phosphate *see* Phosphorus Replacement Products
on page 284

Sodium Phosphate and Potassium Phosphate *see* Potassium
Phosphate and Sodium Phosphate *on page 292*

Sodium Polystyrene Sulfonate (pol ee stye' reen)
Brand Names Kayexalate®; SPS®
Use Treatment of hyperkalemia
Pregnancy Risk Factor C
Usual Dosage

Adult:
Oral: 15 g 1-4 times a day
Rectal: 30-60 every six hours

Children:
Oral: 1 g/kg/dose every six hours
(Continued)

Sodium Polystyrene Sulfonate *(Continued)*

Rectal: 1 g/kg/dose every 2-6 hours (In small children and infants employ lower doses by using the practical exchange ratio of 1 mEq K$^+$ /g of resin as the basis for calculation)

Sodium Sulfacetamide

Brand Names Bleph®-10; Sulamyd® Sodium

Synonyms Sulfacetamide Sodium

Use Treatment and prophylaxis of conjunctivitis due to susceptible bacterial infections

Pregnancy Risk Factor C

Usual Dosage

Ointment: Apply to lower conjunctival sac 1-4 times daily and at bedtime

Solution: 1-3 drops several times a day up to every 2-3 hours

Sodium Sulfacetamide and Prednisolone Acetate

Brand Names Blephamide®; Cetapred®; Metimyd®

Use Steroid-responsive inflammatory ocular conditions where infection is present or there is a risk of infection

Usual Dosage

Ointment: Apply to lower conjunctival sac 1-4 times daily

Solution: 1-3 drops every 2-3 hours

Sodium Sulfacetamide and Sulfur *see* Sulfur and Sodium Sulfacetamide *on page 339*

Sodium Tetradecyl Sulfate

Brand Names Sotradecol®

Use Treatment of small, uncomplicated varicose veins of the lower extremities; endoscopic sclerotherapy in the management of bleeding esophageal varices

Pregnancy Risk Factor C

Usual Dosage I.V.: 0.5-2 mL

Sodium Thiosulfate *(thye oh sul' fate)*

Brand Names Tinver®

Use Used alone or with sodium nitrite or amyl nitrite in cyanide poisoning

Pregnancy Risk Factor C

Usual Dosage Dose should be based on determination as with nitrite; at rate of 2.5-5 mL/minute. See table.

Sodium Versenate® *see* Edetate Disodium *on page 127*

Sodol® *see* Carisoprodol *on page 61*

Solaquin Forte® *see* Hydroquinone *on page 176*

Solarcaine® [OTC] *see* Benzocaine *on page 40*

Solatene® *see* Beta Carotene *on page 43*

Solfoton® *see* Phenobarbital *on page 279*

Solganal® *see* Aurothioglucose *on page 33*

**Variation of Sodium Nitrite and
Sodium Thiosulfate Dose With Hemoglobin Concentration***

Hemoglobin (g/dL)	Initial Dose Sodium Nitrite (mg/kg)	Initial Dose Sodium Nitrite 33% (mL/kg)	Initial Dose Sodium Thiosulfate 25% (mL/kg)
7	5.8	0.19	0.95
8	6.6	0.22	1.10
9	7.5	0.25	1.25
10	8.3	0.27	1.35
11	9.1	0.30	1.50
12	10.0	0.33	1.65
13	10.8	0.36	1.80
14	11.6	0.39	1.95

* Adapted from Berlin DM Jr, "The treatment of cyanide poisoning in children," *Pediatrics*, 1970, 46:793.

Solu-Cortef® *see* Hydrocortisone *on page 174*

Solu-Medrol® *see* Methylprednisolone *on page 231*

Soma® *see* Carisoprodol *on page 61*

Somatrem-Human Growth Hormone (soe' ma trem)
Brand Names Protropin®
Use Long term treatment of growth failure from lack of adequate endogenous growth hormone secretion
Pregnancy Risk Factor C
Usual Dosage Children: I.M.: Up to 0.1 mg (0.26 U)/kg/dose three times per week

Somnos® *see* Chloral Hydrate *on page 68*

Somophyllin® *see* Aminophylline *on page 18*

Somophyllin®-CRT *see* Theophylline *on page 348*

Somophyllin®-DF *see* Aminophylline *on page 18*

Somophyllin®-T *see* Theophylline *on page 348*

Soothe® [OTC] *see* Tetrahydrozoline Hydrochloride *on page 347*

Soprodol® *see* Carisoprodol *on page 61*

Sorbitol (sor' bi tole)
Use Genitourinary irrigant in transurethral prostatic resection or other transurethral resection or other transurethral surgical procedures; diuretic; humectant; sweetening agent
Usual Dosage Hyperosmotic laxative (as single dose, at infrequent intervals):

Adult: > 12 years of age: Rectal enema: 120 mL as 25-30% solution

(Continued)

Sorbitol *(Continued)*

Children: 2-11 years: Rectal enema: 30-60 mL as 25-30% solution

See monograph for Sodium Polystyrene Sulfonate for doses as an adjunct to therapy

Sorbitrate® *see* Isosorbide Dinitrate *on page 194*

Soridol® *see* Carisoprodol *on page 61*

Sotradecol® *see* Sodium Tetradecyl Sulfate *on page 330*

Soyacal® *see* Fat Emulsion *on page 144*

Soyalac® [OTC] *see* Nutritional Formula, Enteral/Oral *on page 258*

Sparine® *see* Promazine Hydrochloride *on page 300*

Spectam® *see* Spectinomycin Hydrochloride *on this page*

Spectazole™ *see* Econazole Nitrate *on page 126*

Spectinomycin Hydrochloride *(spek ti noe mye' sin)*
Brand Names Spectam®; Trobicin®
Use Treatment of uncomplicated gonorrhea
Pregnancy Risk Factor C
Usual Dosage I.M.:

Adult: 2 g deep I.M. or 4 g where antibiotic resistance is prevalent one time; 4 g (10 mL) dose should be given as 2-5 mL injections

Children:
< 45 kg: 40 mg/kg/dose one time
≥ 45 kg: See adult dose
Children > 8 years of age who are allergic to PCNS/cephalosporins may be treated with oral tetracycline

Spectrobid® *see* Bacampicillin Hydrochloride *on page 35*

Spectro-Chlor® *see* Chloramphenicol *on page 69*

Spherulin® *see* Coccidioidin Skin Test *on page 86*

Spironolactone *(speer on oh lak' tone)*
Brand Names Aldactone®
Use Management of edema associated with excessive aldosterone excretion; hypertension; primary hyperaldosteronism; hypokalemia; treatment of hirsutism
Pregnancy Risk Factor C
Usual Dosage Oral:

Adult:
Edema: 25-200 mg/day in 1-2 divided doses
Hypertension: 50-100 mg in 1-2 divided doses
Primary aldosteronism: 100-400 mg in 1-2 divided doses
Hypokalemia: 25-100 mg in 1-2 divided doses

Children: Edema: 1.0-3.3 μg/kg/day in 2-4 divided doses

Spironolactone and Hydrochlorothiazide *see* Hydrochlorothiazide and Spironolactone *on page 172*

Sportscreme® [OTC] *see* Triethanolamine Salicylate *on page 361*

SPS® *see* Sodium Polystyrene Sulfonate *on page 329*

S-P-T *see* Thyroid *on page 354*

SSKI® *see* Potassium Iodide *on page 291*

Stadol® *see* Butorphanol Tartrate *on page 51*

Stanozolol (stan oh' zoe lole)
Brand Names Winstrol®
Use Prophylactic use against angioedema
Pregnancy Risk Factor X
Usual Dosage Adult: Oral: 2 mg three times a day

Staphcillin® *see* Methicillin Sodium *on page 226*

Staticin® *see* Erythromycin, Topical *on page 135*

Stay Trim® Diet Gum [OTC] *see* Phenylpropanolamine Hydrochloride *on page 283*

Stelazine® *see* Trifluoperazine Hydrochloride *on page 362*

Stemetic® *see* Trimethobenzamide Hydrochloride *on page 364*

Stemex® *see* Paramethasone Acetate *on page 270*

Sterapred® *see* Prednisone *on page 295*

Sterculia Gum *see* Indian Gum *on page 184*

Stilbestrol *see* Diethylstilbestrol *on page 112*

Stilphostrol® *see* Diethylstilbestrol *on page 112*

Stimate™ *see* Desmopressin Acetate *on page 101*

St. Joseph® Measured Dose Nasal Solution [OTC] *see* Phenylephrine Hydrochloride *on page 282*

Stoxil® *see* Idoxuridine *on page 181*

Streptase® *see* Streptokinase *on this page*

Streptokinase (strep toe kye' nase)
Brand Names Kabikinase®; Streptase®
Use Thrombolytic agent used in treatment of recent severe or massive deep vein thrombosis, pulmonary emboli, myocardial infarction, and occluded arteriovenous cannulas
Pregnancy Risk Factor C
Usual Dosage Adult:

Thromboses: I.V.: 250,000 IU to start, then 100,000 IU/hour for 24-72 hours depending on location

Myocardial infarction: 20,000 IU to start, then 2000-4000 IU/minute for 60 minutes intracoronary

Cannula occlusion: 250,000 IU into cannula, clamp for two hours, then aspirate

Streptomycin Sulfate (strep toe mye' sin)
Use Combination therapy of active tuberculosis or streptococcal or enterococcal endocarditis
Pregnancy Risk Factor D
Usual Dosage I.M.:

Adult:
TB: 15 mg/kg/day; maximum: 2 g/24 hours, divided every 12 hours
Enterococcal endocarditis: 1 g every 12 hours for two weeks, 400 mg every 12 hours for 40 weeks
Streptococcal endocarditis: 1 g every 12 hours for one week, 500 mg every 12 hours for one week

Children: TB: 20-40 mg/kg/day; maximum 2 g/24 hours, divided every 8-12 hours

Infants: 20-30 mg/kg/day, divided every 12 hours

Streptonase-B® see Diagnostic Test for Streptococci
on page 108

Strepto-Sec® see Diagnostic Test for Streptococci
on page 108

Streptozocin (strep toe zoe' sin)
Brand Names Zanosar®
Use Treat metastatic islet cell carcinoma of the pancreas
Pregnancy Risk Factor C
Usual Dosage Adult and Children: I.V.: 500 mg/m^2 for five days every 4-6 weeks until optimal benefit or toxicity occurs or may be given in single dose 1000 mg/m^2 at weekly intervals for two doses, then increased to 1500 mg/m^2; usual course of therapy is 4-6 weeks

Strifon® Forte DSC see Chlorzoxazone on page 77

Strong Iodine Solution see Iodine on page 188

Strong Iodine Solution see Potassium Iodide on page 291

Sublimaze® see Fentanyl Citrate on page 145

Succinylcholine Chloride (suk sin ill koe' leen)
Brand Names Anectine® Chloride; Anectine® Flo-Pack®; Quelicin®; Sucostrin®
Synonyms Suxamethonium Chloride
Use Used with general anesthesia to produce skeletal muscle relaxation in procedures of short duration
Pregnancy Risk Factor C
Usual Dosage

Adult: I.M., I.V.: 0.6 mg/kg, up to 150 mg total dose

Children: I.M., I.V.: 1-2 mg/kg

Intermittent:
Adult: Initial: 0.3-1.1 mg/kg/dose one time; maintenance: 0.04-0.07 mg/kg/dose at appropriate intervals to maintain the required degree of relaxation

Children: Initial: 1 mg/kg/dose one time; maintenance: 0.3-0.6 mg/kg/dose at intervals of 5-10 minutes as necessary

Neonate: Initial: 2 mg/kg/dose one time; maintenance: 0.3-0.6 mg/kg/dose at intervals of 5-10 minutes as necessary

Note: Pretreatment with atropine may reduce occurrence of bradycardia

Sucostrin® *see* Succinylcholine Chloride *on previous page*

Sucralfate (soo kral' fate)
Brand Names Carafate®
Use Short-term management of duodenal ulcers; suspension may be used topically for treatment of stomatitis due to cancer chemotherapy
Pregnancy Risk Factor B
Usual Dosage Oral:

Stomatitis: 2.5-5 mL, swish and spit or swish and swallow 4 times/day

Adult: 1 g four times a day, one hour before meals or food and at bedtime

Children: Dose not established

Sucrets® [OTC] *see* Hexylresorcinol *on page 169*

Sudafed® [OTC] *see* Pseudoephedrine *on page 307*

Sudafed® 12 Hour [OTC] *see* Pseudoephedrine *on page 307*

Sudafed® Tablet [OTC] *see* Pseudoephedrine *on page 307*

Sudahist® *see* Triprolidine and Pseudoephedrine *on page 365*

Sufedrin® [OTC] *see* Pseudoephedrine *on page 307*

Sufenta® *see* Sufentanil Citrate *on this page*

Sufentanil Citrate (soo fen' ta nil)
Brand Names Sufenta®
Use Analgesic supplement in maintenance of balanced general anesthesia
Restrictions C-II
Pregnancy Risk Factor C/D
Usual Dosage Adult: I.V.:

1-2 μg/kg with NO_2/O_2 for endotracheal intubation

2-8 μg/kg with NO_2/O_2 more complicated major surgical procedures

8-30 μg/kg with 100% O_2 and muscle relaxant produces sleep; at doses of $\geq$ 8 μg/kg maintains a deep level of anesthesia

Sulamyd® Sodium *see* Sodium Sulfacetamide *on page 330*

Sulbactam and Ampicillin *see* Ampicillin and Sulbactam *on page 23*

Sulconazole Nitrate (sul kon' a zole)
Brand Names Exelderm®; Sulcosyn®
Use Treatment of superficial fungal infections of the skin, including tinea cruris, tinea corporis, tinea versicolor and possibly tinea pedis
Usual Dosage Apply once or twice daily

Sulcosyn® *see* Sulconazole Nitrate *on previous page*

Sulfabenzamide, Sulfacetamide, and Sulfathiazole

(sul fa benz' a mide)
Brand Names Gyne-Sulf®; Sultrin™; Trysul®; Vagilia®; V.V.S.®
Use Treatment of *Haemophilus vaginalis* vaginitis
Usual Dosage One (1) applicatorful in vagina twice daily for 4-6 days;
dosage may then be decreased to 1/2-1/4 of an applicatorful twice daily;
one (1) tablet intravaginally twice daily for 4-6 days

Sulfacetamide Sodium *see* Sodium Sulfacetamide
on page 330

Sulfacet-R® *see* Sulfur and Sodium Sulfacetamide
on page 339

Sulfacytine (sul fa sye' teen)

Brand Names Renoquid®
Use Treatment of urinary tract infections
Pregnancy Risk Factor B/D at term
Usual Dosage Adult: Oral: Initially 500 mg, then 250 mg every four hours
for 10 days

Sulfadiazine (sul fa dye' a zeen)

Brand Names Microsulfon®
Use Treatment of urinary tract infections and nocardiosis, rheumatic fever
prophylaxis; adjunctive treatment in toxoplasmosis; uncomplicated at-
tack of malaria
Pregnancy Risk Factor B/D at term
Usual Dosage Oral:

Urinary tract infection:
Adult: 2-4 g to start, then 0.5-1 g every six hours
Children: 2 g/m^2 to start, then 4 g/m^2 in 4-6 divided doses

Rheumatic fever prophylaxis:
Adult and Children: > 30 kg- 1 g/day
Children: < 30 kg- 500 mg/day

Toxoplasmosis:
Adult: 1 g four times a day (every 6 hours) for 3-4 weeks, given with
pyrimethamine 25 mg/day
Children: 25 mg/kg four times a day (every 6 hours) for 3-4 weeks with
pyrimethamine 2 mg/kg/day for three days, then 1 mg/kg/day for 3-4
weeks

Malaria:
Adult: 500 mg four times a day for five days
Children: 25-50 mg/kg four times a day for five days

Sulfadiazine, Sulfamethazine and Sulfamerazine

Brand Names Lantrisul®; Terfonyl®
Synonyms Multiple Sulfonamides; Trisulfapyrimidines
Use Treatment of toxoplasmosis

Pregnancy Risk Factor B/D

Usual Dosage Adult: Oral: 2-4 g to start, then 2-4 g/daily in 3-6 divided doses

Sulfadoxine and Pyrimethamine (sul fa dox' een)

Brand Names Fansidar®

Use Treatment of *Plasmodium falciparum* malaria in patients in whom chloroquine resistance is suspected; malaria prophylaxis for travelers to areas where chloroquine-resistant malaria is endemic

Pregnancy Risk Factor C

Usual Dosage Treatment of acute attack of malaria: A single dose of the following number of Fansidar® tablets is used in sequence with quinine or alone:

Adult: 2-3 tablets

Children:
9-14 years of age: 2 tablets
4-8 years: 1 tablet
< 4 years: 1/2 tablet

Malaria prophylaxis:
The first dose of Fansidar® should be taken one or two days before departure to an endemic area; administration should be continued during the stay and for 4-6 weeks after return

Adult: 1 tablet once weekly; 2 tablets once every two weeks

Children:
9-14 years of age: 3/4 tablet once weekly; 1 1/2 tablets once every two weeks
4-8 years: 1/2 tablet once weekly; 1 tablet once every two weeks
< 4 years: 1/4 tablet once weekly; 1/2 tablet once every two weeks

Sulfamethoprim® *see* Sulfamethoxazole and Trimethoprim
on next page

Sulfamethoxazole (sul fa meth ox' a zole)

Brand Names Gantanol®

Use Treatment of urinary tract infections; acute otitis media in children; acute exacerbations of chronic bronchitis in adults

Pregnancy Risk Factor B/D

Usual Dosage Oral:

Adult: 2 g stat, 1 g twice daily; maximum: 3 g/24 hours

Children: 25-30 mg/kg twice daily; maximum: 3 g/24 hours

Newborn: Not recommended

Sulfamethoxazole and Phenazopyridine

Brand Names Azo Gantanol®

Use Treatment of urinary tract infections complicated with pain

Pregnancy Risk Factor B/D

Usual Dosage Four (4) tablets to start, then 2 tablets twice daily for up to two days, then switch to sulfamethoxazole only

Sulfamethoxazole and Trimethoprim

Brand Names Bactrim™; Bactrim™ DS; Cotrim®; Cotrim® DS; Septra®; Septra® DS; Sulfamethoprim®; Sulfatrim®; Sulfatrim® DS; Sulfoxaprim®; Sulfoxaprim® DS; Trisulfam®; Uroplus® DS; Uroplus® SS

Synonyms Co-trimoxazole; SMX-TMP; TMP-SMX; Trimethoprim and Sulfamethoxazole

Use Treatment of urinary tract infections; acute otitis media in children; acute exacerbations of chronic bronchitis in adults

Pregnancy Risk Factor B/D

Usual Dosage Oral:

Adult: UTI/chronic bronchitis: One (1) double strength tablet every 12 hours for 10-14 days

Children: Acute otitis media:
> 2 months: 8 mg/kg/day trimethoprim and 40 mg/kg/day sulfamethoxazole given in two divided doses every 12 hours for 10 days
10 kg: 5 mL every 12 hours
20 kg: 10 mL every 12 hours
30 kg: 15 mL every 12 hours
40 kg: 20 mL every 12 hours

Sulfamylon® *see* Mafenide Acetate *on page 209*

Sulfanilamide

Brand Names AVC™ Cream; AVC™ Suppository; Vagitrol®

Use Treatment of vulvovaginitis caused by *Candida albicans*

Pregnancy Risk Factor B/D

Usual Dosage One (1) applicatorful once or twice daily continued through one complete menstrual cycle

Sulfasalazine (sul fa sal' a zeen)

Brand Names Azulfidine®; Azulfidine® EN-tabs®

Synonyms Salicylazosulfapyridine

Use Management of ulcerative colitis

Pregnancy Risk Factor B/D

Usual Dosage Oral:

Adult: 1 g 3-4 times daily, 2 g/day maintenance

Children: > 2 years of age: 40-60 mg/kg/day in 3-6 divided doses; maintenance dose is 30 mg/kg in four divided doses; maximum: 2 g/24 hours

Sulfatrim® *see* Sulfamethoxazole and Trimethoprim *on this page*

Sulfatrim® DS *see* Sulfamethoxazole and Trimethoprim *on this page*

Sulfinpyrazone (sul fin peer' a zone)

Brand Names Anturane®

Use Treatment of chronic gouty arthritis and intermittent gouty arthritis

Pregnancy Risk Factor C

Usual Dosage 200 mg twice daily

Sulfisoxazole (sul fi sox' a zole)
Brand Names Gantrisin®
Synonyms Sulfisoxazole Acetyl; Sulphafurazole
Use Treatment of urinary tract infections and nocardiosis
Pregnancy Risk Factor B/D
Usual Dosage

Pelvic inflammatory disease (prepubertal children): Oral: 100 mg/kg/day in four doses in combination with I.V. ceftriaxone or cefuroxime

Adult:
Oral: 2-4 g stat, 4-8 g in divided doses every 4-6 hours
I.M., S.C.: 50 mg/kg stat, then 100 mg/kg/day in divided doses every 8-12 hours
Ointment: Apply a ribbon (1.25-2.5 cm) in conjunctival sac four times daily and at bedtime

Children: > 2 months old:
Oral: 75 mg/kg stat, 120-150 mg/kg/24 hours in divided doses every 4-6 hours; maximum: 6 g/24 hours
I.M., S.C.: 50 mg/kg stat, then 100 mg/kg/day in divided doses every 8-12 hours

Sulfisoxazole Acetyl *see* Sulfisoxazole *on this page*

Sulfisoxazole and Erythromycin *see* Erythromycin and Sulfisoxazole *on page 134*

Sulfisoxazole and Phenazopyridine
Brand Names Azo Gantrisin®
Use Treatment of urinary tract infections and nocardiosis
Pregnancy Risk Factor B/D
Usual Dosage 4-6 tablets to start, then two tablets four times a day for two days, then continue with sulfisoxazole only

Sulfoxaprim® *see* Sulfamethoxazole and Trimethoprim
on previous page

Sulfoxaprim® DS *see* Sulfamethoxazole and Trimethoprim
on previous page

Sulfur and Salicylic Acid
Brand Names Fostex® [OTC]; Sebulex® [OTC]
Synonyms Salicylic Acid and Sulfur
Use Therapeutic shampoo for dandruff and seborrheal dermatitis; acne skin cleanser
Usual Dosage Shampoo is normally used every other day

Sulfur and Sodium Sulfacetamide
Brand Names Sulfacet-R®
Synonyms Sodium Sulfacetamide and Sulfur
Use Aid in the treatment of acne vulgaris, acne rosacea and seborrheic dermatitis
Usual Dosage Apply in a thin film 1-3 times a day

Sulindac (sul in' dak)
Brand Names Clinoril®
Use Management of inflammatory disorders
Pregnancy Risk Factor B/D
Usual Dosage 150-200 mg twice daily

Sulphafurazole see Sulfisoxazole on previous page

Sultrin™ see Sulfabenzamide, Sulfacetamide, and Sulfathiazole on page 336

Sumycin® see Tetracycline on page 346

SuperChar® [OTC] see Charcoal on page 68

Super D® Perles [OTC] see Vitamin A and Vitamin D on page 377

Suprax® see Cefixime on page 63

Suprofen (soo proe' fen)
Brand Names Profenal®
Use Inhibition of intraoperative miosis
Usual Dosage On day of surgery, instill 2 drops in conjunctival sac at 3, 2, and 1 hour prior to surgery; or 2 drops in sac every 4 hours, while awake, the day preceding surgery

Surbex® [OTC] see Vitamin B Complex on page 377

Surbex-T® Filmtabs® [OTC] see Vitamin B Complex With Vitamin C on page 377

Surbex® with C Filmtabs® [OTC] see Vitamin B Complex With Vitamin C on page 377

Surfak® [OTC] see Docusate on page 121

Surgicel® see Cellulose, Oxidized on page 65

Surgilube® [OTC] see Lubricating Jelly on page 208

Surital® see Thiamylal Sodium on page 351

Surmontil® see Trimipramine Maleate on page 364

Sus-Phrine® see Epinephrine on page 131

Sustaire® see Theophylline on page 348

Sutilains (soo' ti lains)
Brand Names Travase®
Use To promote debridement of necrotic debris, as an adjunct in the treatment of 2nd and 3rd degree burns, decubitus ulcers
Pregnancy Risk Factor D
Usual Dosage Apply in a thin layer extending 1/4-1/2 inch beyond the tissue being debrided, thoroughly cleanse irrigated wound, apply loose moist dressing; repeat 3-4 times daily

Suxamethonium Chloride see Succinylcholine Chloride on page 334

Sweet Oil *see* Olive Oil *on page 259*

Syllact® [OTC] *see* Psyllium *on page 308*

Symadine® *see* Amantadine Hydrochloride *on page 16*

Symmetrel® *see* Amantadine Hydrochloride *on page 16*

Synalar® *see* Fluocinolone Acetonide *on page 150*

Synalgos® [OTC] *see* Aspirin *on page 30*

Synalgos®-DC *see* Dihydrocodeine Compound *on page 115*

Synarel® *see* Nafarelin Acetate *on page 244*

Synemol® *see* Fluocinolone Acetonide *on page 150*

Synkayvite® *see* Menadiol Sodium Diphosphate *on page 217*

Synthroid® *see* Levothyroxine Sodium *on page 202*

Synthrox® *see* Levothyroxine Sodium *on page 202*

Syntocinon® *see* Oxytocin *on page 266*

Syroxine® *see* Levothyroxine Sodium *on page 202*

T₃/T₄ Liotrix *see* Liotrix *on page 205*

T₃ Thyronine Sodium *see* Liothyronine Sodium *on page 205*

T₄ Thyroxine Sodium *see* Levothyroxine Sodium *on page 202*

Tacaryl® *see* Methdilazine Hydrochloride *on page 226*

TACE® *see* Chlorotrianisene *on page 72*

Tagamet® *see* Cimetidine *on page 79*

Talwin® *see* Pentazocine *on page 275*

Talwin® Compound *see* Pentazocine and Aspirin *on page 275*

Talwin® NX *see* Pentazocine *on page 275*

Tambocor® *see* Flecainide Acetate *on page 148*

Tamoxifen Citrate (ta mox' i fen)
Brand Names Nolvadex®
Use Palliative or adjunctive treatment of advanced breast cancer
Pregnancy Risk Factor D
Usual Dosage Oral: 10-20 mg twice daily

Tao® *see* Troleandomycin *on page 366*

Tapazole® *see* Methimazole *on page 226*

Taractan® *see* Chlorprothixene *on page 77*

TAT *see* Tetanus Antitoxin *on page 345*

Tavist® *see* Clemastine Fumarate *on page 81*

Tazidime™ *see* Ceftazidime *on page 64*

TCN *see* Tetracycline *on page 346*

Tearisol® [OTC] *see* Artificial Tears *on page 29*

Tebamide® *see* Trimethobenzamide Hydrochloride *on page 364*

T.E.C.® *see* Trace Metals *on page 358*

Tedral® *see* Theophylline, Ephedrine and Phenobarbital *on page 350*

Tegison® *see* Etretinate *on page 143*

Tegopen® *see* Cloxacillin Sodium *on page 85*

Tegretol® *see* Carbamazepine *on page 57*

Tegrin® [OTC] *see* Allantoin and Coal Tar *on page 12*

Teldrin® [OTC] *see* Chlorpheniramine Maleate *on page 74*

Telepaque® *see* Iopanoic Acid *on page 189*

Teline® *see* Tetracycline *on page 346*

Temaril® *see* Trimeprazine Tartrate *on page 363*

Temazepam (te maz' e pam)
Brand Names Restoril®
Use Treatment of anxiety and as an adjunct in the treatment of depression; also may be used in the management of panic attacks
Restrictions C-IV
Pregnancy Risk Factor X
Usual Dosage Adult: Oral: 15-30 mg at bedtime

Temovate® *see* Clobetasol Dipropionate *on page 82*

Tenex® *see* Guanfacine Hydrochloride *on page 164*

Teniposide (ten i poe' side)
Synonyms EPT; VM-26; Vumon
Use Treatment of Hodgkin's and non-Hodgkin's lymphomas, acute lymphocytic leukemia, bladder carcinoma and neuroblastoma
Pregnancy Risk Factor D
Usual Dosage I.V.:

Adult: 50-180 mg/m^2 once or twice weekly for 4-6 weeks

Children: 130 mg/m^2/week, increasing to 150 mg/m^2 after three weeks and to 180 mg/m^2 after six weeks

Tenormin® *see* Atenolol *on page 31*

Tensilon® *see* Edrophonium Chloride *on page 128*

Tenuate® *see* Diethylpropion Hydrochloride *on page 112*

Tepanil® *see* Diethylpropion Hydrochloride *on page 112*

Terazol® 7 *see* Terconazole *on next page*

Terazosin (ter ay' zoe sin)
Brand Names Hytrin®
Use Management of mild to moderate hypertension
Pregnancy Risk Factor C
Usual Dosage Adult: Oral: 1 mg; slowly increase dose to achieve desired blood pressure, up to 20 mg/day

Terbutaline Sulfate (ter byoo' ta leen)
Brand Names Brethaire®; Brethine®; Bricanyl®
Use Bronchodilator in reversible airway obstruction and bronchial asthma
Pregnancy Risk Factor B
Usual Dosage

Adult:
Inhalation (unlabeled use): 5-7 mg (5-7 mL) undiluted every 4-6 hours as necessary
Oral: Initial: 2.5 mg/dose three times/day; maintenance: usually 5 mg/dose or 0.075 mg/kg/dose 3-4 times/day
S.C.: 0.25 mg/dose repeated in 15-30 minutes as necessary for one (1) time only; a total dose of 0.5 mg should not be exceeded within a four hour period

Children: < 12 years of age:
Inhalation (unlabeled use): 0.1-0.3 mg/kg/dose every 2-6 hours as necessary; maximum: 5-7 mL/dose
Oral: Initial: 0.05 mg/kg/dose three times/day, increased gradually as required; maximum: 0.15 mg/kg/dose 3-4 times a day or a total of 5 mg/24 hours
S.C.: 0.005-0.01 mg/kg/dose to a maximum of 0.4 mg/dose every 15-20 minutes for three doses

Terconazole (ter kon' a zole)
Brand Names Terazol® 7
Synonyms Triaconazole
Use Local treatment of vulvovaginal candidiasis
Usual Dosage One applicatorful in vagina at bedtime for 7 consecutive days

Terfenadine (ter fen' a deen)
Brand Names Seldane®
Use Perennial and seasonal allergic rhinitis and other allergic symptoms including urticaria
Pregnancy Risk Factor C
Usual Dosage Oral:

Adult and Children: > 12 years: 60 mg twice daily

Children:
6-12 years: 30-60 mg twice daily
3-6 years: 15 mg twice daily

Terfonyl® see Sulfadiazine, Sulfamethazine and Sulfamerazine on page 336

Teriparatide (ter i par' a tide)
Brand Names Parathar™
Use Diagnosis of hypocalcemia in either hypoparathyroidism or pseudohypoparathyroidism
Pregnancy Risk Factor C
(Continued)

Teriparatide *(Continued)*

Usual Dosage I.V.:

Adult: 200 units over 10 minutes

Children: ≥ 3 years old: 3 units/kg up to 200 units

Terpin Hydrate (ter' pin)

Synonyms ETH; Terpinol

Use Symptomatic relief of cough due to minor bronchial irritations including colds

Pregnancy Risk Factor C

Usual Dosage Oral:

Adult: 170 mg every 3-4 hours

Children:

10-12 years: 85 mg 3-4 times daily

5-9 years: 40-45 mg 3-4 times daily

1-4 years: 20-25 mg 3-4 times daily

Terpin Hydrate and Codeine

Synonyms ETH and C

Use Symptomatic relief of cough

Restrictions C-V

Pregnancy Risk Factor C

Usual Dosage Based on codeine content

Adult: 10-20 mg/dose every 4-6 hours as needed

Children (not recommended): 1-1.5 mg/kg/24 hours divided every four hours to a maximum of 30 mg/24 hours

6-12 years: 2.5-5 mL every 4-6 hours as needed

2-6 years: 1.25-2.5 mL every 4-6 hours as needed

Terpinol *see* Terpin Hydrate *on this page*

Terramycin® IV *see* Oxytetracycline Hydrochloride *on page 266*

Terramycin® Ophthalmic Ointment *see* Oxytetracycline and Polymyxin B *on page 266*

Teslac® *see* Testolactone *on this page*

TESPA *see* Thiotepa *on page 353*

Tessalon® Perles *see* Benzonatate *on page 41*

Tes-Tape® [OTC] *see* Diagnostic Test for Glucose in Urine *on page 107*

Testoject® *see* Testosterone *on next page*

Testoject®-L.A. *see* Testosterone *on next page*

Testolactone (tess toe lak' tone)

Brand Names Teslac®

Use Palliative treatment of advanced disseminated breast carcinoma

Pregnancy Risk Factor C

Usual Dosage Adult: Oral: 250 mg four times daily

Testosterone (tess toss' ter one)

Brand Names Andro®; Andro-Cyp®; Andro-L.A.®; Androlan®; Andronaq®; Andronaq®-L.A.; Andronate®; Andropository®; Andryl®; Delatestryl®; Depotest®; Depo®-Testosterone; Duratest®; Durathate®; Everone®; Histerone®; Testoject®; Testoject®-L.A.; Testrin® P.A.

Synonyms Aqueous Testosterone; Testosterone Cypionate; Testosterone Enanthate

Use Androgen replacement therapy in the treatment of delayed male puberty; postpartum breast pain and engorgement; inoperable breast cancer; male hypogonadism

Pregnancy Risk Factor X

Usual Dosage I.M.:

Male hypogonadism:
  Initiation of pubertal growth: 40-50 mg/m^2/dose monthly until the growth rate falls to prepubertal levels ($\sim$ 5 cm/year)
  During terminal growth phase: 100 mg/m^2/dose monthly until growth ceases
  Maintenance virilizing dose: 100 mg/m^2/dose twice monthly or 50-400 mg/dose every 2-4 weeks

Delayed puberty: Children: 40-50 mg/m^2/dose monthly for six months

Inoperable breast cancer: Adult: 200-400 mg every 2-4 weeks

Testosterone Cypionate see Testosterone on this page

Testosterone Enanthate see Testosterone on this page

Testred® see Methyltestosterone on page 232

Testrin® P.A. see Testosterone on this page

Tetanus and Diphtheria Toxoid see Diphtheria and Tetanus Toxoid on page 118

Tetanus Antitoxin

Synonyms TAT

Use Tetanus prophylaxis or treatment only when tetanus immune globulin (TIG) is not available

Pregnancy Risk Factor D

Usual Dosage

Prophylaxis:
  Adult and Children: I.M., S.C.: > 30 kg: 3000-5000 units
  Children: < 30 kg: 1500 units

Treatment: Adult and Children: Inject 10,000-40,000 units into wound; give 40,000-100,000 units I.V.

Tetanus Immune Globulin, Human

Brand Names Hyper-Tet®

Synonyms TIG

Use Passive immunization against tetanus

Pregnancy Risk Factor C

(Continued)

Tetanus Immune Globulin, Human *(Continued)*

Usual Dosage I.M.:
Adult: 250 units
Children: 4 units/kg

Tetanus Toxoid Adsorbed

Use Active immunity against tetanus
Pregnancy Risk Factor C
Usual Dosage I.M., S.C.: 0.5 mL

Tetanus Toxoid, Fluid

Synonyms Tetanus Toxoid Plain
Use Active immunization against tetanus
Pregnancy Risk Factor C
Usual Dosage Inject 3 doses of 0.5 mL I.M. or S.C. at 4-8 week intervals with fourth dose given about 6-12 months after third dose

Tetanus Toxoid Plain *see* Tetanus Toxoid, Fluid *on this page*

Tetracaine Hydrochloride *(tet' ra kane)*

Brand Names Pontocaine®
Synonyms Amethocaine Hydrochloride
Use Spinal anesthesia; local anesthesia in the eye for various diagnostic and examination purposes; topically applied to nose and throat for various diagnostic procedures
Pregnancy Risk Factor C
Usual Dosage Adult:
Spinal anesthesia: Subarachnoid injection: 5-20 mg; saddle block: 2-5 mg
Ophthalmic: Solution: Use 1-2 drops; ointment: Apply 1/2-1 inch to lower conjunctival fornix
Mucous membranes: Topical solution: Apply as needed

Tetracaine Hydrochloride, Benzocaine Butyl Aminobenzoate and Benzalkonium Chloride *see* Benzocaine, Butyl Aminobenzoate, Tetracaine and Benzalkonium Chloride *on page 41*

Tetracaine With Dextrose

Brand Names Pontocaine® With Dextrose
Use Spinal anesthesia (saddle block)
Usual Dosage Dose varies with procedure, depth of anesthesia, duration desired and physical condition of patient

Tetraclear® [OTC] *see* Tetrahydrozoline Hydrochloride *on next page*

Tetracycline *(tet ra sye' kleen)*

Brand Names Achromycin®; Achromycin® V; Nor-tet®; Panmycin®; Robitet®; Sumycin®; Teline®; Tetracyn®; Tetralan®
Synonyms TCN; Tetracycline Hydrochloride

Use Treatment of susceptible bacterial infections, some gram-positive and gram-negative pathogens. Also some unusual organisms including *Mycoplasma*, *Chlamydia*, and *Rickettsia*; may also be used for acne, exacerbations of chronic bronchitis, and treatment of gonorrhea and syphilis in patients that are allergic to penicillin

Pregnancy Risk Factor D

Usual Dosage

Adult:
Oral: 1-2 g/day in 2-4 divided doses
I.M.: 250-300 mg/day in divided doses every 8-12 hours
I.V.: 250-500 mg every 12 hours, maximum: 500 mg every six hours

Children: > 8 years of age:
Oral: 25-50 mg/kg/day given every six hours, maximum: 3 g/day
I.M.: 15-25 mg/kg/day given every 8-12 hours, maximum: 250 mg/day
I.V.: 20-30 mg/kg/day given every 8-12 hours, maximum: 2 g/day

Tetracycline Hydrochloride *see* Tetracycline *on previous page*

Tetracyn® *see* Tetracycline *on previous page*

Tetrahydrocannabinol, THC *see* Dronabinol *on page 124*

Tetrahydrozoline Hydrochloride (tet ra hye drozz' a leen)
Brand Names Collyrium Fresh® [OTC]; Eye-Zine® [OTC]; Murine® Plus [OTC]; Ocu-Drop® [OTC]; Optigene® [OTC]; Soothe® [OTC]; Tetraclear® [OTC]; Tetra-Ide® [OTC]; Tyzine®; Visine® [OTC]
Synonyms Tetryzoline
Use Symptomatic relief of nasal congestion and conjunctival congestion
Pregnancy Risk Factor C
Usual Dosage

Nasal congestion:
Adult and Children: > 6 years of age: Use 2-4 drops or 0.1% spray nasal mucosa every 4-6 hours as needed
Children: 2-6 years: Use 2-3 drops of 0.05% solution every 4-6 hours as needed

Conjunctival congestion: Adult: 1-2 drops in each eye 2-3 times daily

Tetra-Ide® [OTC] *see* Tetrahydrozoline Hydrochloride *on this page*

Tetralan® *see* Tetracycline *on previous page*

Tetryzoline *see* Tetrahydrozoline Hydrochloride *on this page*

TG *see* Thioguanine *on page 352*

6-TG *see* Thioguanine *on page 352*

T/Gel® [OTC] *see* Coal Tar *on page 85*

T-Gen® *see* Trimethobenzamide Hydrochloride *on page 364*

Tham® *see* Tromethamine *on page 366*

Tham-E® *see* Tromethamine *on page 366*

Theelin® *see* Estrone *on page 137*

Theo-24® see Theophylline *on this page*

Theobid® see Theophylline *on this page*

Theochron® see Theophylline *on this page*

Theoclear® L.A. see Theophylline *on this page*

Theo-Dur® see Theophylline *on this page*

Theolair™ see Theophylline *on this page*

Theon® see Theophylline *on this page*

Theophylline (thee off' i lin)

Brand Names Accurbron®; Aerolate®; Aerolate III®; Aerolate JR®; Aerolate SR® S; Aquaphyllin®; Asmalix®; Bronkodyl®; Constant-T®; Duraphyl™; Elixicon®; Elixophyllin®; Elixophyllin® SR; LaBID®; Lixolin®; Lodrane®; Quibron®-T; Quibron®-T/SR; Respbid®; Slo-bid™; Slo-Phyllin®; Somophyllin®-CRT; Somophyllin®-T; Sustaire®; Theo-24®; Theobid®; Theochron®; Theoclear® L.A.; Theo-Dur®; Theolair™; Theon®; Theophyl-SR®; Theospan®-SR; Theo-Time®; Theovent®; Uniphyl®

Synonyms Theophylline Anhydrous

Use As a bronchodilator in reversible airway obstruction due to asthma or COPD

Pregnancy Risk Factor C

Usual Dosage Dosage should be determined by plasma level monitoring

Acute symptoms requiring rapid theophyllinization in patients not receiving theophylline: To achieve a rapid effect, an initial loading dose is required; dosage recommendations are for theophylline anhydrous. See Table 1.

Infants (preterm up to < six months): There appears to be a delay in theophylline elimination in infants < one year old, especially neonates; both the initial dose and maintenance dosage should be conservative. See Table 2.

Acute symptoms requiring rapid theophyllinization in patients receiving theophylline: Each 0.5 mg/kg of theophylline administered as a loading dose will result in a 1 μg/mL increase in serum theophylline concentration. Ideally, defer the loading dose if a serum theophylline concentration can be obtained rapidly. However, if this is not possible, exercise clinical judgment. When there is sufficient respiratory distress to warrant a small risk, then 2.5 mg/kg of theophylline administered in rapidly absorbed form is likely to increase serum concentration by approximately 5 μg/mL. If the patient is not experiencing theophylline toxicity, this is unlikely to result in dangerous adverse effects. Maintenance doses are as in Table 2.

Chronic therapy: Slow clinical titration is generally preferred. Initial dose: 16 mg/kg/24 hours or 400 mg/24 hours, whichever is less, of anhydrous theophylline in divided doses at six or eight hour intervals; increasing dose: the above dosage may be increased in approximately 25% increments at two to three day intervals so long as the drug is tolerated or until the maximum dose is reached.

Maximum dose (where the serum concentration is not measured): Do not attempt to maintain any dose that is not tolerated. See Table 3.

Table 1

Patient Group	Oral Loading	Followed by	Maintenance
Children 6 mo–9 y	6 mg/kg (7.6)*	4 mg/kg q 4 h x 3 doses (5.1)*	4 mg/kg q 6 h (5.1)*
Children 9–16 y and young adult smokers	6 mg/kg (7.6)*	3 mg/kg q 4 h x 3 doses (3.8)*	3 mg/kg q 6 h (3.8)*
Otherwise healthy nonsmoking adults	6 mg/kg (7.6)*	3 mg/kg q 6 h x 2 doses (3.8)*	3 mg/kg q 8 h (3.8)*
Older patients and patients with cor pulmonale	6 mg/kg (7.6)*	2 mg/kg q 6 h x 2 doses (2.5)*	2 mg/kg q 8 h (2.5)*
Patients with congestive heart failure	6 mg/kg (7.6)*	2 mg/kg q 8 h x 2 doses (2.5)*	1–2 mg/kg q 12 h (1.3–2.5)*

Adapted from *Facts & Comparisons*, 1990, 788–9.
* = Aminophylline dihydrate.

Table 2

Infant	Loading Dose	Maintenance Dose
Preterm (≤ 40 wk postconception*)	1 mg/kg for each 2 µg/mL serum theophylline concentration desired	1 mg/kg q 12 h
Term (birth or 40 wk postconception*) up to 4 wk postnatal		1–2 mg/kg q 12 h
4–8 wk		1–2 mg/kg q 8 h
beyond 8 wk		1–3 mg/kg q 6 h

Adapted from *Facts & Comparisons*, 1990, 788–9.
* Postconception age = gestational age at birth + postnatal age.

Table 3

Age	Maximum Daily Dose
< 9 y	24 mg/kg/d (30.4)*
9–12 y	20 mg/kg/d (25.3)*
12–16 y	18 mg/kg/d (22.8)*
> 16 y	13 mg/kg/d or 900 mg (16.5 or 1100)* (whichever is less)

Adapted from *Facts & Comparisons*, 1990, 788–9.
* = Aminophylline dihydrate.

Exercise caution in younger children who cannot complain of minor side effects. Older adults and those with cor pulmonale. CHF or liver disease may have unusually low dosage requirements; they may experience toxicity at the maximal dosage recommended in Table 3.

Theophylline Anhydrous see Theophylline on page 348

Theophylline, Ephedrine and Hydroxyzine
Brand Names Marax®
Use Possibly effective for controlling bronchospastic disorders
Pregnancy Risk Factor C
Usual Dosage

Adult: One tablet 2-4 times daily

Children:
> 5 years of age: 1/2 tablet 2-4 times a day or 5 mL 3-4 times daily
2-5 years: 1/2 tablet 2-4 times a day or 2.5 mL 3-4 times daily

Theophylline, Ephedrine and Phenobarbital
Brand Names Tedral®
Synonyms Ephedrine, Theophylline and Phenobarbital
Use Prevention and symptomatic treatment of bronchial asthma; relief of asthmatic bronchitis and other bronchospastic disorders
Pregnancy Risk Factor D
Usual Dosage

Adult: 1-2 tablets or 10-20 mL every four hours

Children: > 60 pounds: One tablet or 5 mL every four hours

Theophylline Ethylenediamine see Aminophylline
on page 18

Theophyl-SR® see Theophylline on page 348

Theospan®-SR see Theophylline on page 348

Theo-Time® see Theophylline on page 348

Theovent® see Theophylline on page 348

Thera-Combex® H-P Kapseals® [OTC] see Vitamin B Complex
With Vitamin C on page 377

Thermazene® see Silver Sulfadiazine on page 324

Thiabendazole (thye a ben' da zole)
Brand Names Mintezol®
Synonyms Tiabendazole
Use Systemic infections with pinworm, roundworm, threadworm, whipworm, trichinosis and cutaneous larva migrans (creeping eruption)
Pregnancy Risk Factor C
Usual Dosage Maximum daily dose is 3 g

Adult and Children:
Systemic infections: Oral: 25 mg/kg/day in two doses for two successive days

Cutaneous infestations with larva migrans: 25 mg/kg twice a day for 2-5 days

Thiamazole *see* Methimazole *on page 226*

Thiamine Hydrochloride (thye' a min)
Brand Names Betalin®S; Biamine®

Synonyms Aneurine Hydrochloride; Thiaminium Chloride Hydrochloride; Vitamin B_1

Use Treatment of thiamine deficiency including beriberi, Wernicke's encephalopathy syndrome, and peripheral neuritis associated with pellagra, alcoholic patients with altered sensorium; various genetic metabolic disorders

Pregnancy Risk Factor A/C

Usual Dosage

Adult:

Noncritically ill thiamine deficiency: Oral: 5-30 mg/day for one month

Beriberi: I.M.: 10-20 mg three times a day for two weeks, then switch to 5-10 mg orally every day for one month (oral as therapeutic multivitamin)

RDA: 1.4 mg (male); 1 mg (female)

Children:

Noncritically ill thiamine deficiency: Oral: 10-50 mg/day in divided doses every day for two weeks followed by 5-10 mg/day every day for one month

Beriberi: I.M.: 10-25 mg every day for two weeks, then 5-10 mg orally every day for one month (oral as therapeutic multivitamin)

RDA: Infants/children: 0.3-1.4 mg

Thiaminium Chloride Hydrochloride *see* Thiamine
Hydrochloride *on this page*

Thiamylal Sodium (thye am' i lal)
Brand Names Anestatal®; Surital®

Use Induction of anesthesia; maintenance of anesthesia; agent for inducing a hypnotic state

Restrictions C-III

Usual Dosage Adult: I.V.:

Induction: 2.5 % of intermittent injection

Maintenance: 0.3% intermittent injection or drip

Thiethylperazine Maleate (thye eth il per' a zeen)
Brand Names Norzine®; Torecan®

Use Relief of nausea and vomiting

Pregnancy Risk Factor X

Usual Dosage Adult:

Oral, rectal: 10-30 mg every day in divided doses

I.M.: 2 mL 1-3 times daily

Thioguanine (thye oh gwah' neen)

Synonyms 2-Amino-6-mercaptopurine; TG; 6-TG; 6-Thioguanine; Tioguanine

Use Remission induction in acute myelogenous leukemia; treatment of chronic myelogenous leukemia and granulocytic leukemia

Pregnancy Risk Factor D

Usual Dosage Adult and Children: For induction of remission: Oral:
2 mg/kg/day calculated to nearest 20 mg, may increase, cautiously, to 3 mg/kg/day; if no response in four weeks (dosages are based on clinical and hematological response)
Alternate dosage: 75-200 mg/m^2/day in 1-2 divided doses for 5-7 days or until remission is attained
Maintenance dosage: Varies, but often given as 2 mg/kg/day (dosages of 75-400 mg/m^2 have been used)

6-Thioguanine see Thioguanine on this page

Thiopental Sodium (thye oh pen' tal)

Brand Names Pentothal® Sodium

Use Induction of anesthesia; control of convulsive states

Restrictions C-III

Pregnancy Risk Factor C

Usual Dosage

Increased cranial pressure: 1.5-5 mg/kg/dose, repeat as required to control intracranial pressure

General anesthesia:
Induction: Adult: I.V.: 3-5 mg/kg one time; children: 2 mg/kg one time
Maintenance: Adult: I.V.: 50-100 mg as needed; children: 1 mg/kg as needed (give via rapid infusion over 1-2 minutes, avoid extravasation or intra-arterial injection)

Thioridazine (thye oh rid' a zeen)

Brand Names Mellaril®; Mellaril-S®

Synonyms Thioridazine Hydrochloride

Use Management of manifestations of psychotic disorders; depressive neurosis; alcohol withdrawal; dementia in elderly; behavioral problems in children

Pregnancy Risk Factor C

Usual Dosage Oral:

Adult: Psychosis: Initially, 150-300 mg/day in three divided doses, increase gradually if necessary; maximum: 800 mg/day

Children: 2-12 years of age: 0.5-1 mg/kg/day divided every 6-12 hours, increase gradually if necessary; maximum: 3 mg/kg/day

Short-term treatment of anxiety/depressive states: Range: 20-200 mg/day (usual 25 mg three times/day)

Thioridazine Hydrochloride see Thioridazine on this page

Thiotepa (thye oh tep' a)
Synonyms TESPA; Triethylenethiophosphoramide; TSPA
Use Treatment of superficial tumors of the bladder; palliative treatment of adenocarcinoma of breast or ovary; lymphomas such as Hodgkin's; controlling intracavitary effusions caused by metastatic tumors
Pregnancy Risk Factor D
Usual Dosage

Adult:
I.V.: 0.2-0.4 mg/kg at 1-4 week intervals
Intracavitary: 0.6-0.8 mg/kg

High dose investigational protocol: I.V.: 65-175 mg/m^2 as a single dose

Children: I.V.: 25-65 mg/m^2 as a single dose

Thiothixene (thye oh thix' een)
Brand Names Navane®
Synonyms Tiotixene
Use Management of psychotic disorders
Pregnancy Risk Factor C
Usual Dosage

Adult and Children: > 12 years: Mild to moderate psychosis:
Oral: 2 mg three times a day, up to 20-30 mg/day; more severe psychosis: Initially, 5 mg two times a day, may increase gradually, if necessary; maximum: 60 mg/day
I.M.: 4 mg 2-4 times daily, initially; may increase to optimum 16-20 mg/day; maximum: 30 mg/day; switch to oral dose as soon as feasible

Children: < 12 years: Oral: Approximately 0.25 mg/kg/day (dose not well established)

Thiuretic® *see* Hydrochlorothiazide *on page 172*

Thorazine® *see* Chlorpromazine Hydrochloride *on page 76*

Thrombin, Topical (throm' bin)
Use Hemostasis where ever minor bleeding from capillaries and small venules
Pregnancy Risk Factor C
Usual Dosage Use 1000-2000 units/mL of solution where bleeding is profuse; apply powder directly to the site of bleeding or on oozing surfaces; use 100 units/mL for bleeding from skin or mucosal surfaces

Thymopentin (thye' moe pen tin)
Brand Names Timunox®
Synonyms Thymopoietin; TP5
Use Immunomodulator

Thymopoietin *see* Thymopentin *on this page*

Thypinone® *see* Protirelin *on page 306*

Thyrar® *see* Thyroid *on next page*

Thyro-Block® *see* Potassium Iodide *on page 291*

Thyroglobulin (thye roe glob' yoo lin)
Brand Names Proloid®
Use Replacement or supplemental therapy in hypothyroidism
Pregnancy Risk Factor A
Usual Dosage Oral: 65-200 mg/day

Thyroid (thye' roid)
Brand Names Armour® Thyroid; S-P-T; Thyrar®; Westhroid®
Synonyms Dessicated Thyroid; Thyroid Extract
Use Replacement or supplemental therapy in hypothyroidism
Pregnancy Risk Factor A
Usual Dosage Adult: Oral: 65-145 mg/day

Thyroid Extract *see* Thyroid *on this page*

Thyroid-Stimulating Hormone *see* Thyrotropin *on this page*

Thyrolar® *see* Liotrix *on page 205*

Thyrotropin (thye roe troe' pin)
Brand Names Thytropar®
Synonyms Thyroid-Stimulating Hormone; TSH
Use Diagnostic aid to differentiate thyroid failure; diagnosis of decreased thyroid reserve
Pregnancy Risk Factor C
Usual Dosage I.M., S.C.: 10 IU every day for 1-3 days; follow by a radioiodine study 24 hours past last injection, no response in thyroid failure, substantial response in pituitary failure

Thytropar® *see* Thyrotropin *on this page*

Tiabendazole *see* Thiabendazole *on page 350*

Ticar® *see* Ticarcillin Disodium *on this page*

Ticarcillin and Clavulanic Acid
Brand Names Timentin®
Synonyms Ticarcillin Disodium and Clavulanate Potassium
Use To treat infections of lower respiratory tract, urinary tract, skin and skin structures, bone and joint, and septicemia caused by susceptible organisms
Pregnancy Risk Factor B
Usual Dosage I.V.:

Adult: 3.1 g every 4-6 hours; maximum: 18-24 g/day

Children: < 60 kg: 200-300 mg/kg/day in divided doses every 4-6 hours

Neonates/Infants: Dosages available for ticarcillin (no information available for the ticarcillin/clavulanic acid product)

Ticarcillin Disodium (tye kar sill' in)
Brand Names Ticar®
Use Treatment of susceptible bacterial infections caused by gram-negative and some anaerobic strains

Pregnancy Risk Factor B
Usual Dosage

Adult:
I.M.: 1-4 g every 4-6 hours
I.V.: 1 g every six hours

Children:
I.M.: 50-100 mg/kg/day in divided doses every 6-8 hours
I.V.: 50-300 mg/kg/day in divided doses every 4-8 hours

Ticarcillin Disodium and Clavulanate Potassium see Ticarcillin and Clavulanic Acid on previous page

Ticon® see Trimethobenzamide Hydrochloride on page 364

TIG see Tetanus Immune Globulin, Human on page 345

Tigan® see Trimethobenzamide Hydrochloride on page 364

Tiject® see Trimethobenzamide Hydrochloride on page 364

Timentin® see Ticarcillin and Clavulanic Acid on previous page

Timolol Maleate (tye' moe lole)
Brand Names Blocadren®; Timoptic®
Use Treatment of hypertension and prevention of myocardial infarction; ophthalmic dosage form used to treat elevated intraocular pressure as in glaucoma
Pregnancy Risk Factor C
Usual Dosage

Adult: Oral:
Hypertension: 10-40 mg in two divided doses, up to 60 mg/day
Prevention of MI: 10 mg twice daily initiated within 1-4 weeks after infarction

Adult and Children: Ophthalmic: One drop once or twice daily

Timoptic® see Timolol Maleate on this page

Timunox® see Thymopentin on page 353

Tinactin® [OTC] see Tolnaftate on page 357

Tindal® see Acetophenazine Maleate on page 6

Tinver® see Sodium Thiosulfate on page 330

Tioguanine see Thioguanine on page 352

Tiotixene see Thiothixene on page 353

Tisit® [OTC] see Pyrethrins on page 309

Tissue Plasminogen Activator, Recombinant see Alteplase on page 14

Titralac® Plus Liquid [OTC] see Calcium Carbonate and Simethicone on page 53

TMP see Trimethoprim on page 364

TMP-SMX *see* Sulfamethoxazole and Trimethoprim
on page 338

TobraDex® *see* Tobramycin and Dexamethasone *on this page*

Tobramycin and Dexamethasone
Brand Names TobraDex®
Synonyms Dexamethasone and Tobramycin
Use Treatment of external ocular infection caused by susceptible gram-negative bacteria and steroid response inflammatory conditions of the palpebral and bulbar conjunctiva, lid, cornea, and anterior segment of the globe
Pregnancy Risk Factor D
Usual Dosage 1-2 drops every 4-6 hours (first 24-48 hours may increase frequency to every two hours until signs of clinical improvement are seen)

Tobramycin Sulfate (toe bra mye' sin)
Brand Names Nebcin®; Tobrex®
Use Treatment of susceptible bacterial infections, including gram-negative *Bacillus* and staphylococci in origin. Topically used to treat superficial ophthalmic infections caused by susceptible bacteria.
Pregnancy Risk Factor D
Usual Dosage Use patient's ideal body weight to calculate dosage; obese patients, calculate dose based on estimated lean body weight plus 40% of the excess

Neonate: Monitor blood levels: I.M., I.V.:
< 1 week: 4 mg/kg/day in divided doses every 12 hours
> 1 week: 6 mg/kg/day in divided doses every eight hours
< 1 kg: May only need 2.5 mg/kg every 18 hours or 3 mg/kg every 24 hours

Children: 6-7.5 mg/kg/day (2-2.5 mg/kg every eight hours or 1.5-1.9 mg/kg every six hours)
Cystic fibrosis: 7-10 mg/kg/day given every eight hours

Adult: I.M., I.V.: 3-5 mg/kg/day in divided doses every eight hours

Adult and Children: Ophthalmic:
Mild to moderate infections: 1-2 drops every four hours
Severe infections: Two drops into eye(s) hourly until improvement, then reduce to less frequent intervals

Tobrex® *see* Tobramycin Sulfate *on this page*

Tocainide Hydrochloride (toe kay' nide)
Brand Names Tonocard®
Use Suppress and prevent symptomatic ventricular arrhythmias
Pregnancy Risk Factor C
Usual Dosage Adult: Oral: 1200-1800 mg/day in three divided doses

Tofranil® *see* Imipramine *on page 182*

Tofranil-PM® *see* Imipramine *on page 182*

Tolazamide (tole az' a mide)
Brand Names Ronase®; Tolinase®
Use As an adjunct to diet for the management of mild to moderately severe, stable, noninsulin-dependent (type II) diabetes mellitus
Pregnancy Risk Factor D
Usual Dosage Adult: Oral: 100-1000 mg/day

Tolazoline Hydrochloride (tole az' oh leen)
Brand Names Priscoline®
Synonyms Benzazoline Hydrochloride
Use Persistent pulmonary vasoconstriction and hypertension of the newborn (persistent fetal circulation)
Pregnancy Risk Factor C
Usual Dosage I.V.: 1-2 mg/kg via scalp vein over 10 minutes followed by an I.V. infusion of 1-2 mg/kg/hour

Tolbutamide (tole byoo' ta mide)
Brand Names Orinase®
Use As an adjunct to diet for the management of mild to moderately severe, stable, noninsulin-dependent (type II) diabetes mellitus
Pregnancy Risk Factor D
Usual Dosage Adult:
Oral: 250-2000 mg/day
I.V. bolus: 20 mg/kg

Tolectin® *see* Tolmetin Sodium *on this page*

Tolinase® *see* Tolazamide *on this page*

Tolmetin Sodium (tole' met in)
Brand Names Tolectin®
Use Treatment of rheumatoid arthritis and osteoarthritis, juvenile rheumatoid arthritis
Pregnancy Risk Factor C/D
Usual Dosage Oral:

Adult:
Rheumatoid arthritis: Initially 400 mg three times a day, usual range: 600-1800 mg/day given 3-4 times/day; maximum: 2000 mg/day
Osteoarthritis: Initially 400 mg three times/day, usual range: 600-1600 mg/day given 3-4 times/day; maximum: 600 mg/day

Children: ≥ 2 years of age: Initially 20 mg/kg/day, usual dose range is 15-30 mg/kg/day given 3-4 times/day; maximum: 30 mg/kg/day

Tolnaftate (tole naf' tate)
Brand Names Aftate® [OTC]; Footwork® [OTC]; Fungatin® [OTC]; Genaspor® [OTC]; NP-27® [OTC]; Tinactin® [OTC]; Zeasorb-AF® [OTC]
Use Treatment of tinea pedis, tinea cruris, tinea corporis, tinea manuum; tinea capitis; tinea unguium, tinea versicolor infections
Pregnancy Risk Factor C
Usual Dosage Wash and dry affected area; apply 1-2 drops of solution or
(Continued)
357

Tolnaftate *(Continued)*

a small amount of cream or powder and rub into the affected areas twice daily for 2-3 weeks

Tonocard® *see* Tocainide Hydrochloride *on page 356*

Topicort® *see* Desoximetasone *on page 101*

Topicort®-LP *see* Desoximetasone *on page 101*

TOPV *see* Poliovirus Vaccine, Live, Trivalent *on page 289*

Toradol® *see* Ketorolac Tromethamine *on page 197*

Torecan® *see* Thiethylperazine Maleate *on page 351*

Tornalate® *see* Bitolterol Mesylate *on page 46*

Totacillin® *see* Ampicillin *on page 23*

TP5 *see* Thymopentin *on page 353*

t-PA *see* Alteplase *on page 14*

Trace-4® *see* Trace Metals *on this page*

Trace Metals

Brand Names Chroma-Pak®; Cupri-Pak®; Iodo-Pak®; Iodopen®; Manga-Pak®; Moly-Pak®; Molypen®; M.T.E.-4®; M.T.E.-5®; M.T.E.-6®; Multe-Pak-4®; Neotrace-4®; Pedte-Pak-5®; Pedtrace-4®; P.T.E.-4®; P.T.E.-5®; Sele-Pak®; Selepen®; T.E.C.®; Trace-4®; Zinca-Pak®

Synonyms Chromium; Copper; Iodine; Manganese; Molybdenum; Neonatal Trace Metals; Selenium; Zinc

Use Supplement to TPN solutions

Tracrium® *see* Atracurium Besylate *on page 31*

Tral® *see* Hexocyclium Methylsulfate *on page 169*

Tramisol *see* Levamisole *on page 201*

Trandate® *see* Labetalol Hydrochloride *on page 198*

Tranexamic Acid *(tran ex am' ik)*

Brand Names Amstat®; Cyklokapron®

Use Short-term use (2-8 days) in hemophilia patients during and following tooth extraction

Pregnancy Risk Factor B

Usual Dosage I.V.: 10 mg/kg immediately before surgery, then 25 mg/kg orally 3-4 times daily for 2-8 days

Transamine Sulphate *see* Tranylcypromine Sulfate *on next page*

Transdermal-NTG® *see* Nitroglycerin *on page 253*

Transderm-Nitro® *see* Nitroglycerin *on page 253*

Transderm Scop® *see* Scopolamine *on page 321*

Tranxene® T-Tab™ *see* Clorazepate Dipotassium *on page 84*

Tranylcypromine Sulfate (tran ill sip' roe meen)
Brand Names Parnate®

Synonyms Transamine Sulphate

Use Symptomatic treatment of depressed patients refractory to or intolerant to tricyclic antidepressants or electroconvulsive therapy

Pregnancy Risk Factor C

Usual Dosage Adult: Oral: 10 mg twice a day, increase to a maximum of 30 mg/day after two weeks

Travase® *see* Sutilains *on page 340*

Trazodone (traz' oh done)
Brand Names Desyrel®

Use Treatment of depression

Pregnancy Risk Factor C

Usual Dosage Adult: 150 mg/day in three divided doses increasing by 50 mg/day every 3-4 days if needed, up to a maximum of 400 mg/day (inpatient may receive up to 600 mg/day)

Trecator®-SC *see* Ethionamide *on page 140*

Trendar® [OTC] *see* Ibuprofen *on page 181*

Trental® *see* Pentoxifylline *on page 276*

Tretinoin (tret' i noyn)
Brand Names Retin-A™

Synonyms Retinoic Acid; Vitamin A Acid

Use Treatment of acne vulgaris, photodamaged skin, and some skin cancers

Pregnancy Risk Factor B

Usual Dosage Apply once a day before retiring

Trexan™ *see* Naltrexone Hydrochloride *on page 245*

Triaconazole *see* Terconazole *on page 343*

Triam-A® *see* Triamcinolone *on this page*

Triamcinolone (trye am sin' oh lone)
Brand Names Amcort®; Aristocort® Forte; Aristocort® Intralesional Suspension; Aristocort® Tablet; Aristospan®; Azmacort™; Cenocort®; Cenocort® Forte; Cinonide®; Kenacort® Syrup; Kenacort® Tablet; Kenalog® Injection; Triam-A®; Triamolone®; Tri-Kort®; Trilog®; Trilone®; Trisoject®

Synonyms Triamcinolone Acetonide, Aerosol; Triamcinolone Acetonide, Parenteral; Triamcinolone Diacetate, Oral; Triamcinolone Diacetate, Parenteral; Triamcinolone Hexacetonide; Triamcinolone, Oral

Use For severe inflammation or immunosuppression

Pregnancy Risk Factor C

Usual Dosage

Oral:
   Adult: 4-48 mg/day (depending upon the disease being treated) in 1-4 divided doses

(Continued)

359

Triamcinolone *(Continued)*

Children: 0.117-1.66 mg/kg/day in four divided doses

I.M.:
   Adult: > 12 years of age: 60 mg (of 40 mg/mL), additional 20-100 mg doses (usual 40-80 mg) may be given when signs and symptoms recur; best at six week intervals to minimize HPA suppression
   Children: 6-12 years: 0.03-0.2 mg/kg at 1-7 day intervals

Intralesional (use 10 mg/mL): Adult: 1 mg/injection site, may be repeated one or more times per week depending upon patient response; maximum: 30 mg intralesionally at any one time; may use multiple injections if they are more than 1 cm apart

Intra-articular, intrasynovial, and soft-tissue injection (use 10 or 40 mg/mL): 2.5-40 mg depending upon location, size of joint, and degree of inflammation, repeat when signs and symptoms recur

Inhalation:
   Adult: Usual dose is two sprays 3-4 times daily; severe asthma: Four sprays 3-4 times/day; maximum: 16 sprays/day
   Children: 6-12 years: Usual dose 1-2 sprays 3-4 times/day; maximum: 12 sprays/day; dose is adjusted to patient response

Triamcinolone Acetonide, Aerosol *see* Triamcinolone *on previous page*

Triamcinolone Acetonide, Parenteral *see* Triamcinolone *on previous page*

Triamcinolone and Nystatin *see* Nystatin and Triamcinolone *on page 258*

Triamcinolone Diacetate, Oral *see* Triamcinolone *on previous page*

Triamcinolone Diacetate, Parenteral *see* Triamcinolone *on previous page*

Triamcinolone Hexacetonide *see* Triamcinolone *on previous page*

Triamcinolone, Oral *see* Triamcinolone *on previous page*

Triaminic® Cold Syrup [OTC] *see* Chlorpheniramine and Phenylpropanolamine *on page 73*

Triaminic® Expectorant [OTC] *see* Guaifenesin and Phenylpropanolamine *on page 163*

Triaminicol® Multi-Symptom Cold Syrup [OTC] *see* Chlorpheniramine, Phenylpropanolamine and Dextromethorphan *on page 75*

Triaminic® Oral Infant Drops *see* Pheniramine, Phenylpropanolamine and Pyrilamine *on page 278*

Triamolone® *see* Triamcinolone *on previous page*

Triamterene *(trye am' ter een)*
Brand Names Dyrenium®
   Use Used alone or in combination with other diuretics to treat edema and hypertension; decreases potassium excretion caused by kaliuretic diuretics

Pregnancy Risk Factor B
Usual Dosage Adult: Oral: 100 mg twice daily after meals

Triamterene and Hydrochlorothiazide *see* Hydrochlorothiazide and Triamterene *on page 173*

Triavil® *see* Amitriptyline and Perphenazine *on page 20*

Triazolam (trye ay' zoe lam)
Brand Names Halcion®
Use Short-term treatment of insomnia
Restrictions C-IV
Pregnancy Risk Factor X
Usual Dosage Oral: 0.125-0.25 mg at bedtime

Tribavirin *see* Ribavirin *on page 315*

Trichlormethiazide (trye klor meth eye' a zide)
Brand Names Metahydrin®; Naqua®
Use Management of mild to moderate hypertension; treatment of edema in congestive heart failure and nephrotic syndrome
Pregnancy Risk Factor B
Usual Dosage Oral: 1-4 mg/day

Trichloroacetaldehyde Monohydrate *see* Chloral Hydrate *on page 68*

Tridesilon® *see* Desonide *on page 101*

Tridil® *see* Nitroglycerin *on page 253*

Tridione® *see* Trimethadione *on page 363*

Trientine Hydrochloride (trye' en teen)
Brand Names Cuprid®
Use Treatment of Wilson's disease in patients intolerant to penicillamine
Pregnancy Risk Factor C
Usual Dosage Oral:

Adult: 750-1250 mg/day in divided doses 2-4 times a day

Children: < 12 years of age: 500-750 mg/day in divided doses 2-4 times a day

Triethanolamine Polypeptide Oleate-Condensate
Brand Names Cerumenex®
Use Removal of ear wax
Pregnancy Risk Factor C
Usual Dosage Fill ear canal, insert cotton plug; allow to remain for 15-30 minutes, gently flush with lukewarm water

Triethanolamine Salicylate
Brand Names Myoflex® [OTC]; Sportscreme® [OTC]
Use Relief of pain of muscular aches, rheumatism, neuralgia, sprains, arthritis on intact skin
Usual Dosage Apply to area as needed

Triethylenethiophosphoramide *see* Thiotepa *on page 353*

Trifluoperazine Hydrochloride (trye floo oh per' a zeen)
Brand Names Stelazine®
Use Treatment of psychoses and management of anxiety
Pregnancy Risk Factor C
Usual Dosage Oral:

Adult:
Psychoses: Outpatients: 1-2 mg twice/day; Hospitalized or well supervised patients: Initial dose 2-5 mg twice/day with optimum response in the 15-20 mg/day range; do not exceed 40 mg/day
Anxiety: 1-2 mg twice daily; maximum: 6 mg/day; therapy for anxiety should not exceed 12 weeks

Children: 6-12 years of age: Psychoses: Hospitalized or well supervised patients: Initial dose 1-2 times/day, gradually increase until symptoms are controlled or adverse effects become troublesome; maximum: 15 mg/day

Trifluorothymidine *see* Trifluridine *on this page*

Triflupromazine Hydrochloride (trye floo proe' ma zeen)
Brand Names Vesprin®
Use Treatment of psychoses, nausea, vomiting, and intractable hiccups
Pregnancy Risk Factor C
Usual Dosage

Adult:
I.M.: 5-15 mg every four hours
I.V.: 1 mg

Children: I.M.: 0.2-0.25 mg/kg

Trifluridine (trye flure' i deen)
Brand Names Viroptic®
Synonyms F_3T; Trifluorothymidine
Use For treatment of primary keratoconjunctivitis and recurrent epithelial keratitis caused by herpes simplex virus types I and II
Pregnancy Risk Factor C
Usual Dosage Adult: One drop into affected eye every two hours while awake, to a maximum of nine drops daily, until re-epithelialization of corneal ulcer occurs, then use one drop every four hours for another seven days

Triglycerides, Medium Chain *see* Medium Chain Triglycerides *on page 215*

Trihexane® *see* Trihexyphenidyl Hydrochloride *on this page*

Trihexy® *see* Trihexyphenidyl Hydrochloride *on this page*

Trihexyphenidyl Hydrochloride (trye hex ee fen' i dill)
Brand Names Artane®; Trihexane®; Trihexy®
Synonyms Benzhexol Hydrochloride
Use Adjunctive treatment of Parkinson's disease; also used in treatment of drug-induced extrapyramidal effects and acute dystonic reactions

Pregnancy Risk Factor C
Usual Dosage Oral: 5-15 mg/day in 3-4 divided doses; sustained action capsule given every 12-24 hours

Tri-Immunol® *see* Diphtheria and Tetanus Toxoids and Pertussis Vaccine, Adsorbed *on page 118*

Tri-Kort® *see* Triamcinolone *on page 359*

Trilafon® *see* Perphenazine *on page 277*

Trilisate® *see* Choline Magnesium Salicylate *on page 78*

Trilog® *see* Triamcinolone *on page 359*

Trilone® *see* Triamcinolone *on page 359*

Trimeprazine Tartrate (trye mep' ra zeen)
Brand Names Temaril®
Synonyms Alimenazine Tartrate
Use Perennial and seasonal allergic rhinitis and other allergic symptoms including urticaria
Pregnancy Risk Factor C
Usual Dosage Oral:

Adult: 2.5 mg four times a day (5 mg every 12-hour capsule)

Children:
> 3 years: 2.5 mg at bedtime or three times a day if needed
6 months to 3 years: 1.25 mg at bedtime or three times a day if needed

Trimetaphan Camsilate *see* Trimethaphan Camsylate *on this page*

Trimethadione (trye meth a dye' one)
Brand Names Tridione®
Synonyms Troxidone
Use To control absence (petit mal) seizures refractory to other drugs
Pregnancy Risk Factor D
Usual Dosage Oral:

Adult: 900 mg-2.4 g/day in 3-4 equally divided doses

Children: 300-900 mg/day in 3-4 equally divided doses

Trimethaphan Camphorsulfonate *see* Trimothaphan Camsylate *on this page*

Trimethaphan Camsylate (trye meth' a fan)
Brand Names Arfonad®
Synonyms Trimetaphan Camsilate; Trimethaphan Camphorsulfonate
Use Immediate and temporary reduction of blood pressure in patients with hypertensive emergencies; controlled hypotension during surgery
Pregnancy Risk Factor C
Usual Dosage I.V.:

Severe hypertension and hypertensive emergencies:
Adult: Initial rate: 0.5-1 mg/minute; titrate dose to the desired effect
Children: 50-150 μg/kg/minute
(Continued)

363

Trimethaphan Camsylate *(Continued)*

Hypertension due to acute dissecting aneurysms: Initial rate: 1-2 mg/minute, adjusting as need to keep systolic blood pressure of 100-120 mm Hg

Controlled hypertension during surgery: Initial rate: 3-4 mg/minute adjusted to maintain blood pressure at a desirable level; usual dosage needed 0.3-6 mg/minute

Trimethobenzamide Hydrochloride

(trye meth oh ben' za mide)
Brand Names Bio-Gan®; Stemetic®; Tebamide®; T-Gen®; Ticon®; Tigan®; Tiject®
Use Control of nausea and vomiting
Pregnancy Risk Factor C
Usual Dosage

Adult:
Oral: 250 mg 3-4 times daily
I.M., rectal: 200 mg 3-4 times daily

Children:
Oral, rectal: 13-40 kg: 100-200 mg 3-4 times daily
Rectal: < 13 kg: 100 mg 3-4 times daily

Trimethoprim (trye meth' oh prim)

Brand Names Proloprim®; Trimpex®
Synonyms TMP
Use Treatment of urinary tract infections; acute otitis media in children; acute exacerbations of chronic bronchitis in adults
Pregnancy Risk Factor C
Usual Dosage Adult: Oral: 100 mg every 12-24 hours

Trimethoprim and Polymyxin B

Brand Names Polytrim®
Use Treatment of surface ocular bacterial conjunctivitis and blepharoconjunctivitis
Usual Dosage Instill one or two drops in eye(s) every 4-6 hours

Trimethoprim and Sulfamethoxazole *see* Sulfamethoxazole and Trimethoprim *on page 338*

Trimethylpsoralen *see* Trioxsalen *on next page*

Trimipramine Maleate (trye mi' pra meen)

Brand Names Surmontil®
Use Treatment of various forms of depression, often in conjunction with psychotherapy
Pregnancy Risk Factor C
Usual Dosage Oral: 50-150 mg/day as a single bedtime dose

Trimox® *see* Amoxicillin *on page 21*

Trimpex® *see* Trimethoprim *on this page*

Trinalin® *see* Azatadine and Pseudoephedrine *on page 34*

Trioxsalen (trye ox' sa len)
Brand Names Trisoralen®
Synonyms Trimethylpsoralen
Use In conjunction with controlled exposure to ultraviolet light or sunlight for repigmentation of idiopathic vitiligo; increasing tolerance to sunlight with albinism; enhance pigmentation
Usual Dosage Adult and Children: Oral: > 12 years of age: 10 mg daily as a single dose, 2-4 hours before controlled exposure to UVA or sunlight

Tripelennamine (tri pel enn' a meen)
Brand Names PBZ®; PBZ-SR®
Synonyms Pyribenzamine®; Tripelennamine Citrate; Tripelennamine Hydrochloride
Use Perennial and seasonal allergic rhinitis and other allergic symptoms including urticaria
Pregnancy Risk Factor B
Usual Dosage Adult: Oral: 25-50 mg every 4-6 hours, extended release tablets 100 mg morning and evening; 5 mg/kg/day in 4-6 divided doses, up to 300 mg/day

Tripelennamine Citrate *see* Tripelennamine *on this page*

Tripelennamine Hydrochloride *see* Tripelennamine *on this page*

Tri-Phen-Chlor® *see* Chlorpheniramine, Phenyltoloxamine, Phenylpropanolamine and Phenylephrine *on page 75*

Triple Dye

Triprolidine and Pseudoephedrine (trye proe' li deen)
Brand Names Actifed®; Sudahist®
Synonyms Pseudoephedrine and Triprolidine
Use Temporary relief of nasal congestion, decongest sinus openings, running nose, sneezing, itching of nose or throat and itchy, watery eyes due to common cold, hay fever or other upper respiratory allergies
Pregnancy Risk Factor C
Usual Dosage Oral:

Adult and Children: > 12 years of age:
Syrup: 10 mL every 4-6 hours; do not exceed four doses in 24 hours
Tablet: One every 4-6 hours; do not exceed four doses in 24 hours

Children: 6-12 years:
Syrup: 5 mL every 4-6 hours; do not exceed four doses in 24 hours
Tablet: 1/2 every 4-6 hours; do not exceed four doses in 24 hours

Triprolidine, Pseudoephedrine and Codeine
Brand Names Actifed® With Codeine
Use Symptomatic relief of cough
Restrictions C-V
(Continued)

Triprolidine, Pseudoephedrine and Codeine
(Continued)
Usual Dosage Oral:
- Adult and Children > 12 years: 10 mL four times daily
- Children 7-12 years: 5 mL four times daily
- Children 2-6 years: 2.5 mL four times daily

Tris Buffer *see* Tromethamine *on this page*

Tris(hydroxymethyl)aminomethane *see* Tromethamine *on this page*

Trisoject® *see* Triamcinolone *on page 359*

Trisoralen® *see* Trioxsalen *on previous page*

Trisulfam® *see* Sulfamethoxazole and Trimethoprim *on page 338*

Trisulfapyrimidines *see* Sulfadiazine, Sulfamethazine and Sulfamerazine *on page 336*

Trobicin® *see* Spectinomycin Hydrochloride *on page 332*

Trofan® [OTC] *see* Tryptophan *on next page*

Troleandomycin (troe lee an doe mye' sin)
Brand Names Tao®
Use Treatment of respiratory tract infections caused by susceptible staphylococci or streptococci *Bacillus*
Pregnancy Risk Factor C
Usual Dosage Oral:

Adult: 250-500 mg four times a day for 10 days

Children: 125-250 mg every six hours for 10 days

Tromethamine (troe meth' a meen)
Brand Names Tham®; Tham-E®
Synonyms Tris Buffer; Tris(hydroxymethyl)aminomethane
Use Correction of metabolic acidosis associated with cardiac bypass surgery or cardiac arrest; to correct excess acidity of stored blood that is preserved with acid citrate dextrose; to prime the pump-oxygenator during cardiac bypass surgery; indicated in infants needing alkalinization after receiving maximum sodium bicarbonate (8-10 mEq/kg/24 hours); advantage of THAM® is that it alkalinizes without increasing PCO_2 and sodium
Pregnancy Risk Factor C
Usual Dosage Dose depends on buffer base deficit; tromethamine mL of 0.3 M solution = body weight (kg) x base deficit (mEq/L) x 1.1

Metabolic acidosis with cardiac arrest:
- I.V.: 3.5-6 mL/kg into large peripheral vein systemic acidosis during bypass surgery
- I.V.: 500-1000 mL if needed

Excess acidity of ACD priming blood: 14-70 mL of 0.3 molar solution added to each 500 mL of blood

Tronolane® [OTC] *see* Pramoxine Hydrochloride *on page 293*

Tropicamide (troe pik' a mide)
Brand Names Mydriacyl®
Synonyms Bistropamide
Use Short-acting mydriatic used in diagnostic procedures; as well as pre-operatively and postoperatively
Usual Dosage 1-2 drops (0.5%) 15-20 minutes before exam for refraction use 1-2 drops (1%) into eye(s); repeat in five minutes

Troxidone *see* Trimethadione *on page 363*

Truphylline® *see* Aminophylline *on page 18*

Tryptophan (trip' toe fan)
Brand Names Trofan® [OTC]
Synonyms L-Tryptophan
Use Amino acid therapy; hypnotic agent; antidepressant
Usual Dosage Oral: 500 mg-2 g daily

Trysul® *see* Sulfabenzamide, Sulfacetamide, and Sulfathiazole *on page 336*

TSH *see* Thyrotropin *on page 354*

TSPA *see* Thiotepa *on page 363*

T-Stat® *see* Erythromycin, Topical *on page 135*

Tuberculin (too ber' kyoo lin)
Brand Names Aplisol®; Aplitest®; Mono-Vacc®; SclavoTest®-PPD; Tuberculin Old Tine Test®; Tubersol®
Synonyms Mantoux; Old Tuberculin; OT; PPD; Purified Protein Derivative
Use Skin test in diagnosis of tuberculosis
Pregnancy Risk Factor C
Usual Dosage Adult and Children: Intradermally: 0.1 mL about four inches below elbow

Tuberculin Old Tine Test® *see* Tuberculin *on this page*

Tubersol® *see* Tuberculin *on this page*

Tubocurarine Chloride (too boe kyoor ar' een)
Synonyms d-Tubocurarine Chloride
Use Adjunct to anesthesia to induce skeletal muscle relaxation
Pregnancy Risk Factor C
Usual Dosage I.V.:

Adult and Children: Initial: 0.2-0.4 mg/kg one time; maintenance: 0.04-0.2 mg/kg/dose as needed to maintain paralysis

Neonates: < 1 month old: Initial: 0.3 mg/kg one time; maintenance: 0.15 mg/kg/dose as needed to maintain paralysis

Tucks® [OTC] *see* Witch Hazel *on page 380*

Tuinal® *see* Amobarbital and Secobarbital *on page 21*

Tums® [OTC] *see* Calcium Carbonate *on page 53*

Tussar® SF *see* Chlorpheniramine, Codeine and Guaifenesin *on page 74*

Tussionex® *see* Hydrocodone and Chlorpheniramine Polistirex *on page 173*

Tussi-Organidin® DM *see* Iodinated Glycerol With Dextromethorphan *on page 188*

Tuss-Ornade® *see* Caramiphen and Phenylpropanolamine *on page 57*

Tylenol® [OTC] *see* Acetaminophen *on page 4*

Tylenol® With Codeine *see* Acetaminophen and Codeine *on page 5*

Tylox® *see* Oxycodone and Acetaminophen *on page 264*

Tylox® *see* Oxycodone Hydrochloride *on page 264*

Typhoid Vaccine (tye' foid)
Use Promotes active immunity to typhoid fever for patients exposed to typhoid carrier or foreign travel to typhoid fever endemic area
Pregnancy Risk Factor C
Usual Dosage

Adult and Children: > 10 years of age: S.L.: 0.5 mL; repeat in four weeks

Children: 6 months-10 years: 0.25 mL; repeat in four weeks
Booster: 0.25 mL every three years

Tyropanoate Sodium (tye roe pa noe' ate)
Brand Names Bilopaque®
Use Oral cholecystography
Pregnancy Risk Factor B
Usual Dosage 3 g

Tyzine® *see* Tetrahydrozoline Hydrochloride *on page 347*

Ultracef® *see* Cefadroxil Monohydrate *on page 62*

Ultralente® *see* Insulin, Zinc Suspension, Extended *on page 186*

Ultralente® Iletin®I *see* Insulin, Zinc Suspension, Extended *on page 186*

Ultralente® Purified Beef *see* Insulin, Zinc Suspension, Extended *on page 186*

Ultra Mide® *see* Urea *on next page*

Unasyn® *see* Ampicillin and Sulbactam *on page 23*

Unguentine® [OTC] *see* Benzocaine *on page 40*

Uni-Gine® *see* Ergoloid Mesylates *on page 133*

Unipen® *see* Nafcillin Sodium *on page 244*

Uniphyl® *see* Theophylline *on page 348*

Uni-Pro® [OTC] *see* Ibuprofen *on page 181*

Unna's Boot *see* Zinc Gelatin *on page 382*

Unna's Paste *see* Zinc Gelatin *on page 382*

Urabeth® *see* Bethanechol Chloride *on page 44*

Urea (yoor ee' a)

Brand Names Amino-Cerv™ Vaginal Cream; Aquacare® [OTC]; Carmol® [OTC]; Nutraplus® [OTC]; Rea-Lo® [OTC]; Ultra Mide®; Ureacin®-20 [OTC]; Ureacin®-40; Ureaphil®

Synonyms Carbamide

Use To reduce intracranial pressure and intraocular pressure (30%); promotes hydration and removal of excess keratin in hyperkeratotic conditions and dry skin; mild cervicitis

Pregnancy Risk Factor C

Usual Dosage

Adult:
Topical: Apply 1-3 times daily
Vaginal: One (1) applicator in vagina at bedtime for 2-4 weeks
I.V. infusion: 1-1.5 g/kg by slow infusion (1-2.5 hours); maximum 120 g/24 hours

Children: I.V. slow infusion:
> 2 years of age: 0.5-1.5 g/kg
< 2 years: 0.1-0.5 g/kg

Urea and Hydrocortisone *see* Hydrocortisone and Urea *on page 175*

Ureacin®-20 [OTC] *see* Urea *on this page*

Ureacin®-40 *see* Urea *on this page*

Urea Peroxide *see* Carbamide Peroxide *on page 58*

Ureaphil® *see* Urea *on this page*

Urecholine® *see* Bethanechol Chloride *on page 44*

Uricult® [OTC] *see* Diagnostic Test for Bacteriuria *on page 106*

Urispas® *see* Flavoxate *on page 147*

Uristix® [OTC] *see* Diagnostic Test for Glucose and Protein in Urine *on page 107*

Urobilistix® *see* Diagnostic Test for Urobilinogen *on page 108*

Urodine® *see* Phenazopyridine Hydrochloride *on page 278*

Urofollitropin (yoor oh fol li troe' pin)

Brand Names Metrodin®

Use Induction of ovulation in patients with polycystic ovarian disease and to stimulate the development of multiple oocytes

Usual Dosage Adult: I.M.: 75 IU daily for 7-12 days, used with hCG

Urokinase (yoor oh kin' ase)

Brand Names Abbokinase®; Breokinase®

Use Thrombolytic agent used in treatment of recent severe or massive deep vein thrombosis, pulmonary emboli, myocardial infarction, and occluded arteriovenous cannulas

Pregnancy Risk Factor B

Usual Dosage Adult:

Myocardial infarction: Intracoronary: 6000 IU/minute up to two hours

Deep vein thrombosis: I.V.: 4400 IU/kg/hour for 12 hours

Occluded I.V. catheters: into catheter: 5000 IU, then aspirate; may repeat every five minutes for 1/2 hour, if still occluded cap and leave in catheter for 1/2-1 hour, then aspirate

Clot lysis: (large vessel thrombi): Loading: 4000 IU/kg/dose I.V. over 10 minutes; maintenance: 4000-6000 IU/kg/hour adjusted to achieve clot lysis or patency of affected vessel; doses up to 50,000 IU/kg/hour have been used. Note: Therapy should be initiated as soon as possible after diagnosis of thrombi and continued until clot is dissolved (usually 24-72 hours)

Uro-KP-Neutral® [OTC] *see* Phosphorus Replacement Products *on page 284*

Urolene Blue® *see* Methylene Blue *on page 230*

Uroplus® DS *see* Sulfamethoxazole and Trimethoprim *on page 338*

Uroplus® SS *see* Sulfamethoxazole and Trimethoprim *on page 338*

Ursodeoxycholic Acid *see* Ursodiol *on this page*

Ursodiol (er' soe dye ole)

Brand Names Actigall™

Synonyms Ursodeoxycholic Acid

Use Gallbladder stone dissolution

Pregnancy Risk Factor B

Usual Dosage 8-10 mg/kg/day in 2-3 divided doses

Uticort® *see* Betamethasone *on page 43*

Vagilia® *see* Sulfabenzamide, Sulfacetamide, and Sulfathiazole *on page 336*

Vagitrol® *see* Sulfanilamide *on page 338*

Valergen® *see* Estradiol *on page 135*

Valisone® *see* Betamethasone *on page 43*

Valium® *see* Diazepam *on page 109*

Valpin® 50 *see* Anisotropine Methylbromide *on page 25*

Valproate Sodium *see* Valproic Acid and Derivatives *on next page*

Valproic Acid *see* Valproic Acid and Derivatives *on next page*

Valproic Acid and Derivatives (val proe' ik)

Brand Names Depakene®; Depakote®

Synonyms Dipropylacetic Acid; Divalproex Sodium; DPA; 2-Propylpentanoic Acid; 2-Propylvaleric Acid; Valproate Sodium; Valproic Acid

Use Treatment of simple and complex absence seizures

Pregnancy Risk Factor D

Usual Dosage

    Oral: 15 mg/kg/day; increase by 5-10 mg/kg/day at weekly intervals until therapeutic levels are achieved; maintenance: 30-60 mg/kg/24 hours divided 1-2 times/day

    Rectal: Dilute syrup 1:1 with water for use as a retention enema. Children: Loading: 20 mg/kg/dose one time; maintenance: 10-15 mg/kg/dose given every eight hours, beginning eight hours after administration of the loading dose

Vancenase® see Beclomethasone Dipropionate on page 38

Vancenase® AQ see Beclomethasone Dipropionate on page 38

Vanceril® see Beclomethasone Dipropionate on page 38

Vancocin® see Vancomycin Hydrochloride on this page

Vancoled® see Vancomycin Hydrochloride on this page

Vancomycin Hydrochloride (van koe mye' sin)

Brand Names Lyphocin®; Vancocin®; Vancoled®; Vancor®

Use Treatment of susceptible potentially life-threatening bacterial infections, normally those caused by the Staphylococcus or Streptococcus strains

Pregnancy Risk Factor C

Usual Dosage

    Adult:

        Serious infections: I.V.: 2 g/day in divided doses 2-4 times daily

        Pseudomembranous colitis: Oral: 500 mg every six hours

    Children:

        Serious infections: I.V.: $\leq$ 7 days old: 15 mg/kg every 12 hours 8-30 days; 15 mg/kg every eight hours; older infants and children: 40-45 mg/kg/day, divided into 3-4 doses administered every 6-8 hours

        Pseudomembranous colitis: Oral: 40 mg/kg/day in divided doses 2-4 times daily, maximum: 2 g/24 hours

    Neonates: 10-50 mg/kg/day divided every 8-12 hours; maximum 2 g/24 hours.

    Recommended doses and dose intervals of vancomycin in preterm infants, to maintain mean steady-state peak concentration 30 mg/L (range 25-40 mg/L) and trough concentration 6 mg/L (range < 10 mg/L) See table on next page.

Vancor® see Vancomycin Hydrochloride on this page

Vanoxide® [OTC] see Benzoyl Peroxide on page 41

Vancomycin Hydrochloride

	Postconceptional Age (wk)			
	< 27	27–30	31–36	> 37
Body weight (g)	< 800	800–1200	1200–2000	> 2000
Daily dose (mg/kg)	18	24	36	45
Dose interval (h)	36	24	12/18	12
Dose/injection (mg/kg)	27	24	18/27	22.5

Adapted from James A, Koren G, Milliken J, et al, "Vancomycin pharmacokinetics and dose recommendations for preterm infants," *Antimicrob AG Chemother*, 1967, 31:52–4.
Mean level assigned to 21 mg/L (midinterval concentration between 40 mg/L and 10 mg/L).

Vanoxide-HC® *see* Hydrocortisone Alcohol and Benzoyl Peroxide *on page 175*

Vansil™ *see* Oxamniquine *on page 263*

Vapo-Iso® *see* Isoproterenol *on page 193*

Vaponefrin® *see* Epinephrine *on page 131*

Varicella-Zoster Immune Globulin (Human)

Synonyms VZIG

Use Passive immunization of susceptible immunodeficient patients after exposure to varicella

Usual Dosage I.M.: Administer by deep injection in the gluteal muscle, or in another large muscle mass. Inject 125 units per 10 kg (22 pounds), up to a maximum dose of 625 units (5 vials). The minimum dose is 125 units; do not give fractional doses. Do not inject I.V. See table.

VZIG Dose Based on Weight

Weight of Patient		Dose	
kg	lb	Units	No. of Vials
0–10	0–22	125	1
10.1–20	22.1–44	250	2
20.1–30	44.1–66	375	3
30.1–40	66.1–88	500	4
> 40	> 88	625	5

Vaseline® [OTC] *see* White Petrolatum *on page 379*

VasoClear® [OTC] *see* Naphazoline Hydrochloride *on page 246*

Vasocon-A® *see* Naphazoline and Antazoline *on page 246*

Vasocon Regular® *see* Naphazoline Hydrochloride *on page 246*

Vasodilan® *see* Isoxsuprine Hydrochloride *on page 194*

Vasopressin (vay soe press' in)
Brand Names Pitressin®; Pitressin® Tannate in Oil
Synonyms ADH; Antidiuretic Hormone; Vasopressin Tannate
Use Treatment of diabetes insipidus; prevention and treatment of postoperative abdominal distention, esophageal varices
Pregnancy Risk Factor B
Usual Dosage

Diabetes insipidus: Pitressin® Tannate in Oil
  Adult: I.M., S.C.: 2.5-5 units every 2-3 days
  Children: 1.25-2.5 units every 2-3 days

Diabetes insipidus: Pitressin®
  Adult: I.M., S.C.: 5-10 units 2-3 times daily as needed;
  Intranasal: Administer on cotton pledget or nasal spray
  Abdominal distention: I.M.: 5 mg stat, 10 mg every 3-4 hours
  Children: Injection, aqueous: 2.5-5 units/dose every 6-8 hours

Vasopressin Tannate *see* Vasopressin *on this page*

Vasotec® *see* Enalapril *on page 129*

Vasoxyl® *see* Methoxamine Hydrochloride *on page 228*

V-Cillin K® *see* Penicillin V Potassium *on page 274*

VCR *see* Vincristine Sulfate *on page 376*

Vecuronium (ve kyoo' roe ni um)
Brand Names Norcuron®
Synonyms ORG NC 45
Use Adjunct to anesthesia, to facilitate intubation, and provide skeletal muscle relaxation during surgery or mechanical ventilation
Pregnancy Risk Factor C
Usual Dosage I.V.:

Adult and Children: > 1 year of age: Initial: 0.08-0.1 mg/kg/dose; maintenance: 0.01-0.015 mg/kg/dose every 25-40 minutes as required to maintain paralysis. Note: Children 1-20 years of age may require slightly higher initial doses and slightly more frequent supplementation.

Infants:
  7 weeks - 1 year of age: Initial: 0.08-0.1 mg/kg/dose; maintenance: 0.01-0.015 mg/kg/dose every 40-60 minutes, as required to maintain paralysis
  < 7 weeks old: Not recommended

Veetids® *see* Penicillin V Potassium *on page 274*

Velban® *see* Vinblastine Sulfate *on page 375*

Velosef® *see* Cephradine *on page 67*

Velosulin® *see* Insulin, Regular *on page 186*

Velosulin® Human *see* Insulin, Regular *on page 186*

Velsar® *see* Vinblastine Sulfate *on next page*

Veltane® *see* Brompheniramine Maleate *on page 48*

Venoglobulin®-I *see* Immune Globulin *on page 183*

Ventolin® *see* Albuterol *on page 10*

VePesid® *see* Etoposide *on page 142*

Veracillin® *see* Dicloxacillin Sodium *on page 111*

Verapamil Hydrochloride (ver ap' a mill)

Brand Names Calan®; Isoptin®

Synonyms Iproveratril Hydrochloride

Use Orally used for treatment of angina pectoris and hypertension; parenterally used for supraventricular tachyarrhythmias

Pregnancy Risk Factor C

Usual Dosage

Adult:

Angina: Oral: Initial dose: 80-120 mg twice/day (elderly or small stature): 40 mg twice/day ; range: 240-480 mg/day in 3-4 divided doses

Hypertension: Usual dose is 80 mg three times/day or 240 g (SR) daily; range 240-480 mg/day (no evidence of additional benefit in doses > 360 mg/day)

I.V.: 5-10 mg (approximately 0.075-0.15 mg/kg), second dose of 10 mg (approximately 0.15 mg/kg) may be given 15-30 minutes after the initial dose if patient tolerates, but does not respond to initial dose

Children: I.V.:

1-16 years: 0.1-0.3 mg/kg over two minutes; maximum: 5 mg/dose, may repeat dose once in 30 minutes if adequate response not achieved; maximum for second dose: 10 mg/dose

< 1 year: 0.1-0.2 mg/kg over two minutes

Children: Oral (dose not well established): 240-360 mg/day divided into three doses

Verazinc® [OTC] *see* Zinc Sulfate *on page 382*

Vercyte® *see* Pipobroman *on page 287*

Vermox® *see* Mebendazole *on page 214*

Verrex-C&M® *see* Podophyllin and Salicylic Acid *on page 288*

Versed® *see* Midazolam Hydrochloride *on page 236*

Vesprin® *see* Triflupromazine Hydrochloride *on page 362*

V-Gan® *see* Promethazine Hydrochloride *on page 301*

Vibazine® *see* Buclizine Hydrochloride *on page 49*

Vibramycin® *see* Doxycycline *on page 123*

Vibra-Tabs® *see* Doxycycline *on page 123*

Vicks Sinex® Long-Acting Nasal Solution [OTC] *see* Oxymetazoline Hydrochloride *on page 265*

Vicks Sinex® Nasal Solution [OTC] *see* Phenylephrine Hydrochloride *on page 282*

Vicks Vatronol® *see* Ephedrine Sulfate *on page 130*

Vicodin® *see* Hydrocodone and Acetaminophen *on page 173*

Vicon-C® [OTC] *see* Vitamin B Complex With Vitamin C *on page 377*

Vidarabine (vye dare' a been)

Brand Names Vira-A®

Synonyms Adenine Arabinoside; Ara-A

Use Treatment of herpes simplex encephalitis; treatment of acute kerato-conjunctivitis and epithelial keratitis due to herpes simplex virus

Pregnancy Risk Factor C

Usual Dosage Document HSV infection prior to therapy

Encephalitis: Adult and Children (given I.V. every 24 hours): 15 mg/kg/day for 10 days

Neonatal HSV: 15-30 mg/kg/day for 10-14 days

Herpes Zoster (chickenpox): I.V.: In immunocompromised patients: 10 mg/kg/day for 5-7 days

Keratoconjunctivitis: 1/2 inch of ointment in lower conjunctiva sac five times daily (every three hours while awake) until complete re-epithelialization has occurred, then twice a day for an additional seven days; consider other therapy if no improvement seen after seven days

Vinblastine Sulfate (vin blas' teen)

Brand Names Velban®; Velsar®

Synonyms Vincaleukoblastine; VLB

Use Palliative treatment of Hodgkin's disease; breast cancer, advanced testicular germinal-cell cancers

Pregnancy Risk Factor D

Usual Dosage Varies depending upon clinical and hematological response. Give at intervals of at least seven days and only after leukocyte count has returned to at least 4000/mm³; maintenance therapy should be titrated according to leukocyte count. Dosage should be reduced in patients with recent exposure to radiation therapy or chemotherapy; single doses in these patients should not exceed 5.5 mg/m². 50% dosage reduction is recommended for patients with a direct serum bilirubin exceeding 3 mg/dL.

Adult: I.V.: Initial dose: 3.7 mg/m² as single dose; increase weekly at increments of 1.8 mg/m²; maximum weekly dose: 18.5 mg/m²; usual weekly dose: 5.5-7.4 mg/m²

Children: I.V.: Initial dose: 2.5 mg/m² as single dose; increase weekly at increments of 1.25 mg/m²; maximum weekly dose: 12.5 mg/m²

Vincaleukoblastine *see* Vinblastine Sulfate *on this page*

Vincasar® *see* Vincristine Sulfate *on this page*

Vincristine Sulfate (vin kris' teen)
 Brand Names Oncovin®; Vincasar®
 Synonyms LCR; Leurocristine; VCR
 Use Treatment of leukemias, Hodgkin's disease, neuroblastoma, malignant lymphomas, and other tumors
 Pregnancy Risk Factor C
 Usual Dosage Dosages vary with protocol used; adjustments are made depending upon clinical and hematological response and upon adverse reactions; dosage reduction necessary with significant hepatic impairment

 Adult: I.V.: 1.4 mg/m², up to 2 mg; may repeat every week

 Children: I.V.: 2 mg/m²; may repeat every week; ≤ 10 kg or BSA < 1 m²: 0.05 mg/kg once weekly

Vioform® [OTC] *see* Iodochlorhydroxyquin *on page 189*

Vioform-HC® *see* Iodochlorhydroxyquin and Hydrocortisone *on page 189*

Viokase® *see* Pancrelipase *on page 267*

Viosterol *see* Ergocalciferol *on page 132*

Vira-A® *see* Vidarabine *on previous page*

Virazole® *see* Ribavirin *on page 315*

Virilon® *see* Methyltestosterone *on page 232*

Viroptic® *see* Trifluridine *on page 362*

Viscoat® *see* Chondroitin Sulfate-Sodium Hyaluronate *on page 78*

Visidex® II [OTC] *see* Diagnostic Test for Glucose in Blood *on page 107*

Visine® [OTC] *see* Tetrahydrozoline Hydrochloride *on page 347*

Visken® *see* Pindolol *on page 286*

Vistaril® *see* Hydroxyzine *on page 178*

Vistazine® *see* Hydroxyzine *on page 178*

Vita-C® [OTC] *see* Ascorbic Acid *on page 29*

Vitacarn® *see* Levocarnitine *on page 201*

Vital HN® [OTC] *see* Nutritional Formula, Enteral/Oral *on page 258*

Vitamin A (vye' ta min)
 Brand Names Aquasol A® [OTC]
 Synonyms Oleovitamin A
 Use Treatment and prevention of vitamin A deficiency
 Pregnancy Risk Factor A/X
 Usual Dosage

 Severe deficiency with xerophthalmia:
  Adult: > 8 years of age: 500,000 IU orally for three days, 50,000 IU oral-

ly for 14 days, 10,000-20,000 IU orally for 2 months **or** 50,000-100,000 IU I.M. for three days, 50,000 IU I.M. for 14 days

Children: 1-8 years of age: 5000-10,000 IU/kg orally for five days or until recovery occurs **or** 5000-15,000 IU I.M. for 10 days

Deficiency (without corneal changes):
Adult: > 8 years: 100,000 IU/day orally for three days then 50,000 IU/day for 14 days
Children: 1-8 years: 5000-10,000 IU/kg/day orally for five days, then 17,000-35,000 IU/day for 10 days
Infants: < 1 year: 10,000 IU/kg/day orally for five days, then 7500-15,000 IU/day for 10 days

Malabsorption syndrome (prophylaxis): Adult: > 8 years: Oral: 10,000-50,000 IU/day of water miscible product

Dietary supplement:
Adult: > 10 years: 4000-5000 IU/day
Children: 7-10 years: 3300-3500 IU/day; 4-6 years: 2500 IU/day; 6 months-3 years: 1500-2000 IU/day
Infants: Up to 6 months: 1500 IU

Vitamin A Acid see Tretinoin on page 359

Vitamin A and Vitamin D
Brand Names A and D™ Ointment [OTC]; Balmex® Ointment [OTC]; Clocream® [OTC]; Primaderm® [OTC]; Scott's® Emulsion [OTC]; Super D® Perles [OTC]
Use Temporary relief of discomfort due to chapped skin, diaper rash, minor burns, abrasions, as well as irritations associated with ostomy skin care
Usual Dosage
Oral, oil: Dietary supplement: 2.5 mL daily
Topical: Apply locally with gentle massage as needed

Vitamin B₁ see Thiamine Hydrochloride on page 351

Vitamin B₂ see Riboflavin on page 316

Vitamin B₃ see Niacinamide on page 251

Vitamin B₅ see Pantothenic Acid on page 268

Vitamin B₆ see Pyridoxine Hydrochloride on page 309

Vitamin B₁₂ see Cyanocobalamin on page 92

Vitamin B Complex
Brand Names Apatate® [OTC]; Becotin® [OTC]; Gevrabon® [OTC]; Lederplex® [OTC]; Lipovite® [OTC]; Mega-B® [OTC]; Megatron® [OTC]; Mucoplex® [OTC]; NeoVadrin® B Complex [OTC]; Orexin® [OTC]; Surbex® [OTC]
Usual Dosage Dosage is usually one tablet or capsule daily; please refer to package insert

Vitamin B Complex With Vitamin C
Brand Names Allbee® With C [OTC]; Surbex-T® Filmtabs® [OTC]; Surbex® with C Filmtabs® [OTC]; Thera-Combex® H-P Kapseals® [OTC]; Vicon-C® [OTC]
(Continued)

Vitamin B Complex With Vitamin C *(Continued)*

Use Supportive nutritional supplementation in conditions in which water-soluble vitamins are required like GI disorders, chronic alcoholism, pregnancy, severe burns, and recovery from surgery

Usual Dosage Adult: Oral: One every day

Vitamin C [OTC] *see* Ascorbic Acid *on page 29*

Vitamin D$_2$ *see* Ergocalciferol *on page 132*

Vitamin E

Brand Names Aquasol® E [OTC]; Eprolin® [OTC]; E-Vital® [OTC]; Pheryl-E® [OTC]

Synonyms *d*-Alpha Tocopherol; *dl*-Alpha Tocopherol

Use Prevention and treatment of vitamin E deficiency

Pregnancy Risk Factor A/C

Usual Dosage 1 IU of vitamin E = 1 mg dL-alpha-tocopheryl acetate

Vitamin E deficiency:
   Adult: 60-70 IU/day
   Children (with malabsorption syndrome): Oral: 1 IU/kg daily of water miscible vitamin E to raise plasma tocopherol concentrations to the normal range within two months
   Neonate, premature, low birthweight: Oral: 25 IU daily results in normal levels within one week

Prevention of vitamin E deficiency:
   Adult: 30 IU/day
   Neonate, full term: 5 IU/L of formula
   Neonate, low birthweight: 5 IU/day

Prevention of retinopathy or prematurity or bronchopulmonary dysplasia (BPD) secondary to O_2 therapy: (American Academy of Pediatrics considers this use investigational and routine use is not recommended):
   Retinopathy: 15-30 IU/kg/day to maintain plasma levels between 1.5-2 μg/mL (may need as high as 100 IU/kg)
   BPD: 20 IU/kg I.M. daily; however, a parenteral product with vitamin E alone is no longer commercially available

Cystic Fibrosis, β-thalassemia, sickle cell anemia may require higher daily maintenance doses:
   CF: 100-400 IU/day
   Sickle cell: 450 IU/day
   β-thalassemia: 750 IU/day

RDA: Adult: Female: 12 IU/day; male: 15 IU/day

Vitamin G *see* Riboflavin *on page 316*

Vitamin K$_1$ *see* Phytonadione *on page 285*

Vitamin K$_4$ *see* Menadiol Sodium Diphosphate *on page 217*

Vitaneed® [OTC] *see* Nutritional Formula, Enteral/Oral *on page 258*

Vivactil® *see* Protriptyline Hydrochloride *on page 306*

Vivonex® [OTC] *see* Nutritional Formula, Enteral/Oral *on page 258*

Vivonex® T.E.N. [OTC] *see* Nutritional Formula, Enteral/Oral *on page 258*

V-Lax® [OTC] *see* Psyllium *on page 308*

VLB *see* Vinblastine Sulfate *on page 375*

VM-26 *see* Teniposide *on page 342*

Voltaren® *see* Diclofenac Sodium *on page 111*

VoSol® *see* Acetic Acid *on page 6*

Vosol-HC® *see* Acetic Acid *on page 6*

VP-16 *see* Etoposide *on page 142*

Vumon *see* Teniposide *on page 342*

V.V.S.® *see* Sulfabenzamide, Sulfacetamide, and Sulfathiazole *on page 336*

Vytone® *see* Iodoquinol and Hydrocortisone *on page 189*

VZIG *see* Varicella-Zoster Immune Globulin (Human) *on page 372*

Warfarin Sodium (war' far in)
Brand Names Coumadin®; Panwarfin®
Use Prophylaxis and treatment of thromboembolic disorders
Pregnancy Risk Factor C
Usual Dosage Oral:

Adult: Initial: 10-15 mg/day for 2-5 days, then adjust dose according to results of prothrombin time (PT); maintenance dose: Based on PT determinations, usually 2-10 mg/day

Children and Infants: 0.05-0.34 mg/kg/day; infants < 12 months old may require doses at or near the high end of this range; consistent anticoagulation may be difficult to maintain in children < five years of age

Water for Injection, Bacteriostatic
Use Sterile vehicle containing one or more suitable antimicrobial agents for parenteral preparations
Pregnancy Risk Factor C

4-Way® Long Acting Nasal Solution [OTC] *see* Oxymetazoline Hydrochloride *on page 265*

Wellbutrin® *see* Bupropion *on page 50*

Wellcovorin® *see* Leucovorin Calcium *on page 200*

Westhroid® *see* Thyroid *on page 354*

Westrim® LA [OTC] *see* Phenylpropanolamine Hydrochloride *on page 283*

White Petrolatum
Brand Names Vaseline® [OTC]
Synonyms Petroleum Jelly
Use Soften and soothe sensitive skin, vehicle in dermatological compounding

Whitfield's Ointment [OTC] *see* Benzoic Acid and Salicylic Acid *on page 41*

Wigraine® *see* Ergotamine *on page 133*

Wincillin®-VK *see* Penicillin V Potassium *on page 274*

Winstrol® *see* Stanozolol *on page 333*

Wintomylon® *see* Nalidixic Acid *on page 245*

Wintrocin® *see* Erythromycin *on page 134*

Witch Hazel
Brand Names Tucks® [OTC]
Synonyms Hamamelis Water
Use An after-stool wipe to remove most causes of local irritation; temporary management of vulvitis, pruritus ani and vulva; help relieve the discomfort of simple hemorrhoids, anorectal surgical wounds, and episiotomies
Usual Dosage Apply to anorectal area as needed

Wool Fat *see* Lanolin *on page 199*

Wyamine® Sulfate *see* Mephentermine Sulfate *on page 219*

Wyamycin® E *see* Erythromycin *on page 134*

Wyamycin® S *see* Erythromycin *on page 134*

Wycillin® *see* Penicillin G Procaine, Aqueous *on page 273*

Wydase® *see* Hyaluronidase *on page 170*

Wygesic® *see* Propoxyphene and Acetaminophen *on page 304*

Wymox® *see* Amoxicillin *on page 21*

Wytensin® *see* Guanabenz Acetate *on page 164*

Xanax® *see* Alprazolam *on page 13*

Xerac BP® [OTC] *see* Benzoyl Peroxide *on page 41*

Xero-Lube® [OTC] *see* Saliva Substitute *on page 320*

X-Prep® Liquid [OTC] *see* Senna *on page 322*

X-seb® T [OTC] *see* Coal Tar and Salicylic Acid *on page 85*

Xylocaine® *see* Lidocaine Hydrochloride *on page 204*

Xylocaine® With Epinephrine *see* Lidocaine and Epinephrine *on page 203*

Xylometazoline Hydrochloride (zye loe met az' oh leen)
Brand Names Otrivin® [OTC]
Use Symptomatic relief of nasal and nasopharyngeal mucosal congestion
Pregnancy Risk Factor C
Usual Dosage

Adult and Children: > 12 years of age: 2-3 drops or sprays (0.1%) in each nostril every 8-10 hours

Children: < 12 years: 2-3 drops (0.05%) in each nostril every 8-10 hours

Xylo-Pfan® *see* d-Xylose *on page 125*

Yellow Fever Vaccine
Brand Names YF-VAX®
Use Active immunization against yellow fever
Usual Dosage Single dose S.C. 0.5 mL

Yellow Mercuric Oxide *see* Mercuric Oxide *on page 220*

YF-VAX® *see* Yellow Fever Vaccine *on this page*

Yocon® *see* Yohimbine Hydrochloride *on this page*

Yodoxin® *see* Iodoquinol *on page 189*

Yohimbine Hydrochloride
Brand Names Aphrodyne™; Yocon®; Yohimex™
Use No FDA sanctioned indications
Usual Dosage Adult: Oral: One tablet 3 times daily

Yohimex™ *see* Yohimbine Hydrochloride *on this page*

Yomesan® *see* Niclosamide *on page 251*

Yutopar® *see* Ritodrine Hydrochloride *on page 317*

Zanosar® *see* Streptozocin *on page 334*

Zantac® *see* Ranitidine Hydrochloride *on page 313*

Zarontin® *see* Ethosuximide *on page 140*

Zaroxolyn® *see* Metolazone *on page 233*

Zeasorb-AF® [OTC] *see* Tolnaftate *on page 357*

Zephiran® [OTC] *see* Benzalkonium Chloride *on page 40*

Zeroxin® *see* Benzoyl Peroxide *on page 41*

Zestril® *see* Lisinopril *on page 205*

Zetar® [OTC] *see* Coal Tar *on page 85*

Zidovudine (zye doe' vue deen)
Brand Names Retrovir®
Synonyms Azidothymidine; AZT; Compound S
Use Management of patients with symptomatic HIV infections
Pregnancy Risk Factor C
Usual Dosage 200 mg every four hours

Zinacef® *see* Cefuroxime *on page 65*

Zinc *see* Trace Metals *on page 358*

Zinca-Pak® *see* Trace Metals *on page 358*

Zincate® *see* Zinc Sulfate *on next page*

Zinc Chloride (zink)
Use Astringent, desensitizer for dentin, replacement therapy
Pregnancy Risk Factor C
Usual Dosage Stable adults with fluid loss from small bowel 12.2 mg zinc per liter TPN or 17.1 mg zinc per kg of stool or ileostomy output

Zinc Gelatin
Brand Names Gelucast®
Synonyms Unna's Boot; Unna's Paste; Zinc Gelatin Boot
Use As a protectant and to support varicosities and similar lesions of the lower limbs
Usual Dosage Apply externally as an occlusive boot

Zinc Gelatin Boot *see* Zinc Gelatin *on this page*

Zincon® Shampoo [OTC] *see* Pyrithione Zinc *on page 310*

Zinc Oxide
Synonyms Lassar's Zinc Paste
Use Protective coating for mild skin irritations
Usual Dosage Apply as required

Zinc Oxide, Cod Liver Oil and Talc
Brand Names Desitin® [OTC]
Use Relief of diaper rash, superficial wounds and burns, and other minor skin irritations
Usual Dosage Apply thin layer as needed

Zinc Sulfate
Brand Names Eye-Sed® [OTC]; Orazinc® [OTC]; Verazinc® [OTC]; Zinc-ate®
Use Dietary supplement; relief of minor eye irritation
Pregnancy Risk Factor C
Usual Dosage Oral:

RDA:

Adult: $\geq$ 11 years of age: 65 mg zinc sulfate (15 mg elemental zinc) daily

Children: 1-10 years: 44 mg zinc sulfate (10 mg elemental zinc) daily

Zinc deficiency:

Adult: 100-220 mg zinc sulfate (23-50 mg elemental zinc)/dose three times/day

Children and Infants: 0.3 mg elemental zinc/kg/day or a minimum of 3 mg elemental zinc/day

Zinc Undecylenate
Brand Names Desenex® [OTC]; Kool Foot® [OTC]; Merlenate® [OTC]; Pedi-Dri; Quinsana® Plus [OTC]
Use Antifungal/antibacterial agents for athlete's foot and ringworm exclusive of nails and hairy areas; relief of diaper rash, jock itch, and other minor skin irritation; excessive perspiration and irritation in the groin area
Usual Dosage Powder is used as adjunctive therapy and is good when drying effect is desirable, ointments are used as primary therapy in mild conditions (or as prophylaxis)

Apply twice a day, after cleansing, to the affected area; continue therapy for four weeks (athlete's foot/ringworm) and for two weeks (jock itch)

Zolicef® *see* Cefazolin Sodium *on page 63*

APPENDIX

ANTIDOTE CHART

Antidote	Poison/Drug	Indications/Symptoms
N-Acetylcysteine	Acetaminophen	• Unknown quantity ingested and $<$ 24 h has elapsed since the time of ingestion • $>$ 7.5 g ingested acutely • Serum acetaminophen $>$ 140 μg/mL at 4 h postingestion • Ingested dose $>$ 140 mg/kg
Amyl nitrite, sodium nitrite, sodium thiosulfate	Cyanide	• Begin treatment at the first sign of toxicity if cyanide exposure is known or strongly suspected
Atropine	Organophosphate and carbamate insecticides	• Myoclonic seizures, severe hallucinations, weakness, arrhythmias, excessive salivation, involuntary urination and defecation
	Atropine	• Bradyarrhythmias, heart block
Calcium EDTA (Versenate®)	Lead	• Symptomatic patients, or asymptomatic children with blood levels $>$ 50 μg/dL
Calcium gluconate	Hydrofluoric acid (HF)	• Calcium gluconate gel 2.5% for dermal exposure of HF of $<$ 20% concentration • SC injections of calcium gluconate for dermal exposures of concentrations $>$ 20% or failure to respond to gel
Deferoxamine (Desferal®)	Iron	• If serum iron level exceeds total iron binding capacity (TIBC), or serum iron $>$ 350 μg/dL and TIBC is unavailable, or unable to obtain SI in a seasonable time and patient is symptomatic
Digoxin immune FAB (Digibind®)	Digoxin	• Life-threatening cardiac arrhythmias, progressive bradyarrhythmias, 2nd or 3rd degree heart block unresponsive to atropine, serum digoxin level $>$ 10 ng/mL or potassium levels $>$ 5 mEq/L
Dimercaprol (BAL in Oil®)	Arsenic	• Any symptoms of arsenic exposure
	Lead	• All patients with symptoms, or asymptomatic children with blood levels 70 μg/dL
	Mercury	• Any symptoms due to mercury, and patient unable to take d-penicillamine

(continued)

Antidote	Poison/Drug	Indications/Symptoms
Ethanol	Ethylene glycol or methanol	• Ethylene glycol or methanol blood levels > 20 mg/dL or blood levels not readily available and suspected ingestion of toxic amounts, or any symptomatic patient with a history of ethylene glycol or methanol ingestion
Naloxone	Opiates (heroin, morphine, etc)	• Coma or respiratory depression from unknown cause, or from opiate overdose
D-penicillamine (Cuprimine®)	Arsenic	• Following BAL therapy in symptomatic, acutely poisoned patients
	Lead	• Asymptomatic patients with excess lead burden
	Mercury	• Patient symptomatic from mercury exposure or excessive levels
Physostigmine (Antilirium®)	Atropine and anticholinergics	• Myoclonic seizures, hypertension, severe arrhythmias, hallucinations
	Cyclic antidepressants	• Refractory seizures or arrhythmias unresponsive to conventional therapies
Phytonadione (Vitamin K_1)	Warfarin	• Large acute ingestion of warfarin rodenticides or chronic exposure, or greater than normal prothrombin time
Pralidoxime (Protopam®)	Organophosphate insecticide	• An adjunct to atropine therapy for treatment of profound muscle weakness, respiratory depression, muscle twitching
Pyridoxine (Vitamin B_6)	Isoniazid	• Unknown overdose, or ingested amount > 80 mg/kg
Antivenin polyvalent	Pit viper bites (rattlesnake, cottonmouth, copperhead)	• History of envenomation by a pit viper and experiencing mild moderate, or severe symptoms **Mild:** Local swelling (progressive), pain, no systemic systems **Moderate:** Ecchymosis and swelling beyond the bite site, some systemic symptoms, and/or lab changes **Severe:** Profound edema involving entire extremity, cyanosis, serious systemic involvement, significant lab changes

BODY SURFACE AREA OF ADULTS AND CHILDREN

Calculating Body Surface Area in Children

A.   In a child of average size, find weight and corresponding surface area on the boxed scale to the left. Or, use the nomogram to the right. Lay a straightedge on the correct height and weight points for the child, then read the intersecting point on the surface area scale.

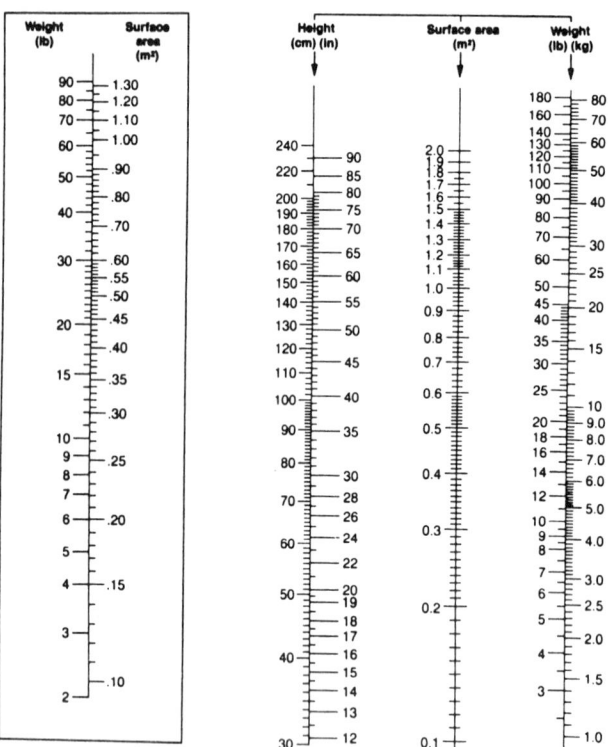

FOR CHILDREN OF NORMAL HEIGHT AND WEIGHT

NOMOGRAM

or

B. Formula: BSA (m²) $= \sqrt{\dfrac{\text{height (cm)} \times \text{weight (kg)}}{3600}}$

CONTROLLED SUBSTANCES

Schedule I = C-I

The drugs and other substances in this schedule have no legal medical uses except research. They have a **high** potential for abuse. They include opiates, opium derivatives and hallucinogens.

Schedule II = C-II

The drugs and other substances in this schedule have legal medical uses and a **high** abuse potential which may lead to severe dependence. They include former "Class A" narcotics, amphetamines, barbiturates and other drugs.

Schedule III = C-III

The drugs and other substances in this schedule have legal medical uses and a **lesser** degree of abuse potential which may lead to **moderate** dependence. They include former "Class B" narcotics and other drugs.

Schedule IV = C-IV

The drugs and other substances in this schedule have legal medical uses and **low** abuse potential which may lead to **moderate** dependence. They include barbiturates, benzodiazepines, propoxyphenes and other drugs.

Schedule V = C-V

The drugs and other substances in this schedule have legal medical uses and **low** abuse potential which may lead to **moderate** dependence. They include narcotic cough preparations, diarrhea preparations and other drugs.

FEVER DUE TO DRUGS

Amphotericin
Antihistamines
Asparaginase
Barbiturates
Bleomycin
Cephalosporins

Iodides
Methyldopa
p-Aminosalicylic acid
Penicillins
Phenolphthalein

Phenytoin
Procainamide
Quinidine
Sulfonamides
Thiouracil

Abstracted from Harrison's *Principles of Internal Medicine*, 11 ed, Braunwald E, ed, New York, NY: McGraw-Hill Book Co, 1987.

DRUGS THAT DISCOLOR THE FECES

Black

Acetazolamide
Aluminum hydroxide
Aminophylline
Amphetamine
Amphotericin B
Bismuth salts
Chlorpropamide
Clindamycin
Corticosteroids
Cyclophosphamide
Cytarabine

Digitalis
Ethacrynic acid
Ferrous salts
Fluorouracil
Hydralazine
Hydrocortisone
Iodide containing
    drugs
Melphalan
Methylprednisolone
Methotrexate

Phenylephrine
Potassium salts
Prednisolone
Procarbazine
Sulfonamides
Tetracycline
Theophylline
Thiotepa
Triamcinolone
Warfarin

Blue

Chloramphenicol
Methylene blue

Green

Indomethacin
Medroxyprogesterone

Yellow

Senna

Pink/Red

Anticoagulants
Aspirin
Barium
Heparin
Oxyphenbutazone
Phenylbutazone
Tetracycline syrup

Black/White Speckling

Aluminum hydroxide
Antibiotics (oral)
Barium

Orange/Red

Phenazopyridine
Rifampin

DRUGS THAT DISCOLOR THE URINE

Black/Brown/Dark

Cascara
Chloroquine
Ferrous sulfate
Metronidazole
Nitrofurantoin
Quinine
Senna

Blue

Methylene blue
Triamterene

Blue/Green

Amitriptyline
Methylene blue

Orange-Yellow

Heparin
Phenazopyridine
Rifampin
Sulfasalazine
Warfarin

Red

Daunorubicin
Doxorubicin
Ibuprofen
Oxyphenbutazone
Phenylbutazone
Phenytoin (pink)
Rifampin
Senna

GUIDELINES FOR DRUG LEVELS COMMONLY MONITORED

Drug	When to Sample	Therapeutic Levels	Usual Half–Life	Potentially Toxic Levels
Antibiotics				
Gentamicin	30 min after 30 min infusion Trough: < 0.5 h before next dose	Peak: 4–10 μg/mL Trough: < 2.0 μg/mL	2 h	Peak: > 12 μg/mL Trough: > 2 μg/mL
Tobramycin			2 h	
Amikacin		Peak: 20–35 μg/mL Trough: < 8 μg/mL	2 h	Peak: > 35 μg/mL Trough: > 8 μg/mL
Vancomycin	Peak: 1 h after 1 h infusion Trough: < 0.5 h before next dose	Peak: 30–40 μg/mL Trough: 5–10 μg/mL	6–8 h	Peak: > 80 μg/mL Trough: > 13 μg/mL
Anticonvulsants				
Carbamazepine	Trough: just before next oral dose In combination with other anticonvulsants	4–12 μg/mL 4–8 μg/mL	15–20 h	> 12 μg/mL
Ethosuximide	Trough: just before next oral dose	40–100 μg/mL	30–60 h	> 100 μg/mL
Phenobarbital	Trough: just before next dose	15–40 μg/mL	40–120 h	> 40 μg/mL
Phenytoin Free phenytoin	Trough: just before next dose Draw at same time as total level	10–20 μg/mL 1–2 μg/mL	Concentration dependent	> 20 μg/mL
Primidone	Trough: just before next dose (Note: Primidone is metabolized to phenobarb, order levels separately)	5–12 μg/mL	10–12 h	> 12 μg/mL
Valproic acid	Trough: just before next dose	50–100 μg/mL	5–20 h	> 100 μg/mL
Bronchodilators				
Aminophylline (I.V.)	30 min after a loading dose and 24 h after starting or changing a maintenance dose given as a constant infusion	10–20 μg/mL	Nonsmoking adult: 8 h Children and smoking adults: 4 h	> 20 μg/mL
Theophylline (P.O.)	Peak levels: not recommended Trough level: just before next dose	10–20 μg/mL		

(continued)

Drug	When to Sample	Therapeutic Levels	Usual Half–Life	Potentially Toxic Levels
Cardiovascular Agents				
Digoxin	Trough: just before next dose (levels drawn earlier than 6 h after a dose will be artificially elevated)	0.5–2 ng/mL	36 h	> 2 ng/mL
Lidocaine	Steady-state levels are usually achieved after 6–12 h	1.2–5.0 µg/mL	1.5 h	> 6 µg/mL
Procainamide	Trough: just before next oral dose I.V.: 6–12 h after infusion started Combined procainamide plus NAPA	4–10 µg/mL NAPA: 6–10 h 5–30 µg/mL	Procain: 2.7–5 h > 30 (NAPA + procain)	> 10 µg/mL
Quinidine	Trough: ust before next oral dose	23.5 µg/mL	6 h	> 10 µg/mL
Other Agents				
Amitriptyline plus nortriptyline	Trough: just before next dose	120–250 ng/mL		
Nortriptyline	Trough: just before next dose	50–140 ng/mL		
Lithium	Trough: just before next dose	0.6–1.6 mEq/mL	18–20 h	> 3 mEq/mL
Imipramine plus desipramine	Trough: just before next dose	150–300 ng/mL		
Desipramine	Trough: just before next dose	50–300 ng/mL		
Methotrexate	By protocol	< 0.5 µmol/L after 48 h		
Cyclosporine	Trough just before next dose	Highly variable Renal: 50–250 ng/mL (RIA) Hepatic: 150–400 ng/mL		

NORMAL LABORATORY VALUES FOR ADULTS

CHEMISTRY

Lab Test		Normal Values
Cardiac Enzymes		
CPK	male	8-150 IU/L
	female	8-110 IU/L
LDH		50-200 IU/L
Chem 14 Panel		
Albumin		3.5-5.5 g/dL
Alk phos	male	34-110 IU/L
	female	24-100 IU/L
Bilirubin, conjugated		0.0-0.2 mg/dL
Bilirubin, total		0.2-1.2 mg/dL
Blood urea nitrogen		8-23 mg/dL
Calcium		8.4-10.3 mg/dL
Creatinine		0.5-1.4 mg/dL
Glucose		65-110 mg/dL
LDH		50-200 IU/L
Phosphorus		2.3-4.5 mg/dL
Protein, total		6.0-8.2 g/dL
SGOT		5-45 IU/L
SGPT		5-45 IU/L
Uric acid	male	3-7 mg/dL
	female	3.6-5 mg/dL

Lab Test	Normal Values
Electrolytes and pH	
Chlorides	100-110 mEq/L
CO_2	26-31 mEq/L
pH	7.35-7.42
Potassium	3.3-5.0 mEq/L
Sodium	138-146 mEq/L
Anion gap	5-14 mEq/L
Other Tests	
Ammonia, plasma	20-60 μg/dL
Amylase, serum	44-128 IU/L
Calcium, ionized	4.6-5.2 mg/dL
Cholesterol	150-250 mg/dL
Iron, serum	50-140 μg/dL
Lactate, serum	1.4-3.9 mEq/L
Lipase	4-28 IU/dL
Magnesium	1.6-3.1 mg/dL
Oncotic pressure	22-28 mm Hg
Osmolality	280-300 mOsm/kg
TIBC	270-390 μg/dL
Triglycerides	50-150 mg/dL

Hematology

Hematocrit	male	40-52%
	female	35-47%
Hemoglobin	male	13.5-17.5 g/dL
	female	11.5-16.0 g/dL
MCH		27-36 pg
MCV		82-100 fL
Platelet count		150-450 K/mcL
RBC	male	4.5-6.2 M/mcL
	female	3.9-5.4 M/mcL
Reticulocyte	male	1-2.5%
count	female	1-3.5%

Sedimentation rate (zeta)	40-54%
Serum ferritin	Over 20 ng/mL
WBC	4.3-10.0 K/mcL
WBC w/differential	
Bands	3-8%
Basophils	0-2%
Eosinophils	1-4%
Lymphocytes	20-45%
Monocytes	1-8%
Neutrophils	40-70%

(continued)

Lab Test   **Normal Values**

Blood Gases

		Arterial	Venous
Base excess		-2.5 - 2.5 mEq/L	0-5 mEq/L
HCO_3		25-30 mEq/L	25-30 mEq/L
O_2 saturation		94-96%	
pCO_2	male	34-45 mm Hg	36-50 mm Hg
	female	31-42 mm Hg	34-48 mm Hg
pH		7.37-7.44	7.35-7.42
pO_2		75-90 mm Hg	

Lab Test   **Normal Values**

Thyroid Function Tests

FTI (free thyroxine index)	0.6-1.3
T_3 resin uptake	26-40%
T_3 (tri-iodothyronine) by RIA	80-180 ng/dL
T_4 (thyroxine) by RIA	4.0-10.0 μg/dL

Weight/Volume Equivalents

1 mg/dL = 10 μg/mL	1 ppm = 1 mg/L
1 mg/dL = 1 mg%	1 μg/mL = 1 mg/L

AVERAGE WEIGHTS AND SURFACE AREAS

**Average Weight and Surface Area of Preterm
Infants, Term Infants and Children**

Age	Average Weight (kg)*	Approximate Surface Area (m²)
Weeks Gestation		
26	0.9-1.0	0.10
30	1.3-1.5	0.12
32	1.6-2.0	0.15
38	2.9-3.0	0.20
40 (term infant at birth)	3.1-4.0	0.25
Months		
3	5.0	0.29
6	7.0	0.38
9	8.0	0.42
Year		
1	10.0	0.49
2	12.0	0.55
3	15.0	0.64
4	17.0	0.74
5	18.0	0.76
6	20.0	0.82
7	23.0	0.90
8	25.0	0.95
9	28.0	1.06
10	33.0	1.18
11	35.0	1.23
12	40.0	1.34
Adult	70.0	1.73

* Weights from age three months and over are rounded off to the nearest kilogram.

POUNDS-KILOGRAMS CONVERSION

1 pound = 0.45359 kilograms
1 kilogram = 2.2 pounds

TEMPERATURE CONVERSION

Centigrade to Fahrenheit = (°C x 9/5) + 32 = °F
Fahrenheit to Centigrade = (°F - 32) x 5/9 = °C

IMMUNIZATION GUIDELINES

Table 1. **Dosage and Administration Guidelines for Vaccines Available in the United States**

Vaccine	Dosage	Route of Administration
DT*	0.5 mL	I.M.
Td*	0.5 mL	I.M.
DTP*	0.5 mL	I.M.
Haemophilus B conjugate vaccine (HbCV)†	0.5 mL	I.M. or S.C. (see package insert)
polysaccharide vaccine (HbPV)	0.5 mL	I.M. or S.C. (see package insert)
Hepatitis B	0.5 mL (infants born to HB$_s$Ag$^+$ mothers)‡,§	I.M.
	0.5 mL (< 10 y)	I.M.
	1.0 mL (> 10 y)	I.M.
Influenza¶	0.25 mL x 2 (6-35 mo)	I.M. (doses 4+ weeks apart)
split virus only in pediatrics	0.5 mL x 2 (3-12 y)	I.M.
	0.5 mL x 1 (> 12 y)	I.M.
Measles#	0.5 mL (> 15 m)	S.C.
MMR#	0.5 mL (> 15 m)	S.C.
Mumps	0.5 mL	S.C.
Pneumococcal polyvalent	0.5 mL (> 2 y)	I.M. or S.C. (I.M. preferred)
Poliovirus (OPV)	0.5 mL	oral
Poliovirus (IPV)•	0.5 mL	S.C.
Rubella	0.5 mL (> 12 m)	S.C.
Tetanus	0.5 mL	I.M.

*DT & DTP for use in children < 7 y. Td contains same amount of tetanus toxoid as DT & DTP, but a reduced dose of diphtheria toxoid. Td for use in children > 7 y.
†The conjugate (HbCV) vaccine is preferred over the polysaccharide (HbPV) vaccine. In children with a high risk for haemophilus influenza type b disease and HbCV is unavailable, an acceptable alternate is to give HbPV at 18 mo with a second dose at 24 mo. Children < 5 y of age who were previously vaccinated with HbPV between 18 & 23 mo of age should be revaccinated with a single dose of HbCV at least 2 mo after the initial dose of HbPV. Either HbCV or HbPV can be administered up to the 5th birthday. However they are generally not recommended for children > 5 y of age.
‡Repeat dose at 1 and 6 months following the initial dose.
§Concurrent hepatitis B immune globulin administration is recommended for infants born to HB$_s$Ag$^+$ mothers (using different administration sites).

¶See package insert for specific dose recommendations for each vaccine.

#During epidemics a 2 dose measles vaccination schedule for preschoolers should be implemented. The first dose should be given at 9 mo or the first contact with a health care provider thereafter. Infants vaccinated befor their first birthday should receive a second dose at about 15 mo of age. Children < 1 y of age should receive single antigen measles vaccine. If 2 vaccinations are not possible, a reasonable alternative is to lower the routine age for MMR to 12 mo.

•The primary series consists of 3 doses. The first two doses should be administered at an interval of 8 wks. The third dose should be given at least 6 and preferably 12 mo after the second dose. A booster dose of 0.5 mL should be given to all children who have completed the primary series, before entering school. However, if the third dose of the primary series is given on or after the 4th birthday a fourth dose is not required before entering school. When polio vaccine is given to persons > 18 y IPV should be given.

Table 2. **Recommended Schedule for Active Immunization of Normal Infants and Children**

Recommended Age	Vaccine(s)	Comments
2 mo	DTP#1*, OPV#1	OPV and DTP can be given earlier in areas of high endemicity
4 mo	DTP#2, OPV#2	6 wk to 2 mo interval desired between OPV doses
6 mo	DTP#3	An additional dose of OPV at this time is optional in areas with a high risk of poliovirus exposure
15 mo	MMR, DTP#4, OPV#3	Completion of primary series of DTP and OPV
18 mo	HbCV	Conjugate preferred over polysaccharide vaccine
4-6 y	DTP#5, OPV#4	At or before school entry
14-16 y	Td	Repeat every 10 y throughout life

*DTP may be used up to the 7th birthday. The first dose can be given at 6 wk of age and at the 2nd & 3rd doses given 4-8 wk after the preceding dose.

Table 3. **Recommended Immunization Schedule for Infants and Children up to the 7th Birthday Not Immunized at the Recommended Time in Early Infancy**

Timing	Vaccine(s)	Comments
First visit	DTP#1, OPV#1 MMR (if child $\geq$ 15 mo) HbCV (if child $\geq$ 18 mo)	DTP, OPV and MMR should be administered simultaneously to children $\geq$ 15 mo. DTP, OPV, MMR and HbCV may be given simultaneously to children aged 18 mo-5 y.
2 mo after DTP#1, OPV#1	DTP#2, OPV#2	
2 mo after DTP#2	DTP#3	An additional dose of OPV at this time is optional in areas with a high risk of poliovirus exposure.
6-12 mo after DTP#3	DTP#4, OPV#3	
Preschool (4-6 y)	DTP#5, OPV#4	Preferably at or before school entry. The preschool doses are not needed if DTP#4 and OPV#3 are given after the 4th birthday.
14-16 y	Td	Repeat every 10 y throughout life

Table 4. **Recommended Immunization Schedule for Persons > 7 y of Age Not Immunized at the Recommended Time in Early Infancy**

Timing	Vaccine(s)	Comments
First visit	Td#1, OPV#1 and MMR	OPV not routinely recommended for persons $\geq$ 18 y
2 mo after Td#1, OPV#1	Td#2, OPV#2	OPV may be given as soon as 6 wk after OPV#1
6-12 mo after Td#2, OPV#2	Td#3, OPV#3	OPV#3 may be given as soon as 6 wk after OPV#2
10 y after Td#3	Td	Repeat every 10 y throughout life

Table 5. **Guidelines for Spacing Live and Killed Antigen Administration**

Antigen Combinations	Recommended Minimum Interval Between Doses
≥ 2 killed antigens	None. May be given simultaneously or at any interval between doses
Killed and live antigens	None. May be given simultaneously or at any interval between doses
≥ 2 live antigens	4 wk minimum interval if not administered simultaneously

Table 6. **Passive Immunization Agents — Immune Globulins**

Immune Globulin	Dosage		Route
Hepatitis B (H-BIG)			
percutaneous inoculation	0.06 mL/k/dose (5 mL max)		I.M.
perinatal	0.5 mL/dose		I.M.
sexual exposure	0.06 mL/k/dose (5 mL max)		I.M.
Immune globulin (Gamastan®)			
hepatitis A prophylaxis	0.02-0.04 mL/k/dose (single exposure)		I.M.
	0.06-0.12 mL/k/dose (continuous exposure) repeat every 4-6 mo		I.M.
hepatitis B (H-BIG preferred)	0.06 mL/k/dose		I.M.
measles	0.25 mL/k/dose (max: 15 mL/dose)		I.M.
	0.5 mL/k/dose (max: 15 mL/dose) (immunocompromised children)		I.M.
Rabies*	20 IU/kg/dose		
Tetanus	250-500 U/dose		I.M.
Varicella-zoster† (VZIG)	0-10 kg	125 U = 1 vial	I.M.
	10.1-20 kg	250 U = 2 vials	I.M.
	20.1-30 kg	375 U = 3 vials	I.M.
	30.1-40 kg	500 U = 4 vials	I.M.
	> 40 kg	625 U = 5 vials	I.M.

*1/2 of dose used locally in wound with the remaining 1/2 of dose given I.M.
†Infants born within 5 days of onset of maternal varicella should receive 125 U I.M. x 1 dose.

Table 7. **Guidelines for Spacing the Administration of Immune Globulin (IG) Preparations and Vaccines**

Immunobiologic Combinations	Recommended Minimum Interval Between Doses
Simultaneous Administration	
IG and killed antigen	None. May be given simultaneously at different sites or at any time between doses.
IG and live antigen	Should generally not be given simultaneously. If unavoidable to do so, give at different sites and revaccinate or test for seroconversion in 3 mo.

Nonsimultaneous Administration

First	Second	
IG	Killed antigen	None
Killed antigen	IG	None
IG	Live antigen	6 wk and preferably 3 mo
Live antigen	IG	2 wk

*The live virus vaccines, oral polio and yellow fever are exceptions to these recommendations. Either vaccine may be administered simultaneously or any time before or after IG without significantly decreasing antibody response.

Table 8. **Recommended for Routine Immunization of HIV-Infected Children — United States**

Vaccine	Known HIV Infection	
	Asymptomatic	Symptomatic
DTP	Yes	Yes
OPV	No	No
IPV	Yes	Yes
MMR	Yes	Yes*
HbVC	Yes	Yes
Pneumococcal	Yes	Yes
Influenza	Not†	Yes

*Should be considered.
†Not contraindicated.

Reference: Children's Hospital of Los Angeles, *Housestaff Manual*, 1990, 424-8.

TABLE OF APOTHECARY-METRIC CONVERSIONS

Exact Equivalents

1 gram (g) = 15.43 grains	0.1 mg = 1/600 gr
1 milliliter (mL) = 16.23 minims	0.12 mg = 1/500 gr
1 minim (𝕞) = 0.06 milliliter	0.15 mg = 1/400 gr
1 grain (gr) = 64.8 milligrams	0.2 mg = 1/300 gr
1 ounce (ʒ) = 31.1 grams	0.3 mg = 1/200 gr
1 fluid ounce (flʒ) = 29.57 mL	0.4 mg = 1/150 gr
1 pint (pt) = 473.2 mL	0.5 mg = 1/120 gr
1 ounce (oz) = 28.35 grams	0.6 mg = 1/100 gr
1 pound (lb) = 453.6 grams	0.8 mg = 1/80 gr
1 kilogram (kg) = 2.2 pounds	1.0 mg = 1/65 gr
1 quart (qt) = 946.4 mL	

Approximate Equivalents*

Liquids

1 teaspoonful = 5 mL
1 tablespoonful = 15 mL

Solids

¼ grain = 15 mg
½ grain = 30 mg
1 grain = 60 mg
1½ grain = 100 mg
5 grains = 300 mg
10 grains = 600 mg

* Use exact equivalents for compounding and calculations requiring a high degree of accuracy.

TABLE OF IDEAL BODY WEIGHTS IN KILOGRAMS*

Height	Male	Female
5' 0"	50.0	45.0
5' 1"	52.3	47.3
5' 2"	54.6	49.6
5' 3"	56.9	51.9
5' 4"	59.2	54.2
5' 5"	61.5	56.5
5' 6"	63.8	58.8
5' 7"	66.1	61.1
5' 8"	68.4	63.4
5' 9"	70.7	65.7
5'10"	73.0	68.0
5'11"	75.3	70.3
6' 0"	77.6	72.6
6' 1"	79.9	
6' 2"	82.2	
6' 3"	84.5	
6' 4"	86.8	

*Calculated from:

IBW (kg) male = 50 kg + 2.3 kg/inch over 5'0"
female = 45 kg + 2.3 kg/inch over 5'0"

CALCULATION OF IDEAL BODY WEIGHT

Adult   (18 years and older)

IBW (male)   = 50 + (2.3 x height in inches over 5 feet)
IBW (female) = 45.5 + (2.3 x height in inches over 5 feet)

* IBW is in kg.

Children

a.   1-18 years

$$IBW = \frac{(height^2 \times 1.65)}{1000}$$

* IBW is in kg.
  Height is in cm.

b.   5 feet and taller

IBW (male)   = 39 + (2.27 x height in inches over 5 feet)
IBW (female) = 42.2 + (2.27 x height in inches over 5 feet)

* IBW is in kg.

ACRONYMS AND ABBREVIATIONS GLOSSARY

ACRONYMS AND ABBREVIATIONS GLOSSARY

A	apical; artery
A1AT	alpha$_1$ antitrypsin
A$_2$	aortic second sound
aa	of each (ana)
AABB	American Association of Blood Banks
AAC	antibiotic associated colitis
AACC	American Association of Clinical Chemistry
AaG	alveolar arterial gradient
AAL	anterior axillary line
AAP	American Academy of Pediatrics
AAPCC	American Association of Poison Control Centers
AAS	acute abdominal series
AAT	alpha antitrypsin
AB	abort; antibiotic
Ab	antibody
ABC	avidin-biotin complex
ABE	acute bacterial endocarditis
ABG	arterial blood gas
ABL	abetalipoprotein
ABLB	alternate binaural loudness balance
ABO	ABO blood group
ABPA	allergic bronchopulmonary aspergillosis
ABR	auditory brainstem response
ABS	alkylbenzene sulfonate
AC	alternating current
Ac	actinium
ac	before meals (ante cibum)
ACA	anticardiolipin antibody; Du Pont chemistry analyzer
ACC	amylase creatinine clearance
ACD	acid-citrate-dextrose
ACE	angiotensin converting enzyme
AChR	acetylcholine receptor antibody
ACLS	advanced cardiac life support
ACOG	American College of Obstetrics and Gynecology
AcP	acid phosphatase
ACT	activated clotting time
ACTH	adrenocorticotropic hormone
ad	right ear; up to (ad)
ADCC	antibody-dependent cell-mediated cytotoxicity
ADH	alcohol dehydrogenase; antidiuretic hormone
ADL	active daily living
ad lib	as desired (ad libitum)
ADM	admission
ADNase	anti-DNAse
ADP	adenosine 5-diphosphate
ADT	adenosine triphosphate; alternate-day treatment
AED	anticonvulsant drugs
AEP	average evoked potential
AF	acid-fast; amniotic fluid; artrial fibrillation
AFB	acid-fast bacillus

AFP	alphafetoprotein
A/G	albumin/globulin ratio
Ag	antigen; silver
AGA	accelerated growth area
AGL	acute glomerular nephritis
AGS	adrenogenital syndrome
AH	antihyaluronidase
AHA	acquired hemolytic anemia; autoimmune hemolytic anemia
AHBC	hepatitis B core antibody
AHF	antihemophilic factor
AHG	antihemophilic globulin
AHT	antihyaluronidase titer
AI	allergy index; aortic insufficiency
AICC	anti-inhibitor coagulant complex
AIDS	acquired immune deficiency syndrome
AIHA	autoimmune hemolytic anemia
AIP	acute intermittent porphyria; average intravascular pressure
AJ	ankle jerk
AK	adenylate kinase; above the knee
Al	aluminum
ALA	aminolevulinic acid
alb	albumin
alk	alkaline
AlkP	alkaline phosphatase
ALL	acute lymphoblastic leukemia; acute lymphocytic leukemia
AlP	alkaline phosphatase
ALPI	alkaline phosphatase isoenzymes
ALS	advanced life support; amyotrophic lateral sclerosis; antilymphocyte serum
ALT	alanine aminotransferase
AM	morning
Am	americium
AMA	against medical advice; American Medical Association; antimitrochondrial antibody
AMI	acute myocardial infarction
AML	acute myeloblastic leukemia
AMP	adenosine monophosphate
AMPS	acid mucopolysaccharide
ANA	antinuclear antibody
ANF	antinuclear factor
ANLL	acute nonlymphocytic leukemia
A & O	alert and oriented
AODM	adult onset diabetes mellitus
AOS	acridine orange staining
A & P	anterior and posterior; assessment and plans
AP	antepartum; anteroposterior
APCA	antiparietal cell antibody
APhA	American Pharmaceutical Association

ACRONYMS AND ABBREVIATIONS GLOSSARY

APP . . . . alum-precipitating pyridine
APTT . . . . . . activated partial thromboplastin time
APUD . . . . . . amine precursor uptake and decarboxylation
aq . . . . water (aqua)
Ar . . . . argon
ARA . . . . antireticulin antibody
ARD . . . . antimicrobial removal device; acute respiratory
                  distress
ARDS . . . . . . adult respiratory distress syndrome
ARF . . . . acute renal failure
Ars . . . . arylsulfatase
ART . . . . arterial line
AS . . . . anal sphincter; ankylosing spondylitis; aortic
                  stenosis
As . . . . arsenic
as . . . . left ear
ASA . . . . acetylsalicylic acid
AsA . . . . arylsulfatase A
ASAP . . . . . . as soon as possible
AsB . . . . arylsulfatase B
ASCP . . . . . . American Society of Clinical Pathologists
ASCVD . . . . arteriosclerotic cardiovascular disease
ASD . . . . atrial septal defect
ASHD . . . . . . arteriosclerotic heart disease
ASHP . . . . . . American Society of Hospital Pharmacists
ASK . . . . antistreptokinase
ASKA . . . . . . antiskeletal antibody
ASLO . . . . . antistreptolysin O
ASMA . . . . antismooth muscle antibody
ASO . . . . . . antistreptolysin O; arterioselerosis obliterans
AST . . . . aspartate aminotransferase
ASVD . . . . . arteriosclerotic vascular disease
At . . . . astatine
AT III . . . . . antithrombin III
ATN . . . . . . acute tubular necrosis
ATP . . . . adenosine triphosphate
ATPase . . . . adenosine triphosphatase
ATS . . . . American Thoracic Society
Au . . . . gold
au . . . . each ear (auris utro)
^{198}Au . . . . . radioisotope of gold
A-V . . . . arteriovenous; atrioventricular; audiovisual
AVA . . . . . . availability
AVM . . . . . . arteriovenous malformation
A & W . . . . alive and well
Ax . . . . axillary

B . . . . boron
Ba . . . . barium

BAC	blood alcohol concentration
BAE	barium enema
BAEP	brainstem auditory evoked potential
BAER	brainstem auditory evoked response
BAL	bronchial alveolar lavage
BAO	basal acid output
BBB	blood brain barrier; bundle branch block
BBPRL	big big prolactin
BBT	basal body temperature
BCG	bacillus Calmette-Guérin
BCP	birth control pills; blood cell profile
bcr	breakpoint cluster region
BD	bronchodilators
BE	bacterial endocarditis; barium enema
Be	beryllium
BEP	brainstem evoked potential
BERA	brainstem evoked response auditory
BF	black female
BFT	bentonite flocculation test
BHB	beta-hydroxybutyrate
BHI	brain heart infusion
Bi	bismuth
bid	twice a day (bis in die)
B-J	Bence Jones
BJ	biceps jerk; bone and joint
BK	below knee
Bk	berkelium
Bl Obs	bladder observation
BLS	basic life support
BM	black male; bone marrow; bowel movement; breast milk
BMR	basal metabolic rate
BNO	bladder neck obstruction
BP	blood pressure
BPH	benign prostatic hypertrophy
BR	bathroom; bedrest
Br	bromine; bromide
BrdU	5-bromodeoxyuridine
BRP	bathroom privileges
BRU	bromide urine
BS	blood sugar; bowel sounds; breath sounds
bsa	body surface area
BSEP	brainstem evoked potential
BSO	bilateral salpingo-oophorectomy
BSP	bromsulfophthalein
BTG	beta thromboglobulin
BTL	bilateral tubal ligation
BUN	blood urea nitrogen
BVL	bilateral vas ligation
BW	birth weight; body weight
Bx	biopsy

ACRONYMS AND ABBREVIATIONS GLOSSARY

C . . . . carbon
c . . . . with (cum)
C₂ . . . . second cervical vertebra
CA . . . . cancer antigen; cardiac arrest; chronological age
Ca . . . . calcium
CAB . . . . coronary artery bypass
CABG . . . . . coronary artery bypass graft
CAC . . . . circulating anticoagulant
CaCO₃ . . . . . calcium carbonate
CAD . . . . coronary artery disease
CAH . . . . chronic active hepatitis
CALLA . . . . . common acute lymphoblastic leukemia antigen
cAMP . . . . . . cyclic AMP
CAPD . . . . . . chronic ambulatory peritoneal dialysis
CAT . . . . computed axial tomography
CBAT . . . . . . Coulter battery
CBC . . . . complete blood count
CBF . . . . cerebral blood flow
CBG . . . . capillary blood gases
CBIL . . . . conjugated bilirubin
CBS . . . . chronic brain syndrome
CBT . . . . computerized body tomography
CC . . . . chief complaint; closing capacity
CCI . . . . corrected count increment
CCK . . . . cholecystokinin
CCU . . . . cardiac care unit; coronary care unit
Cd . . . . cadmium
CDA . . . . congenital dyserythropoietic anemia
CDC . . . . Center for Disease Control
CDP . . . . continuous distending pressure; cytidine
              diphosphate
CDU . . . . cumulative dose unit
Ce . . . . cerium
CEA . . . . carcinoembryonic antigen
CF . . . . cardiac failure; caucasian female; complement
              fixation; cystic fibrosis
Cf . . . . californium
CFU . . . . colony forming units
CGL . . . . chronic granulocytic leukemia
CH . . . . congenital hypothyroidism
CHBHA . . . . congenital Heinz body hemolytic anemia
CHD . . . . congenital heart disease
CHF . . . . congestive heart failure
CI . . . . cardiac index; color index; confidence intervals
CIC . . . . circulating immune complexes
CIE . . . . counterimmunoelectrophoresis
CIF . . . . clone-inhibiting factor
CIN . . . . cervical intraepithelial neoplasia
CIP . . . . cellular immunocompetence profile
CJD . . . . Creutzfeldt-Jakob disease

CK	creatine kinase
Cl	chlorine
CLL	chronic lymphocytic leukemia
CM	caucasian male; contrast media; culture media
Cm	curium
cm	centimeter
cm^2	square centimeter
CMG	cystometrogram
CML	cell mediated lysis; chronic myelogenous leukemia
cmm	square centimeter cm^2
CMP	cardiomyopathy; cervical mucus penetration
CMPT	cervical mucous penetration test
CMV	cytomegalovirus
CMVS	culture midvoid specimen
CN	cyanogen
CNS	central nervous system
CNSHA	congenital nonspherocytic hemolytic anemia
C/O	complaint of
CO	carbon monoxide; cardiac output
Co	cobalt
^{57}Co	radioisotope of cobalt
^{60}Co	radioisotope of cobalt
coag	coagulation
COHb	carboxyhemoglobin
COLD	chronic obstructive lung disease
COP	chronic obstructive pulmonary
COPD	chronic obstructive pulmonary disease
C & P	cystoscopy and pyelogram
CPA	carotid phonoangiography
CPAP	continuous positive airway pressure
CPB	cardiopulmonary bypass
CPD	cyst disease protein; citrate phosphate dextrose
CPDA	citrate phosphate dextrose adenine
CPE	cytopathogenic effects
CPI	coronary prognostic index
CPK	creatine phosphokinase
cpm	counts per minute
CPP	cerebral perfusion pressure
CPPB	continuous positive pressure breathing
CPPD	calcium pyrophosphate dihydrate
CPR	cardiopulmonary resuscitation
CPS	Compendium of Pharmaceuticals and Specialties
cps	cycles per second
CPT	chest physiotherapy
Cr	chromium
^{51}Cr	radioisotope of chromium
CRA	central retinal artery
Cre	creatinine
creat	creatinine
CRF	chronic renal failure; corticotropin releasing factor

CRM . . . . cross reacting material
CRP . . . . C-reactive protein
CRS . . . . catheter related sepsis
CRST . . . . . . calcinosis, Raynaud's phenomenon, sclerodactylia, telangiectasis
CRT . . . . cathode ray tube
C & S . . . . . . culture and sensitivity
CS . . . . cesarean section; coronary sclerosis
Cs . . . . cesium
CS & CC . . . culture, sensitivity and colony count
CSF . . . . cerebrospinal fluid
CSP . . . . chemistry screening profile
CSR . . . . corrected sedimentation rate
CT . . . . circulation time; clotting time; computerized tomography
CTA . . . . Committee on Thrombolytic Agents
CTAB . . . . . . cetyltrimethylammonium bromide
CTD . . . . carpal tunnel decompression; congenital thymic dysplasia
CTM . . . . *Chlamydia* transport media
CTT . . . . computerized transaxial tomography
Cu . . . . copper
CUC . . . . chronic ulcerative colitis
CV . . . . cardiovascular; coefficient of variation; conjugata vera
CVA . . . . cerebrovascular accident
CVE . . . . cerebrovascular evaluation
CVI . . . . cerebral vascular insufficiency; continuous venous infusion
CVP . . . . central venous pressure
CVS . . . . cardiovascular system; clean voided specimen
Cx . . . . cervical; cervix
CXR . . . . chest x-ray

D_5W . . . . 5% dextrose in water solution
DALA . . . . . . delta aminolevulinic acid
DAT . . . . direct antiglobulin test
DB . . . . deep breath
db . . . . decibel
DBI . . . . development at birth index
DBP . . . . diastolic blood pressure
D & C . . . . . . dilatation and curettage
DC . . . . direct current
DCG . . . . . . dynamic electrocardiogram
DCH . . . . delayed and cutaneous hypersensitivity
DD . . . . differential diagnosis
DDD . . . . degenerative disc disease
DDT . . . . dichloro-diphenyltrichloroethane
DDX . . . . differential diagnosis
DEAE . . . . . . diethylaminoethyl

DER . . . . dermatone evoked response
DFA . . . . direct fluorescent antibody
dg . . . . decigram
DH . . . . dermatitis herpetiformis
DHA . . . . dehydroepiandrosterone
DHEA . . . . . . dehydroepiandrosterone
DHEA-S . . . . dehydroepiandrosterone sulfate
DHL . . . . diffuse histiocytic lymphoma
DHS . . . . duration of hospital stay
DHT . . . . dihydrotestosterone
DI . . . . diabetes insipidus
DIC . . . . disseminated intravascular coagulation
diff . . . . differential
DIP . . . . dichlorophenolindophenol
DISIDA . . . . . diisopropyl-iminodiacetic acid
DJD . . . . degenerative joint disease
D-L . . . . Donath-Landsteiner
dL . . . . deciliter
DLCO . . . . . diffusing capacity of the lung for carbon monoxide
DLE . . . . discoid lupus erythematosus
DLF . . . . digoxin-like factors
DM . . . . diabetes mellitus; diastolic murmur
dm . . . . decimeter
DMO . . . . . . dimethyloxazolidinedione
DMSO . . . . . dimethylsulfoxide
DNA . . . . deoxyribonucleic acid
DNase . . . . . deoxyribonuclease
DNBT . . . . . . dinitroblue
DNPH . . . . . dinitrophenylhydrazine
DOA . . . . date of admission; dead on arrival
DOB . . . . date of birth
DOC . . . . . . deoxycorticosterone
DOE . . . . dyspnea on exertion
DOI . . . . date of injury
dos . . . . dose (dosis)
DP . . . . diastolic pressure
DPG . . . . diphosphoglycerate
DPH . . . . diphenylhydantoin
DPT . . . . diphtheria toxoid, pertussis vaccine, tetanus toxoid
DQ . . . . developmental quotient
DR . . . . donor related
Dr . . . . doctor
DRG . . . . diagnostic related group(s)
DSA . . . . digital subtraction angiography
DSD . . . . discharge summary dictated; dry sterile dressing
ds-DNA . . . . double stranded DNA
DSF . . . . disulfiram
DST . . . . dexamethasone suppression test
DT . . . . delirium tremons; duration tetany; dye test
dtd . . . . let such doses be given (dentur tales doses)

ACRONYMS AND ABBREVIATIONS GLOSSARY

DTM . . . . dermatophyte test medium
DTR . . . . deep tendon reflex
dU . . . . deoxyuridine
DVT . . . . deep vein thrombosis
Dx . . . . diagnosis
Dy . . . . dysprosium

EA . . . . early antigen
EAC . . . . external auditory canal
EACA . . . . . . epsilon-aminocaproic acid
EB . . . . Epstein-Barr
EBEA . . . . . . Epstein-Barr early antigen
EBNA . . . . . . Epstein-Barr nuclear antigen
EBV . . . . Epstein-Barr virus
EB-VCA . . . . Epstein-Barr viral capsid antigen
EBVEA . . . . . Epstein-Barr virus, early antigen
EBVNA . . . . Epstein-Barr virus, nuclear antigen
EC . . . . *Escherichia coli*; extracellular
ECA . . . . external carotid artery
ECG . . . . electrocardiogram
ECT . . . . emission computed tomography
EDTA . . . . . . ethylenediaminetetraacetic acid
EDX . . . . electrodiagnosis
EEG . . . . electroencephalography
EENT . . . . . . eyes, ears, nose, throat
EF . . . . ejection fraction; extended-field
EFA . . . . essential fatty acids
EFM . . . . external fetal monitoring
eg . . . . example
EGA . . . . estimated gestational age
EGD . . . . esophagogastroduodenoscopy
EH . . . . enlarged heart; essential hypertension
EHEC . . . . . . enterohemorrhagic *E. coli*
EIA . . . . enzyme immunoassay
EID . . . . electroimmunodiffusion
EIEC . . . . enteroinvasive *E. coli*
EKG . . . . electrocardiogram
ELISA . . . . . . enzyme-linked immunosorbent assay
ELT . . . . euoglobulin lysis time
EM . . . . electron microscopy
EMA . . . . endomysial antibody
EMG . . . . . . electromyogram
EMS . . . . eosinophil myalgia syndrome
ENA . . . . extractable nuclear antigen
ENG . . . . electronystagmography
ENT . . . . ear, nose and throat
EOG . . . . electro-oculogram
eos . . . . eosinophil
EPA . . . . Environmental Protection Agency

EPEC	enteropathogenic *E. coli*
EPIS	episiotomy
EPS	electrophysiologic studies
Eq	equivalent
ER	emergency room; estrogen receptors
Er	erbium
ERA	estrogen receptor assay; evoked response audiometry
ERCP	endoscopic retrograde cholangiopancreatography
ERG	electroretinogram
ERPF	effective renal plasma flow
ERV	expiratory reserve volume
ES	electrical stimulation
Es	Einsteinium
ESP	extrasensory perception
ESR	erythrocyte sedimentation rate
ESRD	end-stage renal disease
EST	electroshock therapy
et	and (et)
ETEC	enterotoxigenic *E. coli*
EtOH	ethyl alcohol
ETT	extrathyroidal thyroxine
EU	Ehrlich unit
EVI	endocardial, vascular, and interstitial

F	fluorine
FA	fatty acid; filterable agent; fluorescent antibody
FAB	French-American-British
FACP	Fellow of the American College of Physicians
FAD	flavin adenine dinucleotide
FAMA	fluorescent antibody to membrane antigen
FANA	fluorescent antinuclear antibody
FAS	fetal alcohol syndrome
FB	finger breadths; foreign bodies
FBC	functional bactericidal concentration
FBP	fibrin breakdown product
FBS	fasting blood sugar
Fc	portion of antibody molecule bound by membrane receptors
FDA	Federal Drug Administration
FDP	fibrin degradation product; fructose diphosphate
Fe	iron
$FeCl_3$	ferric chloride
FEF	forced expiratory flow
FEP	free erythrocyte protoporphyrin
FES	functional electrical stimulation
FETI	fluorescent energy transfer immunoassay
FEV	forced expiratory volume
FF	filtration fraction; force fluids

FFA . . . . free fatty acids
FFP . . . . fresh frozen plasma
fg . . . . femtogram
FH . . . . family history
FHH . . . . . . familial hypocalciuric hypercalcemia
FHR . . . . fetal heart rate
FHS . . . . fetal heart sounds
FIC . . . . functional inhibitory concentration
FIF . . . . forced inspiratory flow
FITC . . . . fluorescein isothiocyanate
FIVC . . . . . . forced inspiratory vital capacity
fL . . . . femtoliter; fluid
Fm . . . . fermium
fmol . . . . femtomole
FMULC . . . . free monoclonal urinary light chains
FNA . . . . fine needle aspiration
FOB . . . . fiberoptic bronchoscopy
FOS . . . . fiberoptic sigmoidoscopy
FP . . . . false-positive
Fr . . . . francium
FRA . . . . fluorescent rabies antibody
FRC . . . . functional residual capacity
FS . . . . frozen section
FSH . . . . follicle stimulating hormone
FSI . . . . foam stability index
FSP . . . . fibrin split products
ft . . . . make (fiat, fiant)
FTA . . . . fluorescent treponemal antibody
FTA-ABS . . . fluorescent treponemal antibody absorption
FTI . . . . free thyroxine index
FTND . . . . . . full-term normal delivery
FUO . . . . fever of undetermined origin
FVC . . . . forced vital capacity
FX . . . . factor X
Fx . . . . fracture

g . . . . gram
G-6-PD . . . . . glucose 6-phosphate dehydrogenase
Ga . . . . gallium
GABA . . . . . gamma-aminobutyric acid
GAL . . . . galactosemia
GAW . . . . . . airway conductance
GAZT . . . . . . glucuronide derivative of azidothymidine
GB . . . . gallbladder
GBM . . . . . . glomerular basement membrane
GC . . . . geriatric chair; gonorrhea culture; gas
                chromatography
GC-MS . . . . . gas chromatography - mass spectrometry
Gd . . . . gadolinium

g/dL . . . . gram percent
GE . . . . gastroesophageal
Ge . . . . germanium
GFR . . . . glomerular filtration rate
GGCT . . . . . ground glass clotting time
GGT . . . . gamma-glutamyltransferase
GH . . . . growth hormone
GHB . . . . glycohemoglobin
GI . . . . gastrointestinal
GIH . . . . gastric inhibitory hormone
GIP . . . . gastric inhibitory polypeptide
GIS . . . . gastrointestinal series
GK . . . . galactokinase
GLC . . . . gas liquid chromatography
GM . . . . geometric mean
GMS . . . . . . Grocott-Gomori methenamine-silver
GnRH . . . . . . gonadotropin releasing hormone
GOT . . . . glutamic-oxaloacetic transaminase
GP . . . . glycoprotein
GPK . . . . guinea pig kidney
GPT . . . . glutamic-pyruvic transaminase
GPUT . . . . . glactose phosphate uridyl transferase
GR . . . . glutathione reductase
GSD . . . . glycogen storage disease
GSH . . . . glutathione; growth stimulating hormone
GSR . . . . galvanic skin response; generalized Schwartzman
              reaction
GSSR . . . . . generalized Sandarelli-Shwartzman reaction
GT . . . . gait training; gamma-glutamyltransferase
GTP . . . . glutamyl transpeptidase
GTT . . . . glucose tolerance test
gtt(s) . . . . . . drop(s) (gutta)
GU . . . . genitourinary; gastric ulcer; gonococcal urethritis
GVHD . . . . . graft versus host disease
GXT . . . . graded exercise test
gyn . . . . gynecological

H . . . . hydrogen
h . . . . hour (hora)
HA . . . . headache
Ha . . . . hahnium
HAA . . . . hepatitis B surface antigen
HABA . . . . . . hydroxybenzeneazobenzoic acid
HAI . . . . hemagglutination inhibition
HANE . . . . . . hereditary angioneurotic edema
HAV . . . . hepatitis A virus
HAVAB . . . . hepatitis A virus antibody
Hb . . . . hemoglobin
HBAB . . . . . . hepatitis B antibody
HB_c . . . . hepatitis B core

HBD . . . . hydroxybutric dehydrogenase
HBDH . . . . . hydroxybutyrate dehydrogenase
HB$_e$Ag . . . . hepatitis B e antigen
HBP . . . . high blood pressure
HB$_s$Ag . . . . hepatitis B surface antigen
HBV . . . . hepatitis B virus
HC . . . . homocystinuria
HCFA. . . . . . Health Care Financing Administration
hCG . . . . human chorionic gonadotropin
HCl. . . . . hydrochloric acid
HCS . . . . human chorionic somatomammotropin
Hct. . . . . hematocrit
HD . . . . Hodgkin's disease
HDL . . . . high density lipoprotein
HDLC. . . . . . high density lipoprotein cholesterol
HDN . . . . hemolytic disease of the newborn
HDP . . . . hydroxydimethylpyrimidine
He . . . . helium
HEMPAS . . . here. erythroblastic multinuclearity with positive
                acidified serum
HEp . . . . human epithelial cells
HES . . . . acute hypereosinophilic syndrome
Hf . . . . hafnium
HFI . . . . hereditary fructose intolerance
HG . . . . herpes gestationis
Hg . . . . mercury
^{197}Hg . . . . . radioisotope of mercury
^{203}Hg . . . . . radioisotope of mercury
HGA. . . . . . . homogentisic acid
Hgb . . . . hemoglobin
HGG . . . . . . human gamma globulin
HGH . . . . . . human growth hormone
HGPRT . . . . hypoxanthine guanine phosphoribosyl transferase
HHC. . . . . . . home health care
HHD . . . . hypertensive heart disease
HHH. . . . . . . hyperornithinemia, hyperammonemia-
                homocitrullinuria
HHM . . . . . . humoral hypercalcemia of malignancy
HHT . . . . head holter traction
HI . . . . hydriodic acid
HIAA . . . . . . hydroxyindoleacetic acid
HIB . . . . *Haemophilus influenzae* B
HIDA . . . . . . acetanilidoiminodiacetic acid
HIP . . . . humoral immunocompetence profile
HIV . . . . human immunodeficiency virus
HK . . . . hexokinase
HLA . . . . human leukocyte antigen
HMO . . . . . . Health Maintenance Organization
HMS. . . . . . . hexose monophosphate shunt
HMW . . . . . . high molecular weight
HMWK . . . . . high molecular weight kininogen

HN . . . . head nurse
H/O . . . . . . history of
HO . . . . house officer
Ho . . . . holmium
HOB . . . . . . head of bed
H & P . . . . . history and physical
HP . . . . hot packs
hpf . . . . high power field
HPFH . . . . . hereditary persistence of fetal hemoglobin
HPI . . . . history of present illness
HPL . . . . . . human placental lactogen
HPLC . . . . . high performance liquid chromatography
HPN . . . . . . home parenteral nutrition
HPP . . . . . . human pancreatic polypeptide
HPPH . . . . . hydroxyphenyl-phenylhydantoin
HPT . . . . . . hyperparathyroidism
HPV . . . . . . human papilloma virus
HR . . . . heart rate; hospital record
hr . . . . hour (hora)
HRANA . . . . histone reactive ANA
HRLM . . . . . high resolution light microscopy
HS . . . . herpes simplex; hereditary spherocytosis
hs . . . . at bedtime (hora somni)
HSV . . . . . . herpes simplex virus
HT . . . . hypertension; hypodermic tablet
HTLV . . . . . human T-lymphotropic virus
HTN . . . . . . hypertension
HTP . . . . . . hydroxytrytophan
HTVD . . . . . hypertensive vascular disease
HUS . . . . . . hemolytic-uremic syndrome; hyaluronidase unit for
                semen
HVA . . . . . . homovanillic acid
Hx . . . . history
Hz . . . . hertz

I . . . . iodine
I-3-AA . . . . . indole-3-acetic acid
^{125}I . . . . radioisotope of iodide
^{131}I . . . . radioisotope of iodide
Ia . . . . antigen
IAA . . . . indole acetic acid
IABP . . . . . . intra-aortic balloon pump
IADH . . . . . inappropriate antidiuretic hormone
IAT . . . . indirect antiglobulin test
Ib . . . . a glycoprotein
IBC . . . . iron binding capacity
IC . . . . immune complexes; inspiratory capacity
ICA . . . . internal carotid artery
ICD . . . . isocitrate dehydrogenase
ICDH . . . . . isocitrate dehydrogenase

ACRONYMS AND ABBREVIATIONS GLOSSARY

ICG	indocyanine green
ICN	intensive care neonatal
ICS	intercostal space
ICSH	interstitial cell stimulating hormone
ICT	indirect Coombs' test
ICU	intensive care unit
ID	identification; immunodiffusion; infectious disease; intradermal(ly)
IDA	iron deficiency anemia; image display and analysis
IDAT	indirect antiglobulin test
IDDM	insulin dependent diabetes mellitus
IDL	intermediate-density lipoprotein
IEF	isoelectric focusing
IEM	inborn errors of metabolism
IEP	immunoelectrophoresis
IF	immunofluorescence; inspiratory force; interstitial fluid; intrinsic factor
IFA	indirect fluorescent antibody
IFIX	immunofixation
Ig	immunoglobulin
IGT	impaired glucose tolerance
IHA	indirect hemagglutination
IIb-IIIa	glycoproteins found on platelet membranes
IIF	indirect immunofluorescence
I.M.	intramuscular
IMD	inherited metabolic disorders
IMP	impression
IMV	intermittent mandatory ventilation
In	indium
INH	isonicotinic acid hydrazide; isoniazid
IOFNA	intraoperative fine needle aspiration
IOL	intraocular lens
IOP	intraocular pressure
IOT	intraocular tension
IP	intraperitoneal(ly)
I-PAO	insulin induced peak acid output
IPG	impedence phlebograph
IPPB	intermittent positive pressure breathing
IR	infrared
Ir	iridium
IRDS	infant respiratory distress syndrome
IRG	immunoreactive glucose
IRGH	immunoreactive growth hormone
IRI	immunoreactive insulin
IRMA	immunoradiometric assay
IRT	immunoreactive trypsinogen
ISD	isosorbide dinitrate
IT	inhalation therapy; intrathecal(ly)
ITP	idiopathic thrombocytopenic purpura
ITT	insulin tolerance test
IU	International unit

IUD . . . . intrauterine device
IUGR . . . . . . intrauterine growth retardation
IUP . . . . intrauterine pregnancy
I.V. . . . . intravenous
IVAC . . . . . . I.V. infusion control device
IVC . . . . inferior vena cava; intravenous cholangiography
IVP . . . . intravenous push; intravenous pyelogram
IVPB . . . . . . intravenous piggyback
IVSD . . . . . . intraventricular septal defect

JVD . . . . jugular-venous distenion
JVP . . . . jugular venous pressure; jugular venous pulse

K . . . . potassium
K-B . . . . Kleihauer-Betke
kcal . . . . kilocalorie
KCl . . . . potassium chloride
KCN . . . . potassium cyanide
kg . . . . kilogram
KGS . . . . . . ketogenic steroids
kL . . . . kiloliter
km . . . . kilometer
KO . . . . keep open
KOH . . . . . . potassium hydroxide
Kr . . . . krypton
KS . . . . ketosteroids; Kaposi's sarcoma
KU . . . . Karmen units
KUB . . . . . . kidney and urinary bladder
KVO . . . . . . keep vein open
KW . . . . Keith-Wagener

L . . . . left; liter; lumbar
L_2 . . . . second lumbar vertebra
LA . . . . left artrium; local anesthetic
La . . . . lanthanum
LAD . . . . . . left anterior descending (artery)
LAI . . . . labioincisal
LAO . . . . . . left anterior oblique
LAP . . . . . . leucine aminopeptidase; leukocyte alkaline
                phosphatase
Lap . . . . . . laparotomy
LATS . . . . . long acting thyroid stimulating hormone
LBBB . . . . . left bundle branch block
LBM . . . . . . lean body mass
LBW . . . . . . low birth weight
LC . . . . lethal concentration
LCI . . . . lung clearance index
LCIS . . . . . . lobular carcinoma *in situ*

LCM	lymphocytic choriomeningitis
LCS	Leydig cell stimulation
LD	lactate dehydrogenase; lethal dose; light difference
LD$_1$	lactate dehydrogenase fraction 1
LDH	lactate dehydrogenase
LDHI	LDH isoenzymes
LDL	low density lipoprotein
LDLC	low density lipoprotein cholesterol
LDV	lactate dehydrogenase virus
LE	lower extremity; lupus erythematosus
LEA	lower extremity arterial
LES	lower esophageal sphincter
LEV	lower extremity venous
LFT	liver function test
LGV	lymphogranuloma venereum
LH	luteinizing hormone
LHRF	luteinizing hormone releasing factor
LHRH	luteinizing hormone releasing hormone
LHV	left ventricular hypertrophy
Li	lithium
LISS	low ionic strength saline
L-J	Löwenstein-Jensen
LKM	liver/kidney microsomes
LKS	liver, kidneys, spleen
LLA	lupus like anticoagulant
LLDH	liver lactate dehydrogenase
LLL	left lower lobe
LLQ	left lower quadrant
LM	light microscopy
LMN	lower motor neuron
LMP	last menstrual period
LMWH	low molecular weight heparin
LOA	left occipital anterior
LOM	limitation of motion
LOS	length of stay
LP	light perception; lumbar puncture
LPC	leukocyte-poor cells
LPO	left posterior oblique
LPRBC	leukocyte-poor red blood cells
LRC	Lipid Research Clinic
L/S	lecithin/sphingomyelin ratio
LSD	lysergic acid diethylamide
LTC	long term care
LTCPs	L-tryptophan-containing products
LTT	lymphocyte transformation test
Lu	lutetium
LUL	left upper lobe
LUQ	left upper quadrant
LVET	left ventricular ejection time
LVH	left ventricular hypertrophy

LVW . . . . lateral vaginal wall
L & W . . . . . living and well
Lw . . . . lawrencium
Lytes . . . . . . electrolytes

M . . . . mix (misce)
m . . . . meter
m^2 . . . . square meter
m^3 . . . . cubic meter
M/A . . . . mood and/or affect
mA . . . . milliampere
MA-1 . . . . . . a type of respirator
MAA . . . . microaggregatedalbumin
MAI . . . . *Mycobacterium avium-intracellulare*
MAO . . . . monoamine oxidase
MAR . . . . mixed antiglobulin reaction
MB . . . . a fraction of creatine kinase
MBC . . . . . . minimum bactericidal concentration; maximum breathing capacity
MBD . . . . . . maximum bactericidal dilution
MBP . . . . myelin basic protein
mc . . . . millicurie
MC-Ab . . . . . monoclonal antibody
mcg . . . . microgram
MCH . . . . . . mean corpuscular hemoglobin
MCHC . . . . . mean cell hemoglobin concentration
mCi . . . . millicurie
MCL . . . . midclavicular line; midcostal line
MCT . . . . medium chain triglycerides
MCTD . . . . . mixed connective tissue disease
MCV . . . . mean corpuscular volume
MD . . . . medical doctor
Md . . . . mendelevium
MDP . . . . mentodextra posterior
MDR . . . . . . minimum daily requirement
MEA . . . . mercaptoethylamine; multiple endocrine adenomatosis
MED . . . . minimal erythemal dose
MEET . . . . . . multistage exercise electrocardiographics test
MEN . . . . . . multiple endocrine neoplasia
mEq . . . . milliequivalent
METS . . . . . metastases
MF . . . . mycosis fungoides
MFC . . . . minimum fungicidal concentration
Mg . . . . magnesium
mg . . . . milligram
$MgCl_2$ . . . . . . magnesium chloride
$MgCO_3$ . . . . . magnesium carbonate
MGP . . . . . . methyl green pyronine

ACRONYMS AND ABBREVIATIONS GLOSSARY

MgSO₄ . . . . . magnesium sulfate
MH . . . . malignant hyperthermia; marital history; menstrual
history; mental health
MHA . . . . . . microhemagglutination
MHA-TP . . . . microhemagglutination *Treponema pallidum*
MHPG . . . . . methoxyhydroxyphenylglycol
MI . . . . myocardial infarction; maturation index
MIC . . . . minimum inhibitory concentration
μg . . . . microgram
μL . . . . microliter
μm^3 . . . . . . cubic micrometer
μ . . . . micron
μm . . . . micrometer
μmol/L . . . . micromolar
μmol . . . . . . micromole
μOsm . . . . . micro-osmolar
μU . . . . microunit
MID . . . . maximum bactericidal dilution
MIF . . . . merthiolate-iodine-formalin; migration inhibitory
factor
MIT . . . . migration inhibition test
mIU . . . . milli International unit
mL . . . . milliliter
MLC . . . . . . mixed leukocyte culture; mixed lymphocyte culture
MLD . . . . . . metachromatic leukodystrophy; minimum lethal dose
MLR . . . . . . mixed lymphocyte reaction
mm . . . . millimeter
mm^2 . . . . square millimeter
mm^3 . . . . cubic millimeter
MMA . . . . . methylmalonic acid
MMC . . . . . minimal medullary concentration
MMEF . . . . . mean midexpiratory flow
MMF . . . . . . maximal midexpiratory flow rate
mm Hg . . . . millimeters of mercury
mmol . . . . . . millimole
mmol/L . . . . millimolar
MMPI . . . . . Minnesota multiple personality inventory
MMT . . . . . . manual muscle test
Mn . . . . manganese
MNS . . . . . . MNS blood group
MO . . . . mesio-occlusal
Mo . . . . molybdenum
mol . . . . mole
mol/L . . . . . . molar
mOsm . . . . . milliosmole
mph . . . . . . miles per hour
MPHD . . . . . methoxyhydroxphenolglycerol
MPS . . . . . . mucopolysaccharidosis
MPV . . . . . . mean plasma volume
MR . . . . moderately resistant

mrad . . . . . . millirad
MRI . . . . magnetic resonance imaging
MRSA . . . . . methicillin-resistant *S. aureus*
MS . . . . mental status; mitral stenosis; multiple sclerosis
MSD . . . . metabolic screening disorders
msec . . . . . . millisecond
MSL . . . . midsternal line
MSLT . . . . . . multiple sleep latency test
MSUD . . . . . maple syrup urine disease
MT . . . . medical technologist
mt . . . . send of such (mitte talis)
MTB . . . . mycobacterium tuberculosis
^{99m}Tc . . . . . . radioisotope of technetium Tc 99m
MTRX . . . . . . methotrexate
MTX . . . . methotrexate
mU . . . . milliunit
MUGA . . . . . multiple gated scan
MV . . . . minute volume
MVP . . . . mitral valve prolapse
MVV . . . . maximum voluntary ventilation
MW . . . . molecular weight
MZ . . . . monozygotic

N . . . . nitrogen; normal
NA . . . . not applicable
Na . . . . sodium
NACI . . . . . National Advisory Committee on Immunization
NaCl . . . . sodium chloride
NaCO$_3$ . . . . . sodium carbonate
NAD . . . . nicotinamide adenine dinucleotide; no acute
              distress; no apparent distress
NADH . . . . . reduced form of NAD
NADP . . . . . . nicotinamide adenine dinucleotide phosphate
NADPH . . . . reduced form of NADP
NaF . . . . sodium fluoride
NaOH . . . . . . sodium hydroxide
NAPA . . . . . . n-acetylprocainamide
NAS . . . . no added salt
NATP . . . . . . neonatal autoimmune thrombocytopenic purpura
Nb . . . . niobium
NBIL . . . . neonatal bilirubin
NBT . . . . nitro blue tetrazolium
NC . . . . nerve conduction
NCA . . . . nonspecific cross reacting antigen
NCEP . . . . . . National Cholesterol Education Program
NCI . . . . National Cancer Institute
NCS . . . . nerve conduction study
NCV . . . . nerve conduction velocity
Nd . . . . neodymium

ACRONYMS AND ABBREVIATIONS GLOSSARY

Ne . . . . neon
ng . . . . nanogram
NGU. . . . . . . nongonococcal urethritis
NH₄Cl . . . . . . ammonium chloride
NH₄OH . . . . . ammonium hydroxide
Ni . . . . nickel
NICU . . . . . . neonatal intensive care unit
NIH . . . . National Institute of Health
NK . . . . natural killer
NKA . . . . no known allergies
NL . . . . normal
nL . . . . nanoliter
nm . . . . nanometer
nmol . . . . nanomole
nmol/L . . . . . millimicromolar
NMR . . . . nuclear magnetic resonance
No . . . . nobelium
noc . . . . in the night (nocturnal)
non rep . . . . do not repeat; no refills
NP . . . . nasopharynx
Np . . . . neptunium
NPO . . . . nothing by mouth
NPT . . . . nocturnal penile tumescence
nr . . . . do not repeat (non repetatur)
NRBCs . . . . . nucleated red blood cells
NRC . . . . National Research Council; Nuclear Regulatory
Commission
NS . . . . normal saline; not seen; not significant
NSA . . . . no salt albumin
NSE . . . . neuron specific enolase
NSR . . . . normal sinus rhythm
NST . . . . nonstress test
NSU . . . . nonspecific urethritis
NSVD . . . . . . normal spontaneous vaginal delivery
N & T . . . . . . nose and throat
NT . . . . nasotracheal
NTI . . . . nonthyroidal illness; nonthyroidal index
N & V . . . . . . nausea and vomiting
NVD . . . . nausea, vomiting, diarrhea
NYD . . . . not yet diagnosed

O . . . . oxygen
OB . . . . obstetrics; occult blood
OBS . . . . organic brain syndrome
OC . . . . on call; oral contraceptive
OCG . . . . . . oral cholecystogram
OCT . . . . ornithine carbamyl transferase
OD . . . . overdose
od . . . . right eye (oculus dexter)
ODC . . . . . . oxygen dissociation curve

ODE . . . . O-desmethylencainide
ODm . . . . . . ophthalmodynamometry
O/E . . . . on examination
OGTT . . . . . . oral glucose tolerance test
OH . . . . hydroxide; hydroxyl
OHCS . . . . . hydroxycorticosteroid
OIF . . . . oil immersion field
OKT . . . . a group of monoclonal antibodies for typing
                 lymphocytes
OM . . . . otitis media
OOB . . . . . . out of bed
OPG . . . . ocular plethysmography
OPV . . . . out patient visit; oral polio vaccine
O.R. . . . . operating room
Os . . . . osmium
os . . . . left eye (oculus sinister)
OT . . . . old tuberculin
OTC . . . . ornithine transcarbamylase
ou . . . . each eye (oculus uterque)
ov . . . . ovarian

P . . . . phosphorus; pulse
^{32}P . . . . radioisotope of phosphorus
p^{50} . . . . half saturation (oxygen)
P & A . . . . . . percussion and auscultation
P & T . . . . . . Pharmacy & Therapeutics
PA . . . . phenylalinine; platelet associated; pernicious
                 anemia; physician's assistant
Pa . . . . protactinium
PABA . . . . . . para-aminobenzoic acid
PAC . . . . . . premature atrial contraction
PAH . . . . phenylalanine hydroxylase
PAI . . . . plasminogen activator inhibitor
PAO . . . . peak acid output
PAP . . . . peroxidase antiperoxidase; pri. atypical pneum.;
                 prostate acid phosphatase
Pap . . . . . . Papanicolaou's stain
PAR . . . . pulmonary arteriolar resistance
PAS . . . . para-aminosalicylic acid; periodic acid Schiff stain
PAT . . . . paroxysmal atrial tachycardia; preadmission testing
Pb . . . . lead
PBC . . . . . . primary biliary cirrhosis
PBG . . . . porphobilinogen
PBI . . . . protein-bound iodine
PBL . . . . peripheral blood lymphocytes
PBS . . . . peripheral blood smear
PC . . . . porto-caval; present complaint
pc . . . . after meals (post cibum)
pc1 . . . . platelet count pretransfusion
pc2 . . . . platelet count post-transfusion

ACRONYMS AND ABBREVIATIONS GLOSSARY

PCA . . . . parietal cell antibody; percutaneous coronary angioplasty
PCE . . . . pseudocholinesterase
PCG . . . . pneumocardiogram
PCH . . . . paroxysmal cold hemoglobinuria
PCHE . . . . . pseudocholinesterase
PCI . . . . prothrombin consumption index
PCP . . . . phencyclidine
PCR . . . . polymerase chain reaction
PCT . . . . prothrombin consumption test
PCV . . . . packed cell volume
PD . . . . postural drainage
Pd . . . . palladium
PDR . . . . *Physician's Desk Reference*
PDW . . . . . platelet distribution width
PE . . . . physical examination; pleural effusion; pulmonary embolism
PEEP . . . . . . positive end-expiratory pressure
PEF . . . . peak expiratory flow
PEFR . . . . . . peak expiratory flow rate
PEFT . . . . . . peak expiratory flow time
PEG . . . . polyethylene glycol
PEP . . . . phosphoenolpyruvate
PERLA . . . . . pupils equal, reactive to light and accommodation
PET . . . . positron emission tomography; pre-eclamptic toxemia
PF . . . . platelet factor
PFK . . . . phosphofructoaldolase
PFS . . . . penile flow study
PFT . . . . pulmonary function test
PG . . . . phosphatidyl glycine
pg . . . . picogram
PGD . . . . . . phosphogluconate dehydrogenase
PGI . . . . phosphoglucose isomerase
PGK . . . . phosphoglycerokinase
PgR . . . . progesterone receptor
pH . . . . measurement of acidity or alkalinity
PHA . . . . phytohemagglutinin activation
pHa . . . . arterial blood pH
PhD . . . . Doctor of Philosophy
PHI . . . . phosphohexoseisomerase
PHP . . . . persistent hyperphenylalaninemia
PHT . . . . peroxide hemolysis test
PI . . . . phosphatidylinositol; protamine insulin; pulmonary infarction
pi . . . . platelet count increment
PID . . . . pelvic inflammatory disease
PK . . . . pyruvate kinase
PKU . . . . phenylketonuria
PM . . . . afternoon
Pm . . . . promethium

PMD . . . . primary myocardial disease; progressive muscular dystrophy
PMH . . . . past medical history
PM-I . . . . platelet membrane antigen
PMN . . . . polymorphonuclear neutrophil
pmol . . . . . . picomole
PMP . . . . previous menstrual period
PM & R . . . . physical medicine and rehabilitation
PMS . . . . premenstrual syndrome
PNH . . . . paroxysmal nocturnal hemoglobinuria
PNP . . . . nonprotein nitrogen
pNPP . . . . . . paranitrophenylphosphate
Pnx . . . . . . pneumothorax
Po . . . . polonium
po . . . . by mouth (per os)
POMR . . . . . problem oriented medical record
POR . . . . . . problem oriented record
PP . . . . postprandial
PPBS . . . . . postprandial blood sugar
PPD . . . . purified protein derivative
PPF . . . . plasma protein fraction
PPG . . . . . . photoplethysmography
PPLO . . . . . . pleuropneumonia-like organisms
ppm . . . . parts per million
ppt . . . . precipitate
Pr . . . . praseodymium; presbyopia
PRA . . . . . . plasma renin activity; progesterone receptor assay
PRBCs . . . . . packed red blood cells
PRG . . . . . . phleborheography
PRL . . . . prolactin
prn . . . . as needed (pro re nata)
PROM . . . . . premature rupture of membranes; prolonged rupture of membranes
PRP . . . . polyribophosphate
PRSM . . . . . peripheral smear
PSA . . . . . . prostate specific antigen
PSIS . . . . posterior/superior iliac spine
PSP . . . . . . phenolsulfonphthalein
PSRO . . . . . . Professional Standards Review Organization
PSS . . . . . . progressive systemic sclerosis
PT . . . . physical therapy; prothrombin time
Pt . . . . platinum
PTA . . . . . . platelet thromboplastin antecedent; prothrombin activity
PTAH . . . . . . phosphotungstic acid hematoxylin
PTC . . . . phenylthiocarbamide; plasma thromboplastin component
PTH . . . . . . parathyroid hormone
PTP . . . . . . prothrombin-proconvertin
PTT . . . . . . partial thromboplastin time
PU . . . . peptic ulcer

ACRONYMS AND ABBREVIATIONS GLOSSARY

Pu . . . . plutonium
PUD . . . . peptic ulcer disease
pulv . . . . a powder (pulvis)
PV . . . . plasma volume
PVA . . . . polyvinyl alcohol
PVC . . . . premature ventricular contraction
PVD . . . . peripheral vascular disease
PVR . . . . pulse volume recording
PVT . . . . paroxysmal ventricular tachycardia
PWM . . . . . . pokeweed mitogen
PYP . . . . pyrophosphate

q . . . . every (quaque)
QBCA . . . . . quantitative buffy coat analysis
qd . . . . every day (quaque die)
qh . . . . every hour (quaque hora)
qhr . . . . every hour (quaque hora)
qid . . . . four times a day (quarter in die)
QNS . . . . quantity not sufficient
qod . . . . every other day
qs . . . . sufficient quantity (quantum sufficiat)
qs ad . . . . . sufficient quantity to make (quantum sufficiat ad)
QTC . . . . quantitative tip culture
qv . . . . as much as you will (quam volveris)

R . . . . respiration; right
RA . . . . rheumatoid arthritis; right atrium
Ra . . . . radium
RAD . . . . radiation absorbed dose
RAF . . . . rheumatoid arthritis factor
RAI . . . . radioactive iodine
RAO . . . . right anterior oblique
RAP . . . . rheumatoid arthritis precipitins
RAW . . . . . . airway resistance
Rb . . . . rubidium
RBC . . . . red blood cell
RC . . . . red cell; retrograde cystogram
RCM . . . . . . radiographic contrast media; right costal margin
RCMI . . . . . . red cell morphology index
rd . . . . rutherford
RDS . . . . respiratory distress syndrome
RDW . . . . . . red cell distribution width
Re . . . . rhenium
REM . . . . . . rapid eye movement
repet . . . . . . to be repeated (repetatur)
RF . . . . renal failure; rheumatoid factor
Rf . . . . rutherfordium
Rh . . . . rhodium; rhesus

RhIG ......Rh$_o$(D) immune globulin
RI ....reticulocyte index
RIA ....radioimmunoassay
RID........radial immunodiffusion
RIPA......radioimmunoprecipitation
RISA......radioiodinated serum albumin
RK ....radial keratotomy
RLL ....right lower lobe
RLQ ......right lower quadrant
RMSF......Rocky Mountain spotted fever
RN ....registered nurse
Rn ....radon
RNA ....ribonucleic acid
RNP ....ribonucleoprotein
R/O ....rule out
RO ....routine order
RODAC ....replicate organism detection and counting
ROM ......range of motion
ROS ....review of symptoms; review of systems
RPF ....renal plasma flow
RPI........reticulocyte production index
rpm ....revolutions per minute
RPO ......right posterior oblique
RPR ......rapid plasma reagin
RPT ......right occipital transverse
RQ ....respiratory quotient
RR ....recovery room; respiratory rate
RRA ......right renal artery
RSV ....respiratory syncytial virus
RTA ......renal tubular acidosis
Ru ....ruthenium
RUG.......right upper quadrant
RUL ....right upper lobe
RUQ......right upper quadrant
RV ....reserve volume
RVH ......right ventricular hypertrophy
RVVT ......Russell viper venom test

S ....sulfur
s ....without (sine)
S$_1$........first heart sound
S$_2$........second heart sound
SA ....surface area; sinoatrial
SACE......serum angiotensin converting enzyme
SAH ......subarachnoid hemorrhage
SAL ......suction assisted lipectomy
Sb ....antimony
SBB ......small bowel biopsy
SBE ......subacute bacterial endocarditis

ACRONYMS AND ABBREVIATIONS GLOSSARY

SBL . . . . serum bactericidal level
SBP . . . . systemic blood pressure; systolic blood pressure
SC . . . . sickle cell; subclavian
Sc . . . . scandium
SCAT . . . . . . sheep cell agglutination test
SCE . . . . sister chromatid exchange
SCID . . . . . . severe combined immunodeficiency
Scl . . . . scleroderma; scleroderma antibody
S-D . . . . strength duration
SD . . . . senile dementia; spontaneous delivery; standard
                    deviation
SDFP . . . . . . single donor frozen plasma
SDS . . . . same day surgery
Se . . . . selenium
SEM . . . . scanning electron microscopy; standard error of the
                    mean
SEP . . . . serum electrophoresis; somatosensory evoked
                    potential
SER . . . . somatosensory evoked response
SG . . . . specific gravity
SGPT . . . . . . serum glutamic pyruvic transaminase
SH . . . . serum hepatitis
SHBG . . . . . sex hormone binding globulin
SI . . . . Système International (SI) units
Si . . . . silicon
SIADH . . . . . syndrome of inappropriate antidiuretic hormone
SIDS . . . . sudden infant death syndrome
Sig . . . . mark, write (signa)
SISI . . . . short increment sensitivity index
SK . . . . streptokinase
SKAB . . . . . . skeletal antibody
SKSD . . . . . . streptokinase-streptodornase
SL . . . . sublingual(ly)
SLCG . . . . . . sulfolithoecholylglycine
SLE . . . . systemic lupus erthyematosus
Sm . . . . samarium; Smith antigen
SMA . . . . sequential/serial multiple analysis; smooth muscle
                    antibody
Sn . . . . tin
SNF . . . . skilled nursing facility
SOAP . . . . . . subjective, objective, assessment and plans
SOB . . . . short of breath
SOD . . . . superoxide dismutase
sos . . . . if there is need (si opus sit)
SPC . . . . standard plate count
SPCA . . . . . . serum prothrombin conversion accelerator
SPECT . . . . . single-photon emission tomography
SPEP . . . . . . serum protein electrophoresis
SPI . . . . selective protein index
SPS . . . . sodium polyanetholsulfonate; sulfite polymyxin
                    sulfadiazine

SQ	subcutaneous(ly)
SR	sedimentation rate; sustained release; systems review
Sr	strontium
SRAW	specific airway resistance
SRIF	somatotropin releasing inhibiting factor
SS	*Salmonella-Shigella*; saturated solution; subaortic stenosis
ss	one-half (semis)
SS-A	Sjögren's syndrome A antibody
SS-B	Sjögren's syndrome B antibody
SS-DNA	single stranded DNA
SSEP	somatosensory evoked potential
SSKI	saturated solution of potassium iodide
SSPE	subacute sclerosing panencephalitis
stat	st once (statim)
STD	skin test dose; sexually transmitted disease
STH	somatotropic hormone
STI	systolic time intervals
STIC	serum trypsin inhibitory capacity
STP	standard temperature and pressure
STS	serologic test for syphillis
supp	suppository (suppositorium)
SW	short wave
Sx	signs; symptom(s)
syr	syrup (syrupus)

T	temperature
T & A	tonsillectomy and adenoidectomy
TA	thyroglobulin autoprecipitins
Ta	tantalum
TAb	therapeutic abortion
tab	tablet (tabella)
TAD	tricyclic antidepressant drug
TAH	total abdominal hysterectomy
tal	such
tal dos	such doses
TAT	thematic apperception test; toxin-antitoxin
TB	tuberculosis
Tb	terbium
TBA	to be administered; to be admitted
TBG	thyroxine binding globulin
TBGI	thyroid binding globulin index
TBI	thyroid binding index; thyroxine binding index
TBM	tuberculous meningitis
TBPA	thyroxine binding prealbumin
TBW	total body water
T & C	type and crossmatch
TC	throat culture; total cholesterol

Tc	technetium
TCA	trichloracetic acid
TCBS	thiosulfate citrate bile salts sucrose
TCM	tissue culture medium
TCT	thrombin clotting time
TDM	therapeutic drug monitoring
TdT	terminal deoxynucleotidyl transferase
Te	tellurium
TEAC	tetraethylammonium chloride
TeBG	testosterone-estradiol-binding globulin
TEE	transesophageal echocardiography
TENS	transcutaneous electrical nerve stimulation
TET	treadmill exercise test
TG	triglyceride
TGT	thromboplastin generation test
TGV	thoracic gas volume
Th	thorium
th	thoracic
THA	transient hemispheric attack
THb	total hemoglobin
THC	tetrahydrocannabinol
TI	total iron
Ti	titanium
TIA	transient ischemic attack
TIBC	total iron binding capacity
tid	three times a day (ter in die)
TIUV	total intrauterine volume
TK	transketolase
TKO	to keep open
TL	tubal ligation
Tl	thallium
TLA	translumbar aortogram
TLC	thin layer chromatography; total lung capacity
Tm	thulium
TMB	transient monocular blindness
TMJ	temporomandibular joint
TMP	trimethoprim
TMP-SMX	trimethoprim-sulfomethoxazole
TNS	transcutaneous nerve stimulation
TOS	thoracic outlet syndrome
TP	total protein
TPA	*Treponema pallidum* agglutination
TPC	telescoping plugged catheter
TPI	*Treponema* immobilization test; triose phosphate isomerase
TPN	total parenteral nutrition
TPP	thiamine pyrophosphate
TPR	temperature, pulse, respiration
TRAP	tartrate resistance leukocyte acid phosphatase
TRH	thyroid releasing hormone
TRIC	trachoma inclusion conjunctivitis

trig . . . . triglycerides
TRIS . . . . . . tris(hydroxymethyl)aminomethane
trit . . . . triturate (tritura)
TRP . . . . tubular reabsorption of phosphorus
TS . . . . total solids
TSB . . . . trypticase soy broth
TSH . . . . thyroid stimulating hormone
TSI . . . . thyroid stimulating immunoglobulin
tsp . . . . teaspoon
TT . . . . thrombin time
TTP . . . . thrombotic thrombocytopenic purpura
TU . . . . thiouracil; Todd unit; toxic unit; tuberculin unit
TUR . . . . transurethral resection
TURP . . . . . . transurethral resection of prostate
TV . . . . total volume
TVC . . . . triple voiding cystogram
Tx . . . . therapy; treatment

U . . . . uranium
UA . . . . uric acid; urinalysis
UB12BC . . . unsaturated B_{12} binding capacity
UBBC . . . . . unsaturated vitamin B_{12} binding capacity
UBC . . . . . . unsaturated binding capacity
UCG . . . . . . urinary chorionic gonadotropin
ud . . . . as directed (ut dictum)
UDP . . . . . . uridine diphosphate
UDPG . . . . . uridinediphosphoglucose
UEA . . . . upper extremity arterial
UES . . . . upper esophageal sphincter
UFC . . . . urinary free cortisol
UGI . . . . . . upper GI
UIBC . . . . . . unbound iron binding capacity
U-I-S . . . . . . uroporphyrinogen-I-synthetase
UK . . . . urokinase
UMN . . . . . . upper motor neuron
ung . . . . ointment (unguentum)
URI. . . . . upper respiratory infection
U.S. . . . . United States
US . . . . ultrasound
USAN. . . . . . United States Adopted Names
USP . . . . United States Pharmacopeia
ut dict . . . . . as directed (ut dictum)
UTI . . . . urinary tract infection
UUN . . . . . . urine urea nitrogen
UV . . . . ultraviolet

V . . . . vanadium
VA . . . . visual activity

ACRONYMS AND ABBREVIATIONS GLOSSARY

VBG . . . . venous blood gases
VC . . . . vena cava; vital capacity
VCA . . . . viral capsid antigen
VCA-EB . . . . viral capsid antigen, Epstein-Barr
VCG . . . . vectorcardiogram
VCT . . . . venous clotting time
VCU . . . . voiding cystourethrogram
VCUG . . . . . voiding cystourethrogram
VD . . . . venereal disease
VDRL . . . . . . Venereal Disease Research Laboratory; test for
              syphilis
VE . . . . visual efficiency
VEP . . . . visual evoked potential
VER . . . . visual evoked response
VF . . . . ventricular fibrillation; vision field
VIP . . . . vasoactive intestinal polypeptide
VLDL . . . . . . very low density lipoprotein
VLM . . . . visceral larva migrans
VMA . . . . vanillylmandelic acid
vo . . . . verbal order
VP . . . . venous pressure
VS . . . . vital signs
VSD . . . . ventricular septal defect
VSS . . . . vital signs stable
VSV . . . . vesicular stimatitis virus
VT . . . . ventricular tachycardia
VTM . . . . virus transport media
vW . . . . von Willebrand
vWD . . . . von Willebrand's disease
vWF . . . . von Willebrand factor
V-Z . . . . varicella-zoster
VZIG . . . . . . varicella-zoster immune globulin
VZV . . . . varicella-zoster virus

W . . . . tungsten
wa . . . . while awake
WB . . . . weight bearing; whole blood
WBC . . . . white blood cell
WD . . . . well developed
WDHA . . . . . watery diarrhea-hypokalemia-achlorhydria
WDHH . . . . . watery diarrhea-hypokalemia-hypochlorhydria
W-F . . . . Weil-Felix
WF . . . . white female
WM . . . . white male
WN . . . . well nourished
WNL . . . . within normal limits
WP . . . . whirlpool
WPW . . . . . . Wolff-Parkinson-White syndrome

WSR . . . . . . Westergren sedimentation rate

Xe . . . . xenon
XO . . . . gonadal dysgenesis of Turner type

Y . . . . yttrium
y . . . . year
YAG . . . . . . yttrium-argon-garnet - a type of laser
Yb . . . . ytterbium

Z-E . . . . Zollinger-Ellison
ZIG . . . . zoster immune globulin
ZIP . . . . zoster immune plasma
Zn . . . . zinc
ZPP . . . . zinc protophorhyrin
Zr . . . . zirconium
ZSR . . . . zeta sedimentation rate

INDICATIONS
INDEX

AIDS *see* ACQUIRED IMMUNODEFICIENCY SYNDROME (AIDS)

AIDS RELATED COMPLEX (ARC) *see* ACQUIRED
  IMMUNODEFICIENCY SYNDROME (AIDS)

ALCOHOLISM *see* CIRRHOSIS

ALCOHOL WITHDRAWAL

ALDOSTERONISM *see* CUSHING'S SYNDROME

ALKALOSIS

ALLERGIC DISORDERS (NASAL)

ALLERGIC DISORDERS (OPHTHALMIC)

ALLERGY

ALOPECIA

INDICATIONS INDEX

ANXIETY

APLASTIC ANEMIA *see* ANEMIA (APLASTIC)

APPENDICITIS

ARIBOFLAVINOSIS

ARRHYTHMIAS

ARSENIC POISONING

ARTERIOSCLEROSIS *see* MYOCARDIAL INFARCTION

ARTERITIS (TEMPORAL)

ARTHRITIS *see* ARTHRITIS (RHEUMATOID), BEHÇET'S SYNDROME, LYME DISEASE, SPONDYLITIS (ANKYLOSING), SYSTEMIC LUPUS ERYTHEMATOSUS (SLE)

ARTHRITIS (GONOCOCCAL)

ARTHRITIS (JUVENILE)

ARTHRITIS (PSORIATIC)

ARTHRITIS (RHEUMATOID)

ASBESTOSIS *see* CARCINOMA (LUNG)

ASCARIASIS

ASCITES *see* CIRRHOSIS, CONGESTIVE HEART FAILURE

ASPERGILLOSIS

ASPIRIN POISONING *see* ACIDOSIS (METABOLIC)

ASTHMA

ASTHMATIC BRONCHITIS *see* BRONCHITIS (ASTHMATIC)

ATELECTASIS

ATHLETE'S FOOT *see* TINEA (PEDIS)

ATOPIC DISEASE *see* ALLERGY

ATROPHIC GASTRITIS *see* ANEMIA (MEGALOBLASTIC)

(Continued)

BITES (INSECT) *(Continued)*

BLADDER *see* CYSTITIS

BLASTOMYCOSIS

BLEEDING

BLEPHARITIS

BLEPHAROCONJUNCTIVITIS

BLOOD INCOMPATIBILITY *see* TRANSFUSION REACTION

BONE *see* OSTEOMALACIA, OSTEOPOROSIS, PAGET'S DISEASE OF BONE

BONE MARROW *see* MACROGLOBULINEMIA OF WALDENSTRÖM, MYELOMA

BOWEL CLEANSING

BOWEL PERFORATION *see* ABDOMINAL PAIN

BOWEL STERILIZATION

BRADYCARDIA

BRAIN ABSCESS

BRAIN TUMOR *see* TUMOR (BRAIN)

BRANHAMELLA CATARRHALIS

BREAST *see* CARCINOMA (BREAST)

(Continued)

BRONCHITIS (CHRONIC) *(Continued)*

BRONCHOGENIC TUMORS *see* CARCINOMA (LUNG)

BRONCHOSPASM

BRUCELLOSIS

BRUISING *see* BLEEDING

BULLOUS SKIN DISEASE

BURNS

BURSITIS

(Continued)

(Continued)

CARCINOMA (PROSTATE) *(Continued)*

CARCINOMA (RENAL)

CARCINOMA (SKIN)

CARCINOMA (SQUAMOUS)

CARCINOMA (STOMACH)

CARCINOMA (TESTIS)

CARCINOMA (THYROID)

CARDIAC ARRHYTHMIAS *see* ARRHYTHMIAS

CARDIAC DECOMPENSATION

CARDIOMYOPATHY

CARTILAGE DISORDERS *see* ARTHRITIS (RHEUMATOID), SPONDYLITIS (ANKYLOSING)

CATARACT

CAT SCRATCH DISEASE

CAUSALGIA

CELIAC DISEASE

CELLULITIS (*B. MELANINOGENICUS*)

CELLULITIS (*PSEUDOMONAS*)

CELLULITIS (*S. AUREUS*, METHICILLIN-RESISTANT)

CELLULITIS (*S. EPIDERMIDIS*, METHICILLIN-RESISTANT)

CENTRAL NERVOUS SYSTEM *see* CONVULSIONS, DEMENTIA, MULTIPLE SCLEROSIS

CERVICAL CARCINOMA *see* CARCINOMA (CERVIX)

CERVICITIS

INDICATIONS INDEX

COCCIDIOIDOMYCOSIS

COLD SENSITIVITY *see* RAYNAUD'S DISEASE, SCLERODERMA

COLITIS

COLITIS (ULCERATIVE)

COLLAGEN DISEASES *see* ARTHRITIS (RHEUMATOID), DERMATOMYOSITIS, SCLERODERMA, SYSTEMIC LUPUS ERYTHEMATOSUS (SLE)

COLON CARCINOMA *see* CARCINOMA (COLORECTAL)

COMA *see* BARBITURATE POISONING, BROMIDE INTOXICATION

COMPLEMENT *see* SYSTEMIC LUPUS ERYTHEMATOSUS (SLE)

CONGESTION (NASAL)

(Continued)

(Continued)

DEMYELINIZATION *see* MULTIPLE SCLEROSIS

DENGUE FEVER

DEPRESSION

DEPRESSION (ACUTE) *see* ANEMIA (MEGALOBLASTIC)

DEPRESSION (RESPIRATORY)

DERMATITIS

DERMATITIS HERPETIFORMIS

DERMATOMYCOSIS

INDICATIONS INDEX

(Continued)

EDEMA

EDEMA (BRAIN)

ELECTROLYTES *see* ADDISON'S DISEASE, BARTTER'S SYNDROME, BROMIDE INTOXICATION, CONGESTIVE HEART FAILURE, CUSHING'S SYNDROME, DIABETES INSIPIDUS

EMBOLISM

EMBOLISM (ARTERIAL)

EMPHYSEMA

(Continued)

EPILEPSY (AKINETIC)

EPILEPSY (COMPLEX PARTIAL)

EPILEPSY (CORTICAL FOCAL) *see* EPILEPSY (SIMPLE PARTIAL)

EPILEPSY (GRAND MAL) *see* EPILEPSY (TONIC-CLONIC)

EPILEPSY (JACKSONIAN) *see* EPILEPSY (SIMPLE PARTIAL)

EPILEPSY (LENNOX-GASTAUT)

EPILEPSY (MIXED SEIZURE)

EPILEPSY (MYOCLONIC)

EPILEPSY (PETIT MAL) *see* EPILEPSY (ABSENCE)

EPILEPSY (PSYCHOMOTOR) *see* EPILEPSY (COMPLEX PARTIAL)

EPILEPSY (SIMPLE PARTIAL)

EPILEPSY (TONIC-CLONIC)

EPISCLERITIS
(Continued)

ESOPHAGEAL REFLUX

ESOPHAGEAL VARICES

ESOPHAGITIS

ESOTROPIA

EWING'S SARCOMA

EXANTHEM see MEASLES (RUBELLA), MEASLES (RUBEOLA)

EXCHANGE TRANSFUSION see HEMOLYTIC DISEASE OF THE NEWBORN

FACTOR VIII DEFICIENCY

FACTOR IX DEFICIENCY

FARMER'S LUNG

FATTY ACID DEFICIENCY

FECES see DIARRHEA, MALABSORPTION

FETOMATERNAL HEMORRHAGE see HEMOLYTIC DISEASE OF THE NEWBORN

FEVER UNDETERMINED ORIGIN (FUO) *see* ACTINOMYCOSIS,
CYSTITIS, CYSTITIS (HEMORRHAGIC), HISTOPLASMOSIS,
HODGKIN'S DISEASE, MALARIA, NOCARDIOSIS,
PHARYNGITIS, TUBERCULOSIS, TYPHOID

GLAUCOMA (SECONDARY)

GLIOMA

GLYCOSURIA *see* DIABETES MELLITUS

GLYCOSURIA (RENAL) *see* DIABETES MELLITUS

GOITER

GOLD POISONING

GONORRHEA

GOUT

(Continued)

HEADACHE *see* MIGRAINE

HEADACHE (SINUS)

HEADACHE (TENSION)

HEADACHE (VASCULAR)

HEART *see* CARDIOMYOPATHY, CONGESTIVE HEART FAILURE, MYOCARDIAL INFARCTION, RHEUMATIC FEVER

HEART BLOCK

HEAVY METAL POISONING

HELMINTHIASIS

HEMATEMESIS *see* CIRRHOSIS, DUODENAL ULCER, GASTRIC ULCER

HEMATURIA *see* CYSTITIS

HEMOCHROMATOSIS *see* CIRRHOSIS

HEMOFLAGELLATES *see* TRYPANOSOMIASIS

HEMOLYTIC DISEASE OF THE NEWBORN

β-HEMOLYTIC *STREPTOCOCCUS*

(Continued)

HYPERTENSION *(Continued)*

HYPERTENSION (OCULAR)

HYPERTENSION (PAROXYSMAL)

HYPERTHERMIA (MALIGNANT)

HYPERTHYROIDISM

HYPERTRIGLYCERIDEMIA *see* HYPERLIPIDEMIA

(Continued)

IMPETIGO

IMPOTENCE

INAPPROPRIATE ANTIDIURETIC HORMONE see SYNDROME
OF INAPPROPRIATE SECRETION OF ANTIDIURETIC
HORMONE (SIADH)

INFARCT OF MYOCARDIUM see MYOCARDIAL INFARCTION

INFECTION

INFECTIOUS HEPATITIS see HEPATITIS A

INFERTILITY (FEMALE)

INFERTILITY (MALE)

INFLAMMATORY BOWEL DISEASE see COLITIS, DIARRHEA

INFLUENZA A INFECTION

INSECTS see BITES (INSECT)

INSOMNIA

INTRACRANIAL PRESSURE

INTRAOCULAR PRESSURE

INDICATIONS INDEX

LEGIONNAIRES' DISEASE

LEISHMANIASIS

LEPROSY

LEUKEMIA (ACUTE LYMPHOCYTIC)

LEUKEMIA (ACUTE MONOCYTIC)

LEUKEMIA (ACUTE MYELOCYTIC)

LEUKEMIA (ACUTE MYELOMONOCYTIC)

LEUKEMIA (CHRONIC LYMPHOCYTIC)

LEUKEMIA (CHRONIC MYELOCYTIC)

LEUKEMIA (CHRONIC MYELOGENOUS)

LEUKEMIA (ERYTHROID)

LEUKEMIA (GRANULOCYTIC)

INDICATIONS INDEX

MITRAL VALVE PROLAPSE

MIXED CONNECTIVE TISSUE DISEASE (MCTD) *see* SYSTEMIC LUPUS ERYTHEMATOSUS (SLE)

MONOCLONAL GAMMOPATHY *see* MACROGLOBULINEMIA OF WALDENSTRÖM, MYELOMA

MONOCYTIC LEUKEMIA *see* LEUKEMIA (MONOCYTIC)

MORAXELLA LACUNATA

MORAXELLA LACUNTA

MOTION SICKNESS

MUCOVISCIDOSIS *see* CYSTIC FIBROSIS

MULTIPLE ENDOCRINE ADENOMATOSIS *see* PHEOCHROMOCYTOMA

MULTIPLE MYELOMA *see* MYELOMA

MULTIPLE SCLEROSIS

MUMPS

MUSCARINE POISONING

MUSCLE SPASM

MUSCULAR DYSTROPHY *see* AMYOTROPHIC LATERAL SCLEROSIS (ALS)

MYASTHENIA GRAVIS

MYCOBACTERIOSIS see TUBERCULOSIS

MYCOBACTERIUM MARINUM

MYCOSIS (FUNGOIDES)

MYDRIASIS

MYELOBLASTIC LEUKEMIA see LEUKEMIA (MYELOBLASTIC)

MYELOCYTIC LEUKEMIA see LEUKEMIA (MYELOCYTIC)

MYELOMA

MYELOPROLIFERATIVE DISEASES see LEUKEMIA (GRANULOCYTIC)

MYOCARDIAL INFARCTION

(Continued)

OSTEOARTHRITIS *(Continued)*

OSTEODYSTROPHY

OSTEOMALACIA

OSTEOMYELITIS

OSTEOPOROSIS

PARROT FEVER *see* PSITTACOSIS

PEDICULOSIS CAPITIS *see* LICE

PEDICULOSIS CORPORIS *see* LICE

PEDICULOSIS PUBIS *see* LICE

PEMPHIGOID *see* BULLOUS SKIN DISEASE

(Continued)

PNEUMONIA (MYCOPLASMAL)

PNEUMONIA (PNEUMOCOCCAL)

PNEUMONIA (*PNEUMOCYSTIS CARINII*)

PNEUMONIA (*PROTEUS*)

PNEUMONIA (PSEUDOMONAL)

PNEUMONIA (STAPHYLOCOCCAL)

PNEUMONIA (STREPTOCOCCAL)

PRIMARY ALDOSTERONISM *see* CONN'S SYNDROME

PRIMARY BILIARY CIRRHOSIS *see* CIRRHOSIS (PRIMARY BILIARY)

PROSTATE *see* CARCINOMA (PROSTATE)

PROSTATIC CARCINOMA *see* CARCINOMA (PROSTATE)

(Continued)

(Continued)

(Continued)

SINUSITIS *(Continued)*

SJÖGREN'S SYNDROME *see* ARTHRITIS (RHEUMATOID)

SKIN CARCINOMA *see* CARCINOMA (SKIN)

SKIN INFECTION

SKIN ULCER

SLE *see* SYSTEMIC LUPUS ERYTHEMATOSUS (SLE)

SMALL INTESTINE *see* ABDOMINAL PAIN, CARCINOID (INTESTINAL TRACT), CELIAC DISEASE, DIARRHEA, MALABSORPTION

SOMATOTROPIN DEFICIENCY *see* GROWTH HORMONE DEFICIENCY

SPASTICITY

SPERM AGGLUTINATING ANTIBODIES *see* INFERTILITY (MALE)

SPLEEN *see* CIRRHOSIS

SPLENOMEGALY *see* GAUCHER'S DISEASE

SPONDYLITIS *see* ARTHRITIS (RHEUMATOID), SPONDYLITIS (ANKYLOSING)

SPONDYLITIS (ANKYLOSING)

SPOROTRICHOSIS

SPRUE *see* CELIAC DISEASE, MALABSORPTION

SQUAMOUS CARCINOMA *see* CARCINOMA (SQUAMOUS)

STAPHYLOCOCCAL INFECTION

STAPHYLOCOCCUS AUREUS

STAPHYLOCOCCUS AUREUS (NON-PENICILLINASE PRODUCING)

(Continued)

STAPHYLOCOCCUS EPIDERMIDIS (PENICILLINASE PRODUCING)

STARVATION *see* DIARRHEA, MALABSORPTION

STEVENS-JOHNSON SYNDROME

(Continued)

STEVENS-JOHNSON SYNDROME *(Continued)*

STOMACH *see* ABDOMINAL PAIN, GASTRIC ULCER

STOMACH CARCINOMA *see* CARCINOMA (STOMACH)

STOMATITIS

STRABISMUS

STREPTOCOCCAL INFECTION

STREPTOCOCCUS (ANAEROBIC)

STREPTOCOCCUS BOVIS

STREPTOCOCCUS (GROUP B)

STREPTOCOCCUS PYOGENES

STREPTOCOCCUS PYOGENES (GROUPS A,C,G)

(Continued)

THYROIDITIS *see* HASHIMOTO'S THYROIDITIS, THYROID

THYROTOXICOSIS *see* HYPERTHYROIDISM

INDICATIONS INDEX

INDICATIONS INDEX

INDICATIONS INDEX

ZOSTER *see* HERPES ZOSTER

NOTES

NOTES

NOTES

NOTES

Can you or your organization use another copy of the

Quick Look Drug Book?

Complete the reply card on the following page
or for more information call

Lexi-Comp at (216) 650-6506

or

Williams & Wilkins at (800) 638-0672